AF782022

Mood Disorders: Clinical Assessment and Management

Mood Disorders: Clinical Assessment and Management

Editor: Leon Chapman

FOSTER
ACADEMICS
www.fosteracademics.com

www.fosteracademics.com

FOSTER ACADEMICS

Cataloging-in-Publication Data

Mood disorders : clinical assessment and management / edited by Leon Chapman.
p. cm.
Includes bibliographical references and index.
ISBN 978-1-63242-633-8
1. Affective disorders. 2. Affective disorders--Diagnosis. 3. Affective disorders--Treatment.
I. Chapman, Leon.
RC537 .M66 2019
616.852 7--dc23

© Foster Academics, 2019

Foster Academics,
118-35 Queens Blvd., Suite 400,
Forest Hills, NY 11375, USA

ISBN 978-1-63242-633-8 (Hardback)

This book contains information obtained from authentic and highly regarded sources. Copyright for all individual chapters remain with the respective authors as indicated. All chapters are published with permission under the Creative Commons Attribution License or equivalent. A wide variety of references are listed. Permission and sources are indicated; for detailed attributions, please refer to the permissions page and list of contributors. Reasonable efforts have been made to publish reliable data and information, but the authors, editors and publisher cannot assume any responsibility for the validity of all materials or the consequences of their use.

Trademark Notice: Registered trademark of products or corporate names are used only for explanation and identification without intent to infringe.

Printed and bound in China.

Contents

Preface

Disruption of a person's mood and the occurrence of manic and depressive episodes can be attributed to a mood disorder. Such a disorder can be depressive, bipolar, substance-induced or triggered by a medical condition. Mood disorders may be grouped under two sections, namely bipolar and related disorders, and depressive and related disorders. There are several treatment avenues for the management of mood disorders, such as behavioral antidepressants, cognitive and interpersonal therapies as well as prescription of antipsychotics and mood stabilizers. Lithium compounds may also be prescribed to reduce the risk of suicide and other causes of mortality in people with mood disorders. This book aims to shed light on some of the unexplored aspects of mood disorders. It presents researches and studies performed by experts across the globe on the clinical assessment and management of mood disorders. It attempts to assist those with a goal of delving into this field.

This book unites the global concepts and researches in an organized manner for a comprehensive understanding of the subject. It is a ripe text for all researchers, students, scientists or anyone else who is interested in acquiring a better knowledge of this dynamic field.

I extend my sincere thanks to the contributors for such eloquent research chapters. Finally, I thank my family for being a source of support and help.

Editor

Hyperhomocysteinemia Is a Result, Rather than a Cause, of Depression under Chronic Stress

Shen Chengfeng[1¶], Liu Wei[3¶], Wang Xinxing[2,3*¶], Wu Lei[3], Zhan Rui[2], Qian Lingjia[2*]

1 Tianjin Centers for Disease Control and Prevention, Tianjin, China, **2** Beijing Institute of Basic Medical Sciences, Beijing, China, **3** Institute of Health & Environmental Medicine, Tianjin, China

Abstract

Background: Although the accumulation of homocysteine (Hcy) has been implicated in the pathogenesis of depression, whether Hcy is directly involved and acts as the primary cause of depressive symptoms remains unclear. The present study was designed to clarify whether increased Hcy plays an important role in stress-induced depression.

Results: We employed the chronic unpredictable mild stress model (CUMS) of depression for 8 weeks to observe changes in the plasma Hcy level in the development of depression. The results showed that Wistar rats exposed to a series of mild, unpredictable stressors for 4 weeks displayed depression-like symptoms such as anhedonia (decreased sucrose preferences) and a decreased 5-Hydroxy Tryptophan (5-HT) concentration in the hippocampus. At the end of 8 weeks, the plasma Hcy level increased in the CUMS rats. The anti-depressant sertraline could decrease the plasma Hcy level and improve the depression-like symptoms in the CUMS rats. RhBHMT, an Hcy metabolic enzyme, could decrease the plasma Hcy level significantly, although it could not improve the depressive symptoms in the CUMS rats.

Conclusions: The results obtained from the experiments did not support the hypothesis that the increased Hcy concentration mediated the provocation of depression in CUMS rats, and the findings suggested that the increased Hcy concentration in the plasma might be the result of stress-induced depression.

Editor: Yong-hui Dang, Xi'an Jiaotong University School of Medicine, China

Funding: The work was supported by research grant from the National Natural Science Foundation of China (grant no. 81372124, 81000584). The funders had no role in study design, data collection and analysis, decision to publish, or preparation of the manuscript.

Competing Interests: The authors have declared that no competing interests exist.

* Email: wxxemail@sohu.com (QL); wxxchf@gmail.com (WX)

¶ These authors are joint first authors on this work.

Background

Depressive disorders are among the most frequent types of mental illnesses. Stress is involved in the etiology of depression [1]. Although dysfunction of the hypothalamic-pituitary-adrenal (HPA) axis and sympathetic nervous system, associating stress with depression, have been discussed, the pathological mechanisms remain unclear. Homocysteine (Hcy) is a thiol amino acid that is generated from the metabolism of methioline, which has been associated with many diseases such as cardiovascular disease and depression [2–4]. High concentrations of Hcy in the plasma or serum have been found in depressive patients. It was reported that approximately 20–50% of patients with severe depression had increased total Hcy levels in the plasma [5,6]. Furthermore, Tolmunen et al. [7] determined in a cross-sectional study that the subjects in the upper tertile for serum total Hcy had a more than two-fold higher risk of being depressed compared with the subjects in the lowest tertile for serum total Hcy. A further study confirmed that being in the lowest quartile of Hcy was associated with fewer depressive symptoms after adjusting for sex, physical health, smoking, and other variables. A high level of Hcy correlates to depressive symptoms in community-dwelling middle-aged individuals [8]. Therefore, as demonstrated by the epidemiological studies described above, an elevated Hcy concentration in plasma is very common in depression. Although the accumulation of Hcy has been implicated in the pathogenesis of depression [9], whether Hcy is directly involved and acts as primary cause of depressive symptoms is unclear [10], and there is little evidence from animal experiments.

The Hcy level in plasma or serum could be influenced by many factors such as age, vitamin deficiency, renal function, and a common mutation in the methylenetetrahydrofolate reductase (MTHFR) gene that impairs Hcy metabolism. Subjects with the TT genotype have a higher Hcy level [11]. Aside from the factors mentioned above, Stoney et al.. demonstrated that acute psychological stress could induce rapid and significant elevations in the plasma total Hcy concentration in a sample of women between 40 and 63 years of age [12]. Oliveira et al.. found that with exposure to restraint stress, a model of psychological stress in rats, the total plasma Hcy concentration increased significantly [13]. Our previous results supported this finding. Setnika reported that foot shock stress also increased the plasma Hcy in female rats that were in either estrus or diestrus, although it did not increase the plasma Hcy in male rats [14]. These studies indicated that the Hcy concentration might be affected by some stressful manipulations.

Because stress has been thought to be one of etiological factors in depression [1], we suspected that hyperhomocysteinemia is a result or a cause of depression induced by stress. To demonstrate this hypothesis, we first established a rat stress model of depression using the chronic unpredictable mild stress (CUMS) described by Willner and colleagues [15]; we then observed the depression-like symptoms and the changes in the plasma Hcy level in CUMS rats and evaluated the effects of the antidepressant sertraline on the depression-like symptoms and the changes in the Hcy level in CUMS rats. These results would be significant for the understanding of the mechanism of stress-induced depression and could provide information regarding the treatment of depression.

Methods

Agents

The following materials were used: 7-fluorobenzene-2-oxy-1, 3-diazolic-4-ammonium sulfate SBD-F (SBD-F, sigma, USA), N-acetyl-L-cysteine (NAC, sigma, USA), serotonin (5-HT, sigma, USA), dihydroxybenzylamine (DHBA, sigma, USA), and sertraline hydrochloride tablets purchased from HuiRui Inc, China. All of the other reagents used were of analytical or chromatographic grade.

Animals

This study was conducted with the approval of the Animal Care and Use Committee of the Beijing Institute of Basic Medical Sciences, China. The protocol was approved by the Committee on the Ethics of Animal Experiments of the Beijing Institute of Basic Medical Sciences (Permit Number: 2012-D-3098). All of the surgical procedures were performed under sodium pentobarbital (1%, 1 ml/100 g weight, i.p.) anesthesia, and efforts were made to minimize suffering.

Male Wistar rats (200–220 g, Tianjin, China) were used for the experiment, and 8 rats were treated in each group. The rats were acclimated to the surroundings for 1 week prior to the start of experiment. The animals were maintained on a 12 h light/dark cycle under a controlled temperature of 25±2°C. Food and water were available for the duration of the experiments unless otherwise noted. All of the animal handling procedures were performed in strict accordance with the guide for the use and care of laboratory animals.

Sucrose Preference Tests and Body Weight Measurements

Anhedonia, which is a central feature of depression, was defined as a reduction in sucrose preference. The methods were similar to those described by Muscat and Willner et al. [15–17]. Rats were trained for adaptation to the taste of a sucrose solution (1%) prior to the start of the experiment. After removing the food and water from each rat's cage for a period of 20 hours, the rats were exposed to water and a 1% sucrose solution in pre-weighed plastic bottles, which were placed on the cages; the animals were allowed to consume the fluids for a period of 1 h. The bottles were then removed and weighed to determine the amount (in grams) of fluid consumed by rats. The tests were conducted, and the body weights were measured before commencing the CUMS protocol (baseline) and every 2 weeks for 8 weeks. Sucrose preference was calculated according to the following formula: %sucrose preference = (sucrose intake/total fluid intake) × 100.

Protocol of Chronic Unpredictable Mild Stress (CUMS)

CUMS is employed to mimic negative life events to which human beings are exposed and to produce anhedonia in rats, which is an important indicator of the establishment of the CUMS animal model [15–18]. According to the rat sucrose preference in the baseline test, the rats were divided into 2 groups: control and CUMS animals. Except for the control rats, the other animals were kept in individual cages. The experimental protocol and CUMS procedure were a variation of methods described by Grippo et al. [19,20]. The CUMS procedure was carried out for a total of 8 weeks. The stressors for CUMS include continuous overnight illumination, 40°C cage tilt along the vertical axis, paired housing, soiled cage (200 ml water spilled into the bedding of each cage), restraint in a small cage (equipped with breathing holes), exposure to an empty water bottle for 1 hour immediately following a period of acute 1-hour water deprivation, and food deprivation. All of the stressors were applied individually and continuously, day and night. The control animals were left undisturbed in their home cages with the exception of general handling (i.e., regular cage cleaning and measuring body weight).

Open field test

Locomotor activity and exploratory behavior were evaluated using an open field test. The open field apparatus was a plywood box measuring 100 cm ×100 cm. All of the walls were painted black. The floor was divided into 25 equal squares. The rats were placed individually in one corner of the apparatus, and their ambulation (number of squares crossed) and immobility frequency were observed for 3 m. An open field test score was calculated as the sum of ambulation and immobility frequency [21].

Forced Swimming Test

A forced swimming test was performed in accordance with the method of Elizete et al.. [22]. The test was performed after 24 hours of treatment. The rats were placed into a cylinder with a diameter of 40 cm containing a column of 17 cm of water at 27°C. The animals were trained 24 hours before the forced swimming test. Then, the rats were exposed to the same experimental conditions for 5 min. A rat was judged to be not moving if it remained floating in the water, in an upright position, with only a small amount of movement to keep its head above water. The immobility time was recorded.

Pharmacological treatment

According to their sucrose preference following 4 weeks of CUMS, the rats were divided into eight groups; a control group that was orally administered water, a control group that received sertraline hydrochloride (Po, 10 mg/kg·day), a control group that received RhBHMT (IV, 0.04 mg/kg·day), a control group that received L-methionine (IG, 1 g/kg·day), the CUMS group, a CUMS with sertraline-treated group, a CUMS with RhBHMT-treated group and a CUMS with L-methionine-treated group. Sertraline is a selective serotonin reuptake inhibitor (SSRI) and appears to be a safe and efficacious treatment for depression [23–25]. RhBHMT is a recombinant human betaine-homocysteine S-methyltransferase that could promote Hcy methyltransferase metabolism specifically and decrease the plasma Hcy level. The CUMS procedures were performed for a total of 8 weeks.

Preparation of Blood Samples and Tissue Collection

Before the initiation of the experiment and every two weeks for 8 weeks, blood was collected from the medial angle of the rat eye into precooled plastic vials containing 0.2 ml of an $EDTANa_2$

solution (60 mg/ml) and centrifuged at 900 g for 20 min at 4°C. The plasma was extracted, transferred to plastic tubes and stored at −80°C until the Hcy assays were performed [13,26].

Immediately after the body weight measurements and sucrose preference tests, all of the animals were left without any treatment until the following morning. They were brought into an adjacent room and then decapitated, and the whole brains were quickly removed onto an ice-plate and washed with 0.9% saline solution. The hippocampus was carefully dissected for the 5-HT assays.

Determination of 5-HT in the hippocampus

The 5-HT levels were determined in the hippocampus using a modification of previous methods [27]. Briefly, the brain tissues were homogenized with an ultrasonic homogenizer in an ice-cold solution (15 μl/mg tissue) of 0.09 M perchloric acid containing 5 mM sodium bisulfite, 0.04 mM EDTA and dihydroxybenzylamine as the internal standard. The homogenate was then centrifuged at 14000× *g* for 20 min at 4°C. The obtained supernatant was subjected to chromatography on a C18 model column (4.6 mmi.d.×250 mm, 10 μm microparticles). The chromatography system consisted of an apparatus and a LC6A electrochemical detector. The measurements were performed at an electrode potential of +0.7 V versus the Ag/AgCL reference electrode.

Measurement of the plasma Hcy concentration

The total plasma Hcy values were determined using high-performance liquid chromatography (HPLC) with fluorimetric detection and isocratic elution [28]. This method involves the reduction of thiol groups, protein precipitation and derivatization with 7-fluorobenzene-2-oxy-1, 3-diazolic-4-ammonium sulfate–SBD-F. The HPLC system included a WATERS LC2695 apparatus and a WATERS 2475 fluorescence detector. Chromatographic separation was performed using a C18 model SymmetryShield RP18 column (3.9 mmi.d.×150 mm, 5 μm microparticles). The fluorescence of the separated compounds was detected with a detector adjusted for excitation at 390 nm and emission at 470 nm. The Hcy content was calculated with a calibration curve using a known Hcy concentration and N-acetyl-L-cysteine (NAC) as the internal standard.

Statistical analyses

The values are presented as the means ± SE for the indicated experiments and were analyzed by mixed-design ANOVA, one-way ANOVA and Student's *t*-tests, where appropriate. A probability value of $P<0.05$ was considered statistically significant.

Results

Unpredictable chronic mild stress induces the comorbidity of depression-like behavior and hyperhomocysteinemia in rats

The changes in the body weight in the control and CUMS groups across time (baseline through 8 weeks CUMS) are shown in Fig. 1A. The analysis yielded a main effect of time [$F(4,110)=271.89$, $P<0.001$], group [$F(1,110)=52.78$, $P<0.001$] and a significant group by time interaction [$F(4,110)=5.86$, $P<0.001$]. After 2 weeks of CUMS throughout the protocol, significantly decreased body weights in the CUMS rats were observed compared with the decreases in the control groups (Week 2: $P=0.003$, Week 4: $P=0.017$, Week 6: $P=0.002$, Week 8: $P<0.001$). The sucrose preference test was used to evaluate anhedonia, which is the most important index for the establishment of the CUMS model. As shown in Fig. 1B, an ANOVA yielded significant main effects of group [$F(1,98)=11.41$, $P=0.001$]. A comparison of the means in sucrose preference revealed a significant difference between the control and CUMS groups at 4, 6 and 8 weeks ($P=0.049$, $P=0.048$, $P=0.001$, respectively), which indicated that the rats in the CUMS group showed depression-like behavior. The total open field test scores are shown in Fig. 1C. The open field test score of the CUMS rats decreased significantly compared with the score of the control group after 4, 6 and 8 weeks of CUMS [$F(2,73)=7.42$, $P=0.001$]. As shown in Fig. 1D, the immobility time of the CUMS rats was increased significantly after 6 and 8 weeks of CUMS [$F(2,71)=8.36$, $P<0.001$].

Changes of the 5-HT level in different brain areas were typically found in the CUMS rats, which supported the establishment of a CUMS depression model. Fig. 1E presents the 5-HT concentrations of the hippocampus of both groups. An ANOVA was performed on the 5-HT level in the hippocampus. Consistent with our expectations, the analysis yielded significant main effects of group [$F(1,20)=26.66$, $P<0.001$], which indicated a decreased 5-HT concentration in the hippocampus in the CUMS rats after 4 weeks of CUMS (Week 4: $P=0.003$, Week 8: $P=0.007$).

The plasma Hcy concentrations are displayed in Fig. 1F. An ANOVA yielded significant main effects of group [$F(1,40)=13.66$, $P<0.001$]. After exposure to CUMS for 6 weeks, the plasma Hcy concentration in the CMS group increased in the CUMS rats; however, this result did not reach statistical significance ($P>0.05$). At the end of the 8-week CUMS exposure, the plasma Hcy concentration was significantly increased [$t(10)=13.66$, $P=0.004$].

Sertraline inhibits depression-like behavior and the plasma Hcy concentration in CUMS rats

The alterations in the sucrose preference, total open field test scores, 5-HT level in the hippocampus and plasma Hcy concentration after CUMS following sertraline treatment are analyzed in Fig. 2. At the end of 8 weeks of CUMS, significant differences in the sucrose preference, total open field test scores and 5-HT level of the hippocampus between the groups were revealed [sucrose preference: $F(3,36)=17.813$, $P<0.001$, total open field test scores: $F(3,26)=16.582$, $P<0.001$, 5-HT level: $F(3,20)=16.357$, $P<0.001$]. The sucrose preference, total open field test scores, immobility time of the forced swimming test and 5-HT level of the hippocampus in the CUMS+sertraline rats were increased compared with the CUMS rats [sucrose preference: $t(19)=4.26$, $P<0.001$, total open field test scores: $t(13)=4.35$, $P<0.001$, Immobility time: $t(12)=3.86$, $P<0.001$, 5-HT level: $t(10)=3.53$, $P=0.005$]. The plasma Hcy concentration between the groups was significantly different [$F(3,20)=17.115$, $P<0.001$]; this concentration was lower in the CUMS+sertraline rats compared with the CUMS rats [$t(10)=4.23$, $P=0.002$].

RhBHMT suppresses the plasma Hcy level, although it has no effect on depression-like behavior

The changes in the Hcy level in the plasma are described in Fig. 3. At the end of 8 weeks of CUMS, a significant difference in the plasma Hcy concentration was revealed [$F(3,27)=16.723$, $P<0.001$]. RhBHMT is a recombinant human betaine-homocysteine S-methyltransferase. In our previous study, we demonstrated that RhBHMT could effectively suppress the level of plasma Hcy in hyperhomocysteinemia rats induced by a methionine diet. In the present study, the plasma Hcy concentration in the CUMS+RhBHMT group rats were decreased compared with the CUMS

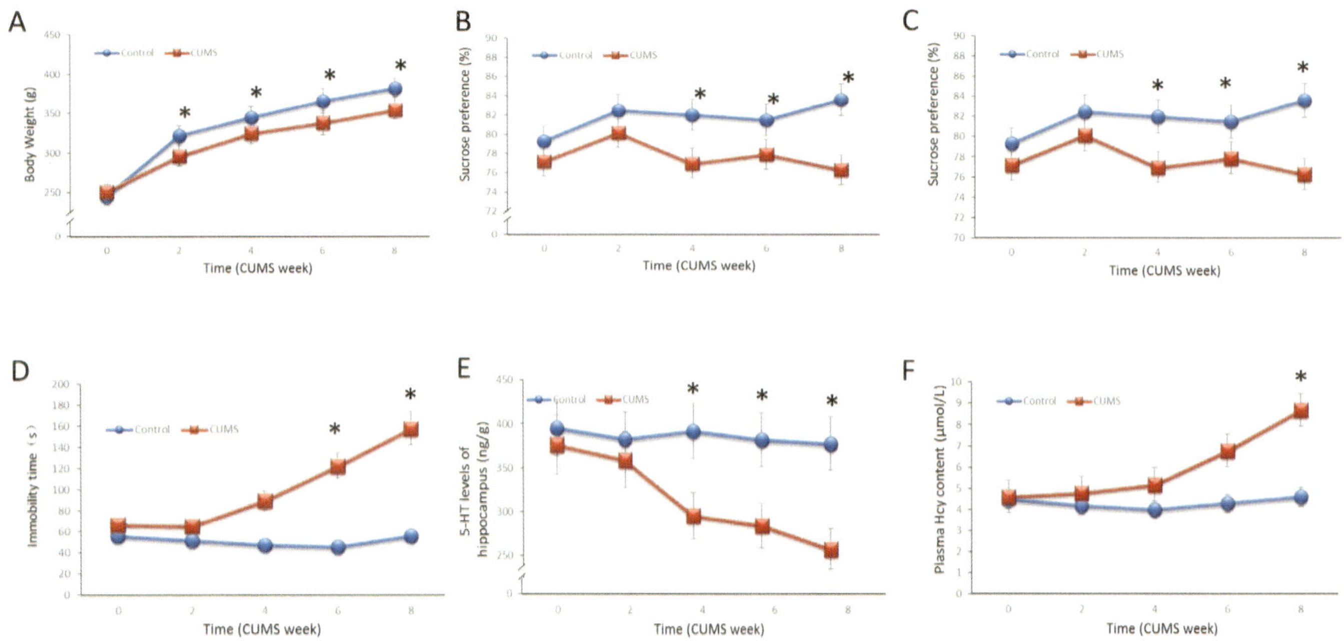

Figure 1. Unpredictable chronic mild stress induces the comorbidities of depression-like behavior and hyperhomocysteinemia in rats. The depression-like behavior of CUMS rats was measured at 2, 4, 6 and 8 weeks. **A.** The rats were weighed weekly, and the weights are shown. **B.** A 2-bottle sucrose preference test was used to measure the rats' preferences for sweetened solution over water. Preference was calculated as the percentage of sucrose solution consumed compared with the total fluid intake: %sucrose preference = (sucrose intake/total fluid intake) $\times$ 100. **C.** Exploratory behavior was evaluated as described in the Materials and Methods section. **D.** The immobility time was detected by manual measurements. **E.** 5-HT level in the hippocampus was detected using liquid chromatography (Waters E2695). **F.** The total plasma Hcy values were determined by high-performance liquid chromatography (HPLC) with fluorimetric detection and isocratic elution. Values represent the group mean $\pm$ structural equation modeling (SEM) (n = 8 rats per group). *$P<0.05$ compared with control, repeated measures ANOVA followed by Tukey's multiple comparison tests.

rats [t(14) = 3.98, $P<0.001$]. The effects of RhBHMT on the body weight, open field test, sucrose preference and 5-HT level of the hippocampus are shown in Fig. 4. However, RhBHMT could not improve the depressive symptoms in the CUMS rats. These results illustrate that reducing the plasma Hcy level had no significant effect on depression-like behavior of rats exposed to CUMS. The Hcy level of plasma was determined during the 24-h period (measured every 4 hours) after RhBHMT treatment (Fig. S1). The Hcy level was not significantly increased in the RhBHMT intervention gap.

Methionine treatment does not have an effect on depression-like behavior

The changes in the Hcy level in the plasma are described in Fig. 3. Methionine treatment increased the level of Hcy in the plasma significantly compared with the control group [t(13) = 4.39, $P<0.001$]. The effects of methionine on the body weight, open field test, sucrose preference, immobility time of the forced swimming test and 5-HT level of the hippocampus are shown in Fig. 5. Methionine did not have an effect on the depressive symptoms in CUMS rats.

Discussion

As supported by some studies, depression is association with an increased Hcy concentration, which could be affected by some stressful manipulations. The present study attempted to elucidate whether the increased Hcy concentration mediated the association underlying stress and depression. The results demonstrated that an increased plasma Hcy level was found at the end of 8 weeks of CUMS exposure; the results did not support the hypothesis that the increased Hcy concentration was one of possible intermediate mechanisms for the provocation of CUMS-induced depression because decreased sucrose preference following CUMS 4 weeks occurred prior to the increase of plasma Hcy concentration. Our study also demonstrated that the anti-depressant sertraline could decrease the plasma Hcy level while improving the depression-like symptoms in this stress model of depression, which indicated that the increased Hcy concentration might be the result of depression in the CUMS model.

The CUMS model is available to the study the pathogenesis, biological mechanisms, and treatments for depression and is focused on the behavioral sign of anhedonia (a central feature of depression characterized by an impaired responsiveness to pleasurable stimuli), which could be examined by sucrose preference tests [17,18,29]. In the present study, the rats displayed reduced sucrose preference after exposure to CUMS for 4 weeks, and this result reflected the occurrence of depression-like behavior, which is similar to previous studies [16,19,20]. Although decreased body weight was observed, it was previously reported that there was no significant relationship between the effects of CUMS on sucrose intake and decreases in body weight [30]. The 5-HT level in the hippocampi were reduced in the CUMS rats, which also supported the occurrence of depression [31].

Regarding the Hcy assay, we expected to see elevated plasma Hcy levels in CUMS rats compared with control groups, and our results were consistent with this expectation. Modest increases in the plasma Hcy levels in the rats exposed to CUMS 6 weeks were found; however, this increase did not reach statistical significance. The plasma Hcy level at the end of 8 weeks of CUMS increased

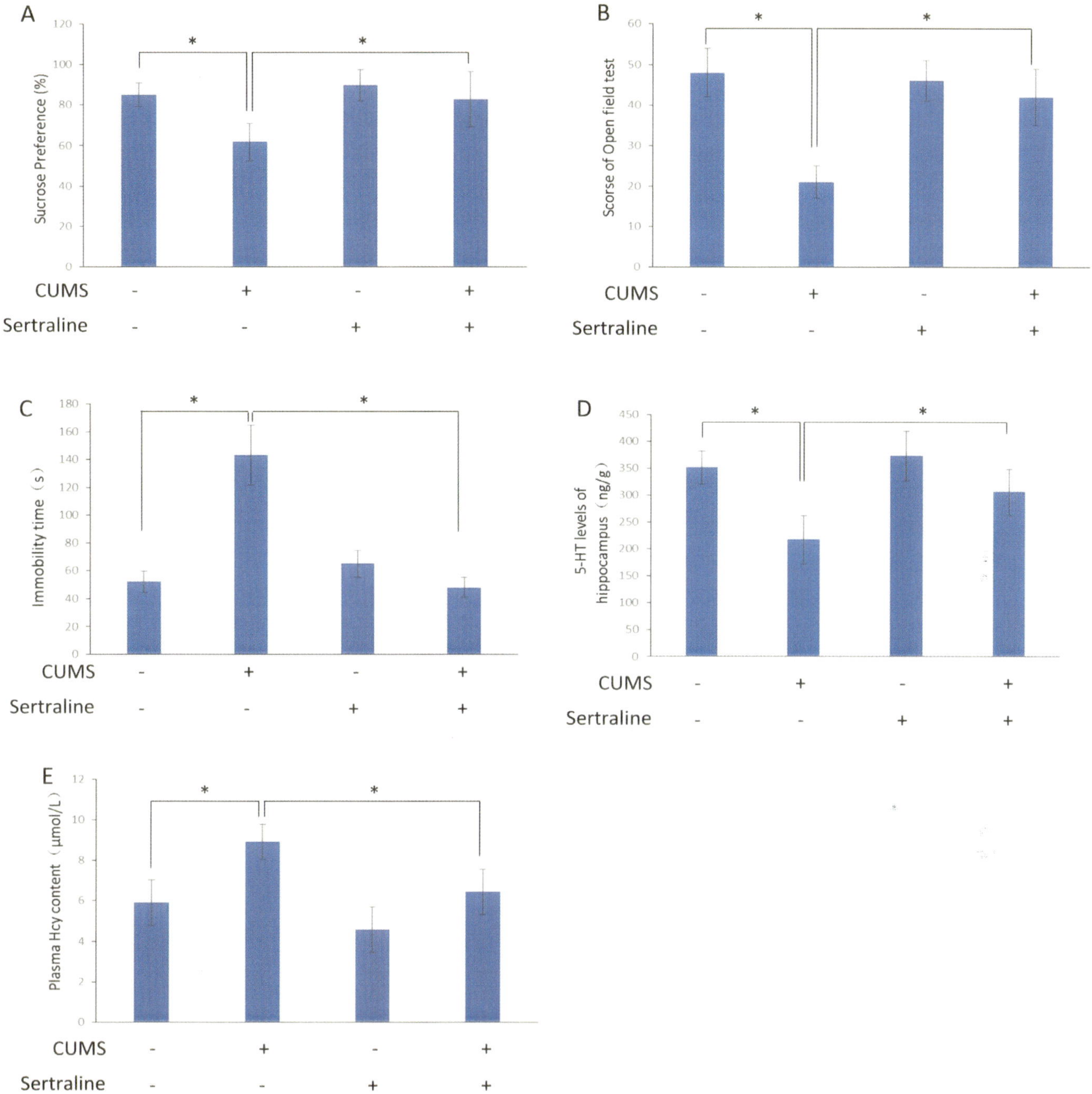

Figure 2. Sertraline inhibits depression-like behavior and plasma Hcy content in CUMS rats. Sucrose preference, open field test scores, 5-HT level in the hippocampus and total plasma Hcy were measured as described in Figure 1. **A.** Sertraline inhibited the decline of sucrose preference induced by CUMS. **B.** Sertraline inhibited the decline of the open field test score induced by CUMS. **C.** Sertraline decreased the immobility time of the forced swimming test induced by CUMS. **D.** Sertraline inhibited the decline in the 5-HT level in hippocampus induced by CUMS. **E.** Sertraline inhibited the increase in the plasma Hcy level induced by CUMS. Values represent the group mean ± structural equation modeling (SEM) (n = 8 rats per group). *$P<0.05$, repeated measures ANOVA followed by Tukey's multiple comparison tests.

significantly, and this increase occurred after depression-like behavior appeared in the CUMS rats. Some studies reported that there was no association between an increased Hcy level and the propensity of developing depressive behavior [32,33]. However, according to some investigations, the thermolabile variant of MTHFR was significantly more common in the group with a history of depressive disorders. The higher Hcy level induced by the MTHFR C677T genotype variant is associated with an increased risk of depressive episodes [34]. Kohen et al.. [35] reported that in a prospective clinical trial, folic acid supplementation could significantly improve the cognitive and depressive status test scores of the majority of volunteers. This result might be related to the fact that folic acid supplementation could lower the Hcy levels. However, these effects were not observed in the present

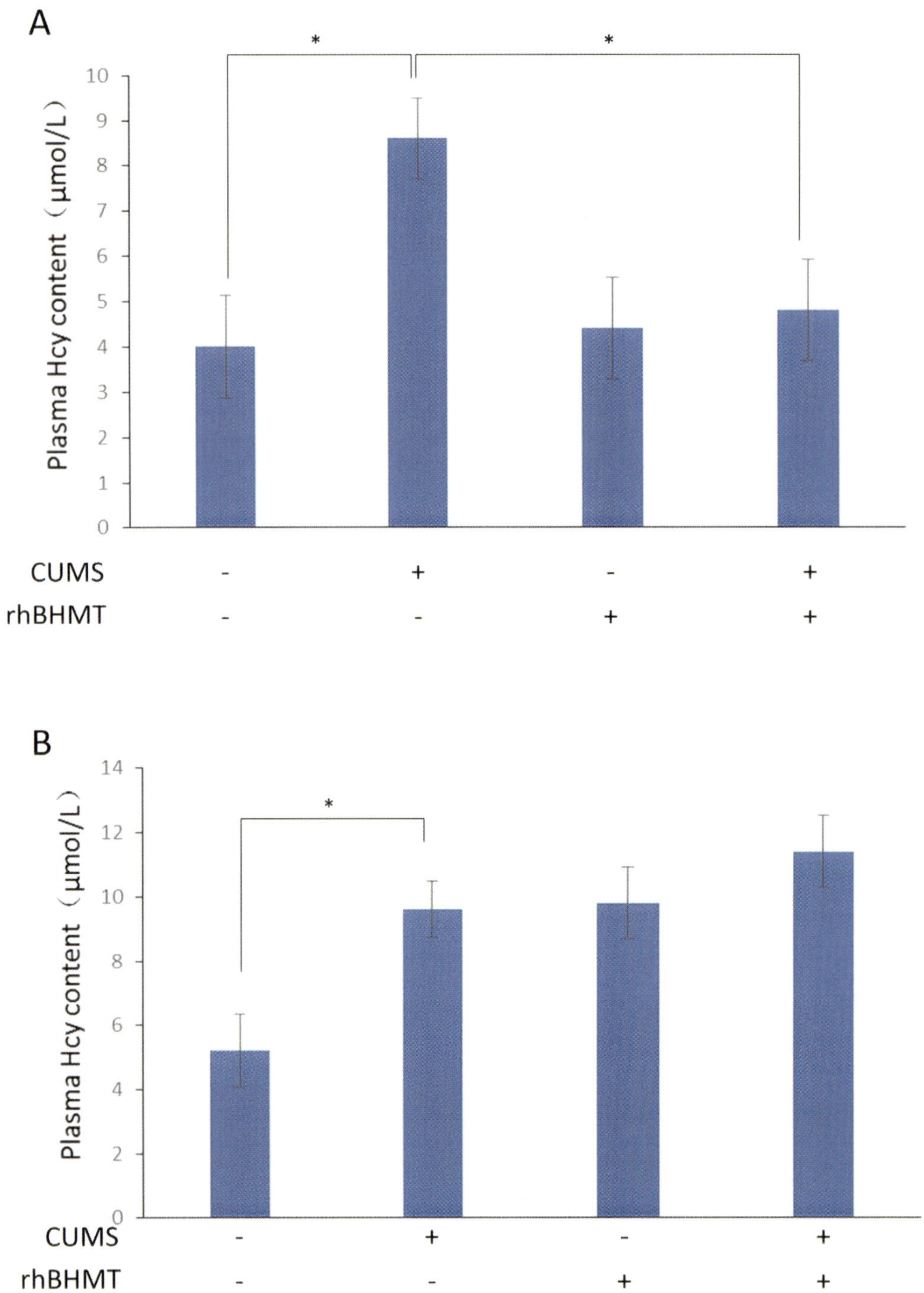

Figure 3. RhBHMT suppress plasma Hcy level in CUMS rats. Total plasma Hcy levels were measured as described in the Methods section. **A.** RhBHMT inhibited the plasma Hcy level induced by CUMS rats. **B.** Methionine increased the plasma Hcy level compared with the control group. Values represent the group mean ± structural equation modeling (SEM) (n = 8 rats per group). **P*<0.05, repeated measures ANOVA followed by Tukey's multiple comparison test.

study, which was consistent with the results of Watanabe et al.. They determined that there was no relationship among folate, homocysteine levels and depression in women during early pregnancy [36]. The reasons for these inconsistencies are unclear. Tiemeier reported that the higher rates of depressive disorders in subjects with high Hcy levels are due to differences in cardiovascular factors and physical comorbidities [33]. The results in the current study appeared to reflect that the high plasma Hcy level was the result of depression, although it was not the reason, or that depression-like changes and elevated plasma levels were produced by the common pathological mechanisms initiated by CUMS.

To clarify these uncertainties, the anti-depressant sertraline [25] and the anti-hyperhomocysteinemia agent RhBHMT were employed. The results demonstrated that sertraline improved the depression-like behavior and also decreased the elevated plasma Hcy concentration in the CUMS rats. However, RhBHMT only

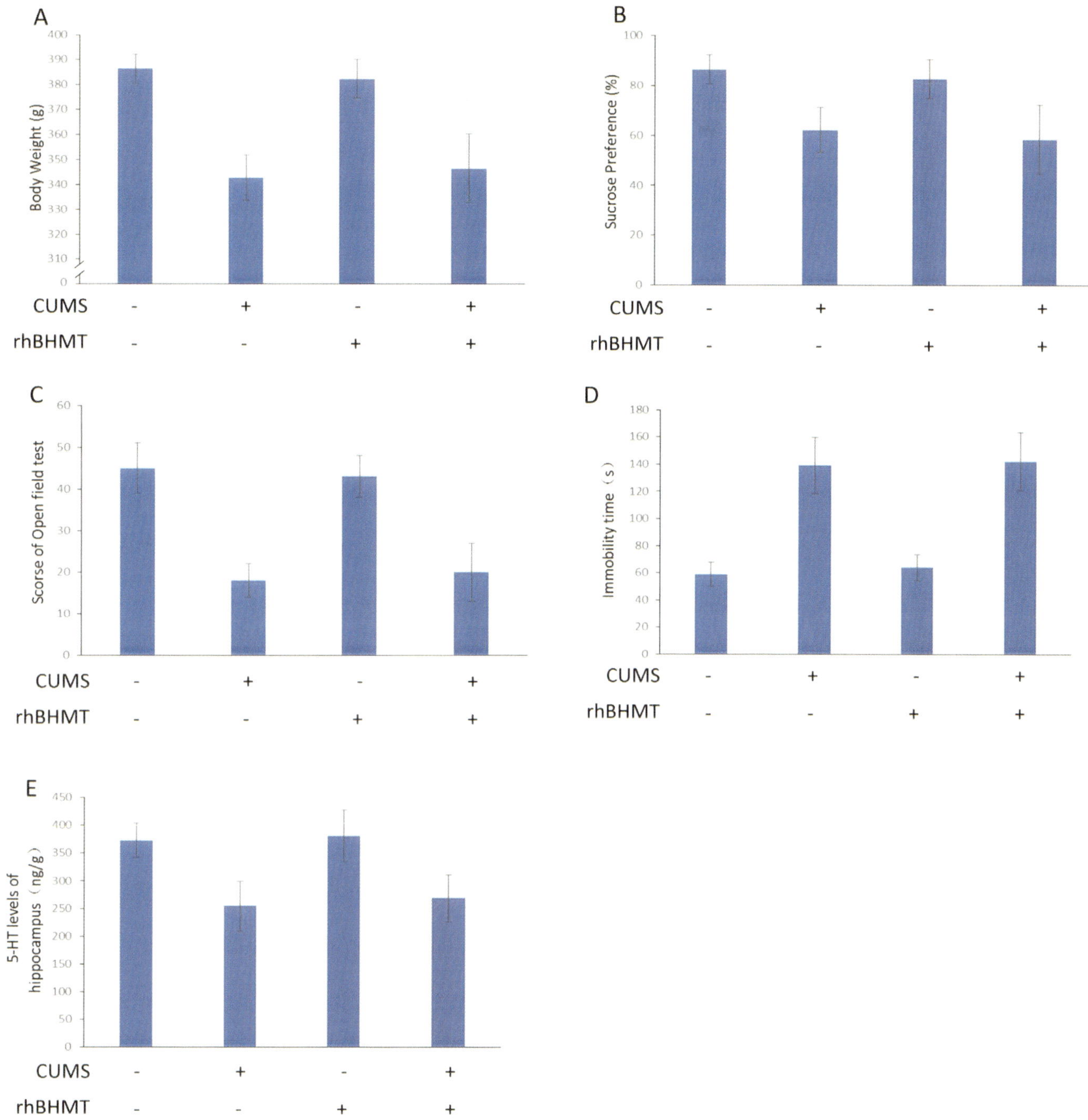

Figure 4. Effect of RhBHMT on depression-like behavior in CUMS rats. Body weight, sucrose preference, open field test scores, immobility time of the forced swimming test, 5-HT level in the hippocampus and total plasma Hcy were measured as described in Figure 1. RhBHMT had no effect on the body weight, sucrose preference, open field test scores, immobility time of the forced swimming test and 5-HT level in the hippocampus of the CUMS rats. Values represent the group mean ± structural equation modeling (SEM) (n = 8 rats per group). *$P<0.05$, repeated measures ANOVA followed by Tukey's multiple comparison test.

suppressed the plasma Hcy level and had no effect on the depression-like behavior. This result suggested that the increased Hcy concentration in plasma might be the result of, although not the cause of, depression. In recent reports of investigational observations, the effects of SSRI antidepressants on immune function and the effects of anticytokine pharmacological agents were demonstrated [37]. However, the conclusion of a direct effect of sertraline on Hcy metabolism could not be drawn. This study could not rule out the possibility either. Further research about how sertraline affects the plasma Hcy level is needed. An increase in the total Hcy plasma concentration (the sum of protein-bound, free and disulfide fractions) is now recognized as an risk factor for many diseases, such as cardiovascular disease [3,4]. The present study also demonstrated that a high Hcy concentration might be

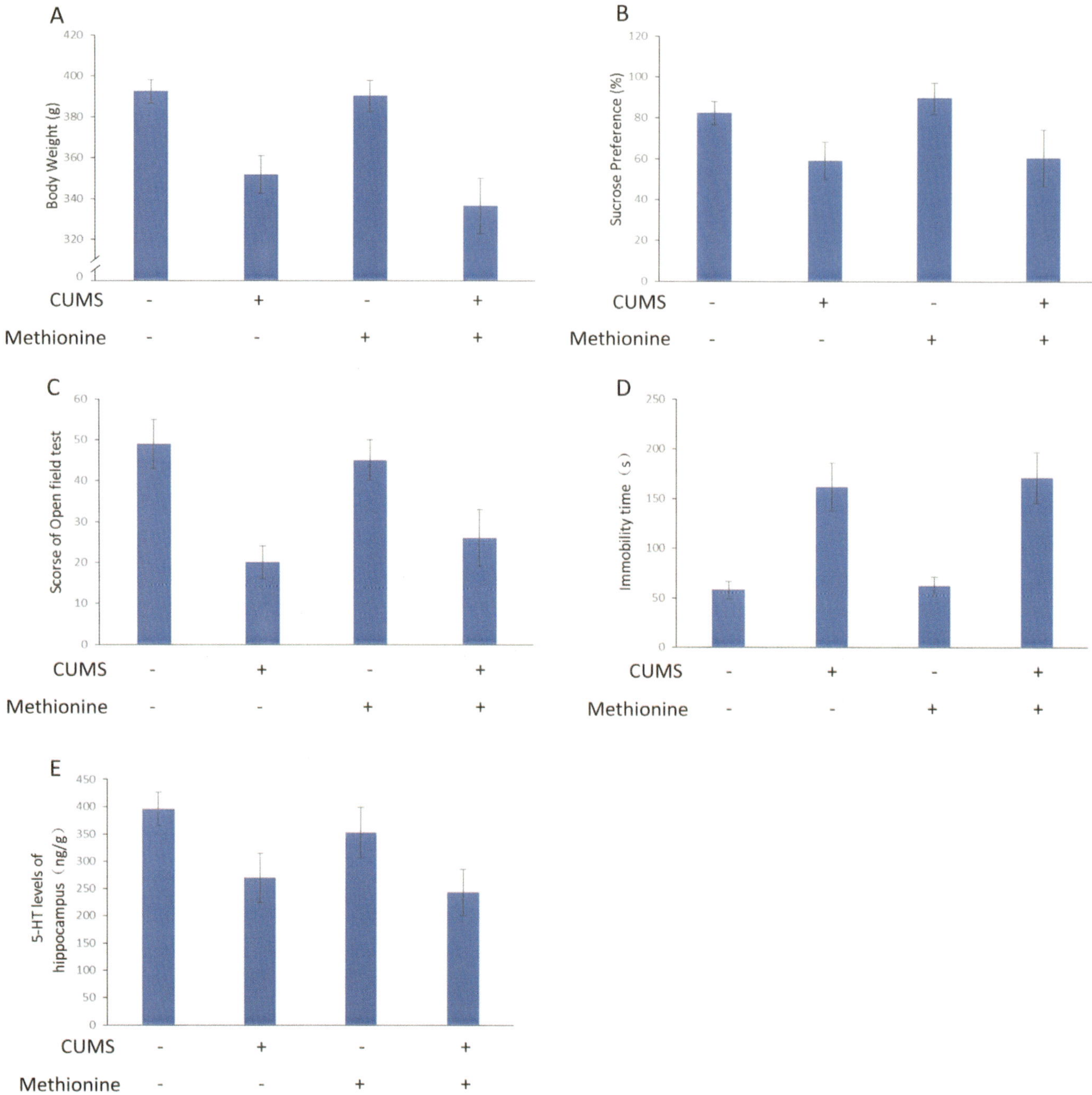

Figure 5. Effect of methionine on depression-like behavior in CUMS rats. Body weight, sucrose preference, open field test scores, immobility time of the forced swimming test, 5-HT level in the hippocampus and total plasma Hcy were measured as described in Figure 1. Methionine had no effect on the body weight, sucrose preference, open field test scores, immobility time of the forced swimming test and 5-HT level in the hippocampus of CUMS rats. Values represent the group mean ± structural equation modeling (SEM) (n = 8 rats per group). *$P<0.05$, repeated measures ANOVA followed by Tukey's multiple comparison tests.

an intermediate factor between depression and other diseases. Considering the damaging effect of a high Hcy concentration, it is very important to decrease the elevated plasma Hcy concentration in patients with depression in clinical treatment; sertraline and RhBHMT might be the drugs for the treatment of depressive patients with high plasma Hcy levels.

Conclusions

The anti-depressant sertraline could decrease the plasma Hcy level while improving the depression-like changes in the CUMS rats. However, RhBHMT suppressed the plasma Hcy level, although it had no effect on the depression-like behavior. These findings might help clarify the mechanisms underlying the association between increased Hcy concentration and stress-induced depression; the results did not support the hypothesis that the increased Hcy concentration mediated the provocation of depression in CUMS rats. The results suggested that the increased Hcy concentration in plasma might be the result of depression in CUMS rats.

Supporting Information

Figure S1 Effect of rhBHMT on total plasma Hcy in CUMS rats. Total plasma Hcy were measured as described in Figure 1. The Hcy level of plasma was determined during the 24-h period (measured every 4 hours) after RhBHMT treatment. The Hcy level was decreased after 4 hours and not significantly increased in the RhBHMT intervention gap. Values represent the group mean ± structural equation modeling (SEM) (n = 8 rats per group). $*P<0.05$ compared with control, repeated measures ANOVA followed by Tukey's multiple comparison tests.

Acknowledgments

The authors thank Wang Dezheng for their assistance with the statistical analysis. We also thank two anonymous reviewers for their patient review and critical reading of our manuscript.

Author Contributions

Conceived and designed the experiments: SC WX QL. Performed the experiments: LW WX WL ZR. Analyzed the data: SC. Contributed reagents/materials/analysis tools: QL SC. Wrote the paper: SC WX LW.

References

1. Alfonso J, Frasch AC, Flugge G (2005) Chronic stress, depression and antidepressants: effects on gene transcription in the hippocampus. Reviews in the Neurosciences 16: 43–56.
2. Lentz SR (1997) Homocysteine and vascular dysfunction. Life sciences 61: 1205–1215.
3. Nygård O, Vollset S, Refsum H, Brattström L, Ueland P (1999) Total homocysteine and cardiovascular disease. Journal of internal medicine 246: 425–454.
4. Budge MM, De Jager C, Hogervorst E, Smith AD, Memory TOPTI (2002) Total plasma homocysteine, age, systolic blood pressure, and cognitive performance in older people. Journal of the American Geriatrics Society 50: 2014–2018.
5. Fava M, Borus JS, Alpert JE, Nierenberg AA, Rosenbaum JF, et al. (1997) Folate, vitamin B_{12}, and homocysteine in major depressive disorder. The American journal of psychiatry.
6. Bottiglieri T, Laundy M, Crellin R, Toone BK, Carney MW, et al. (2000) Homocysteine, folate, methylation, and monoamine metabolism in depression. Journal of Neurology, Neurosurgery & Psychiatry 69: 228–232.
7. Tolmunen T, Hintikka J, Voutilainen S, Ruusunen A, Alfthan G, et al. (2004) Association between depressive symptoms and serum concentrations of homocysteine in men: a population study. The American journal of clinical nutrition 80: 1574–1578.
8. Sachdev PS, Parslow RA, Lux O, Salonikas C, Wen W, et al. (2005) Relationship of homocysteine, folic acid and vitamin B12 with depression in a middle-aged community sample. Psychological medicine 35: 529–538.
9. Plante GE (2005) Depression and cardiovascular disease: a reciprocal relationship. Metabolism 54: 45–48.
10. Bottiglieri T (2005) Homocysteine and folate metabolism in depression. Progress in Neuro-Psychopharmacology and Biological Psychiatry 29: 1103–1112.
11. Kelly CB, McDonnell AP, Johnston TG, Mulholland C, Cooper SJ, et al. (2004) The MTHFR C677T polymorphism is associated with depressive episodes in patients from Northern Ireland. Journal of Psychopharmacology 18: 567–571.
12. Stoney CM (1999) Plasma homocysteine levels increase in women during psychological stress. Life sciences 64: 2359–2365.
13. de Oliveira AC, Suchecki D, Cohen S, D'Almeida V (2004) Acute stressor-selective effect on total plasma homocysteine concentration in rats. Pharmacology Biochemistry and Behavior 77: 269–273.
14. Setnik B, de Souza FG, d'Almeida V, Nobrega JN (2004) Increased homocysteine levels associated with sex and stress in the learned helplessness model of depression. Pharmacology Biochemistry and Behavior 77: 155–161.
15. Willner P, Towell A, Sampson D, Sophokleous S, Muscat R (1987) Reduction of sucrose preference by chronic unpredictable mild stress, and its restoration by a tricyclic antidepressant. Psychopharmacology 93: 358–364.
16. D'Aquila P, Newton J, Willner P (1997) Diurnal variation in the effect of chronic mild stress on sucrose intake and preference. Physiology & behavior 62: 421–426.
17. Muscat R, Papp M, Willner P (1992) Reversal of stress-induced anhedonia by the atypical antidepressants, fluoxetine and maprotiline. Psychopharmacology 109: 433–438.
18. Willner P (1997) Validity, reliability and utility of the chronic mild stress model of depression: a 10-year review and evaluation. Psychopharmacology 134: 319–329.
19. Grippo AJ, Beltz TG, Johnson AK (2003) Behavioral and cardiovascular changes in the chronic mild stress model of depression. Physiology & behavior 78: 703–710.
20. Grippo AJ, Moffitt JA, Johnson AK (2002) Cardiovascular alterations and autonomic imbalance in an experimental model of depression. American Journal of Physiology-Regulatory, Integrative and Comparative Physiology 282: R1333–R1341.
21. Xinxing W, Wei L, Lei W, Rui Z, Baoying J, et al. (2014) A neuroendocrine mechanism of co-morbidity of depression-like behavior and myocardial injury in rats. PloS one 9: e88427.
22. Reis EDM, Neto FWS, Cattani VB, Peroza LR, Busanello A, et al. (2014) Antidepressant-Like Effect of Ilex paraguariensis in Rats. BioMed Research International 2014.
23. Strik JJ, Honig A, Lousberg R, Lousberg AH, Cheriex EC, et al. (2000) Efficacy and safety of fluoxetine in the treatment of patients with major depression after first myocardial infarction: findings from a double-blind, placebo-controlled trial. Psychosomatic Medicine 62: 783–789.
24. Sauer WH, Berlin JA, Kimmel SE (2001) Selective serotonin reuptake inhibitors and myocardial infarction. Circulation 104: 1894–1898.
25. Meijer WE, Heerdink E, Leufkens HG, Herings RM, Egberts AC, et al. (2004) Incidence and determinants of long-term use of antidepressants. European journal of clinical pharmacology 60: 57–61.
26. Li J-M, Kong L-D, Wang Y-M, Cheng CH, Zhang W-Y, et al. (2003) Behavioral and biochemical studies on chronic mild stress models in rats treated with a Chinese traditional prescription Banxia-houpu decoction. Life sciences 74: 55–73.
27. Harro J, Tõnissaar M, Eller M, Kask A, Oreland L (2001) Chronic variable stress and partial 5-HT denervation by parachloroamphetamine treatment in the rat: effects on behavior and monoamine neurochemistry. Brain research 899: 227–239.
28. Pfeiffer CM, Huff DL, Gunter EW (1999) Rapid and accurate HPLC assay for plasma total homocysteine and cysteine in a clinical laboratory setting. Clinical Chemistry 45: 290–292.
29. Vollmayr B, Henn FA (2003) Stress models of depression. Clinical Neuroscience Research 3: 245–251.
30. Griffiths J, Shanks N, Anisman H (1992) Strain-specific alterations in consumption of a palatable diet following repeated stressor exposure. Pharmacology Biochemistry and Behavior 42: 219–227.
31. Gamaro G, Manoli L, Torres I, Silveira R, Dalmaz C (2003) Effects of chronic variate stress on feeding behavior and on monoamine levels in different rat brain structures. Neurochemistry international 42: 107–114.
32. Penninx BW, Guralnik JM, Ferrucci L, Fried LP, Allen RH, et al. (2000) Vitamin B12 deficiency and depression in physically disabled older women: epidemiologic evidence from the Women's Health and Aging Study. American Journal of Psychiatry 157: 715–721.
33. Tiemeier H, van Tuijl HR, Hofman A, Meijer J, Kiliaan AJ, et al. (2002) Vitamin B12, folate, and homocysteine in depression: the Rotterdam Study. American Journal of Psychiatry 159: 2099–2101.
34. Almeida OP, Flicker L, Lautenschlager NT, Leedman P, Vasikaran S, et al. (2005) Contribution of the MTHFR gene to the causal pathway for depression, anxiety and cognitive impairment in later life. Neurobiology of aging 26: 251–257.
35. Loria-Kohen V, Gómez-Candela C, Palma-Milla S, Amador-Sastre B, Hernanz A, et al. (2013) A pilot study of folic acid supplementation for improving homocysteine levels, cognitive and depressive status in eating disorders. Nutricion Hospitalaria 28.
36. Watanabe H, Suganuma N, Hayashi A, Hirowatari Y, Hirowatari T, et al. (2010) No relation between folate and homocysteine levels and depression in early pregnant women. Bioscience trends 4.
37. Parissis JT, Fountoulaki K, Paraskevaidis I, Kremastinos D (2005) Depression in chronic heart failure: novel pathophysiological mechanisms and therapeutic approaches.

2

The Efficacy of Mindfulness-Based Cognitive Therapy as a Public Mental Health Intervention for Adults with Mild to Moderate Depressive Symptomatology

Wendy T. M. Pots[1,2]*, Peter A. M. Meulenbeek[1,3], Martine M. Veehof[1], Jorinde Klungers[3], Ernst T. Bohlmeijer[1]

1 University of Twente, Department of Psychology, Health & Technology, Enschede, the Netherlands, **2** Dimence, Community Mental Health Center, Almelo, the Netherlands, **3** GGNET, Community Mental Health Center, Warnsveld, the Netherlands

Abstract

Objective: Although there has been growing evidence for the efficacy of mindfulness-based cognitive therapy (MBCT) for different clinical populations, its effectiveness as a public mental health intervention has not been studied. The present study evaluates a community-based MBCT intervention for adults with mild to moderate depressive symptomatology in a large multi-site, pragmatic randomized controlled trial.

Method: The participants with mild to moderate depressive symptomatology were recruited from the general population and randomized to the MBCT intervention (n = 76) or to a waiting list control group (n = 75). Participants completed measures before and after the intervention. Participants in the experimental condition also completed these measures at a 3-month follow-up.

Results: In the experimental condition significant reductions in depression, anxiety, and experiential avoidance, and improvements in mindfulness and emotional- and psychological mental health were found, compared to the waiting list (effect sizes Cohen's d = 0.31–0.56). These effects were sustained at the 3-month follow-up. The likelihood of a clinically significant change in depressive symptoms was significantly higher for the MBCT group [odds ratio (OR) 3.026, $p<0.01$ at post-treatment; NNT = 5.10].

Discussion: MBCT as a public mental health intervention for adults with mild to moderate depressive symptoms seems effective and applicable in a natural setting.

Editor: Gabriel S. Dichter, UNC Chapel Hill, United States of America

Funding: The study was funded by University of Twente (www.utwente.nl). The funder had no role in study design, data collection and analysis, decision to publish, or preparation of the manuscript.

Competing Interests: The authors have declared that no competing interests exist.

* Email: w.t.m.pots@utwente.nl

Introduction

Minor depression is a highly prevalent disorder with a large negative impact on quality of life and yielding high economic costs [1]. Offering interventions for people with depressive symptomatology is a necessary public mental health strategy complementary to the treatment of depression in inpatient and outpatient settings [2]. One such effective strategy is to pro-actively offer treatments for people with mild to moderate symptoms of depression [3,4]. However, a public mental health intervention needs to be attractive for people who don't suffer from severe symptoms of depression yet [5]. Using a positive framework and promoting positive mental health as well as reducing psychological distress offers opportunities to attract more people [6–8]. Mindfulness-based cognitive therapy (MBCT) may be such an intervention, as it focuses on promoting positive mental health instead of only focusing on the reduction of psychological distress. MBCT is an 8-week group-based training that combines meditation exercises with cognitive techniques. It was originally designed for prevention of relapse in people with recurrent depression [9]. In patients with three or more previous episodes of depression, MBCT significantly reduced the risk of relapse compared to the treatment as usual [10–12]. Moreover, in a recently published randomized controlled trial Williams et al. [13] found evidence that the number of episodes is a marker for those with greater vulnerability due to a history of childhood trauma and adversity. Strauss et al. [14] conducted a meta-analysis on mindfulness based interventions for people diagnosed with a current episode of an anxiety or depressive disorder and found that MBCT can also be effective for people who are currently depressed. MBCT targets processes such as avoidance of negative emotions and engaging with maladaptive thinking and rumination, that maintain depressive symptomatology in general [15,16]. Mindfulness is often referred to as intentionally paying attention to present moment experiences in a non-judgemental way [17]. Awareness and acceptance of negative experiences will reduce experiential avoidance (EA) [15]. EA has been defined as the unwillingness to remain in contact with experiences such as feelings, thoughts, and bodily sensations, as an attempted means of behavioral regulation [15]. Psychological flexibility is the counterpart of experiential avoidance. As EA could be seen as an important factor that maintains depressive symptomatology, MBCT may also be effective as a public mental health intervention for people with depressive symptomatology. This fits with a growing interest in adapting MBCT to other psychiatric disorders, such as anxiety disorders, and bipolar disorder, but also treatment-resistant major depressive disorder (for a recent review see Chiesa & Serretti [18]). Research into the potential mechanisms of action in MBCT is in its infancy. In a recent review Chiesa and Serretti [19] suggested that mindfulness-based interventions may enhance positive emotion regulation strategies, as well as self-compassion levels, and decrease rumination and experiential avoidance. They suggested that these changes are associated with several clinical benefits, including the reduction of stress and depression levels, as well as the enhancement of positive emotions. Recently, Kaviani et al. [20] found that MBCT can be effective in a non-clinical population of female students in Iran. Also, Cavanagh et al. [21] adapted MBCT as a brief online intervention and found it to be effective in a non-clinical population of students. To our knowledge, there is no research on the effectiveness of a community-based MBCT intervention for adults with depressive symptomatology. In order to modify the original MBCT as a public mental health intervention a few changes were made in time-investment. We expected a community-based MBCT with a reduced weekly time-investment to be more acceptable for the target group.

The aim of this study was to evaluate the effect of mindfulness-based cognitive therapy modified as a public mental health intervention for depressive symptomatology, in a sample of self-referred adults with mild to moderate depressive symptomatology, and offered by community mental health centers. We evaluated the effect with respect to various psychological variables, such as depression, anxiety and positive mental health. We hypothesized that changes in depressive symptoms would be mediated by psychological flexibility and mindfulness. To strengthen the trial's external validity, the intervention was studied in its natural setting.

Method

The protocol for this trial and supporting CONSORT checklist are available as supporting information; see Checklist S1 and Protocol S1. This study was approved by the METiGG, a medical ethics committee for research in mental health settings in the Netherlands. In addition, this study has been registered in the Nederlands Trial Register, the Primary Dutch register for clinical trials (NTR2096).

Design

A pragmatic, multi-site, randomized controlled trial was conducted comparing MBCT with a control condition. Participants were randomly assigned after receiving their written consent, either to MBCT or to the waiting list control, by means of a centrally conducted randomization process executed by an independent researcher. The randomization was carried out for the two groups with stratification on gender, using a computer generated random sequence of numbers. The control condition consisted of a waiting list, where wait-listed people were free to use other kinds of care. The wait-listed participants knew that they could start the training after the experimental condition had completed the intervention, i.e. after 3 months. The study is pragmatic as it mimics the Dutch health care system as closely as possible in terms of patient recruitment, conducting intake, offering interventions, and monitoring outcomes.

Participants and procedure

Participants were recruited from November 2009 until October 2010, through advertisements in regional newspapers, information booklets and general practitioners. Four Dutch community mental health centers, from both urban and rural areas, participated in the study. In the advertisements, distributed within the regions of the participating community mental health services, the target group was described as adults who were hindered by depressive symptoms. Applicants were referred to a specifically developed website, where they could find detailed information about the study. When interested, they were sent an information letter and an informed consent form. For screening, the standard procedures employed by the mental health institutions were used. The community mental health centers were responsible for the procedure, and the in- and exclusion criteria were examined by experienced mental health nurses on the basis of a checklist, under supervision of a clinical psychologist. The inclusion criteria were: adults of 18 years and over, presenting depressive symptoms. Applicants were excluded if diagnosed with a current severe major depressive episode (MDE; eight or nine out of a total of nine symptoms) or when having a moderate to high suicide risk, according to the Dutch version of the Mini International Neuropsychiatric Interview (MINI) [22,23]. Other exclusion criteria were: receiving psychological or pharmacological treatment for mental complaints within the last three months, and presence of other severe mental or social problems warranting treatment or likely to interfere with participation in the group course. People meeting one of the exclusion criteria were advised to seek regular treatment.

Power analysis

A sample of 60 participants per condition at post-intervention was needed to detect an effect size of 0.50 (Cohen's d) for the primary outcome with a statistical power of $(1-\beta)=0.80$ in a two-tailed test ($p<0.05$). Taking into account a drop-out rate of 20%, 150 eligible participants were needed.

Measures

Measurements were taken at baseline (T0), and at post-treatment after 3 months (T1). In order to study the stability of the effect of MBCT, the patients in the experimental group received a follow-up measurement (T2) at 6 months after baseline. For the control condition, the measurement at 6 months is a post-treatment measurement. All measurements had good psychometric properties and are frequently applied in international studies.

The primary outcome measure was depressive symptomatology, measured by the Dutch version of the Center of Epidemiological Studies - Depression Scale (CES-D; 20 items, score 0–60) [24]. Higher scores mean more depressive symptoms [24,25].

Secondary outcome measures were anxiety symptoms and positive mental health. Anxiety was measured by the Hospital

Anxiety and Depression Scale - Anxiety subscale (HADS-A; 7 items, score 0–21) [26] for assessing the presence and severity of anxiety symptoms. Higher scores mean more anxiety symptoms [26,27]. Positive mental health was measured by the Mental Health Continuum - Short Form (MHC-SF) [28], that measures emotional well-being (3 items; score 0–15), social well-being (5 items; score 0–25) and psychological well-being (6 items; score 0–30). Higher scores indicate greater emotional, social, and psychological well-being [28,29].

Measures of proposed processes of change included measures of EA and mindfulness. The Acceptance and Action Questionnaire-II (AAQ-II; 10 items, score 10–70) [30] was used to measure the willingness to be in contact with aversive internal experiences, to accept these events, and to pursue values in the presence of the experiences. Higher scores indicate lower levels of EA or higher levels of psychological flexibility [30,31]. The Five Facet Mindfulness Questionnaire (FFMQ) [32] was used to measure mindfulness in five sub-dimensions: (1) observing (8 items), defined in terms of noticing or attending to internal and external experiences; (2) describing (8 items), defined in terms of labelling internal experiences with words; (3) acting with awareness (8 items), defined in terms of attending to one's activities of the moment (opposite of acting on automatic pilot); (4) non-judging of inner experience (8 items), defined in terms of taking a non-evaluative stance toward thoughts and feelings; and (5) and non-reactivity to inner experience (7 items), defined in terms of allowing thoughts and feelings to come and go, without getting caught up in or carried away by them. Facet scores range from 8 to 40 (except for the non-reactivity, which ranges from 7 to 35), with higher scores indicating more mindfulness [32,33].

To evaluate the level of satisfaction of the participants after the intervention, a self-developed evaluation questionnaire was used, including a question on how the participants evaluated the program using a scale from 1(very poor) to 10 (excellent).

Waiting list control

Participants in the control condition participated in the MBCT training after a 3-month waiting list period. Participants were instructed to seek help from their general practitioner, family or other sources, as they normally would, should they encounter symptomatic deterioration or other difficulties during the waiting list period.

Intervention

In this study MBCT was delivered according to the guidelines of Segal et al. [9]. The original training was adapted to suit a public mental health approach. The intervention was aimed at people with mild to moderate symptoms of depression. In order to lower the threshold for people without severe distress to participate in MBCT, the participants were asked to practice meditations for 15 minutes a day instead of the original 45 minutes a day, and the sessions were limited to 1, 5 hours instead of the original 2, 5 hours. To ensure that all of the elements of the original course were preserved, the eight-session training was extended to 11 sessions. Key themes of the sessions included awareness (sessions 1, 2, 3), acceptance (sessions 5, 7, 9, 10) and disengaging from thoughts (sessions 4, 6, 8), with the last session (session 11) focusing on evaluation and integration. The training teaches skills to become more aware of, and to relate differently to thoughts, feelings and bodily sensations. A core feature of the training is to learn to become aware of, and disengage from habitual dysfunctional (cognitive) routines, to stop reacting automatically to internal experiences, and to act more 'mindfully'. During the period of the training, the program consisted of daily homework exercises. The exercises were aimed at increasing attention to present moment experiences in a non-judgmental way, together with exercises designed to integrate application of awareness skills into daily life. To support homework assignments, participants received weekly homework registration forms, guided (taped) and unguided meditations, and information in a booklet. Group sizes varied between eight and 15 participants.

Therapists

The MBCT instructors were all experienced psychologists and mental health nurses, with extensive former training in the original MBCT protocol by Segal [9] and Group psychotherapy. The trainers were also experienced meditators, with meditation experience ranging from 2 to 15 years.

Statistical analyses

The statistical analyses were performed using SPSS 18. The data was analyzed on an intention-to-treat (ITT) basis. Missing values at baseline, post-intervention and follow-up were imputed with the use of SPSS Missing Value Analysis on the continuous measures with the expectation-maximization (EM) method. This method computes missing values based on maximum likelihood estimates using observed data in an iterative process [34]. The total percentage of missing data (T0-T1-T2) was 5%, due to unanswered items (0,6%) and incomplete assessments (4,4%). A comparison of results based on the imputed intention-to-treat sample versus the observed data revealed similar outcomes. Therefore, only the results from the intention-to-treat analyses are reported.

Independent sample t-tests and chi-square tests were conducted to examine differences between the two groups at baseline on sociodemographic variables and outcome measures. Analysis of covariance (ANCOVA) was conducted with depressive symptoms post-treatment as the dependent variable, treatment group as the independent variable, and five covariates consisting of pre-treatment depression score and four dummy-coded variables for each treatment site. The same analyses were conducted for the secondary measures. Analysis of variance (ANOVA) was conducted with process measures post-treatment as the dependent variable and treatment group as the independent variable. Assumptions for performing parametric analysis of (co)variance were all met. To investigate whether the effects in the intervention condition were maintained at follow-up paired-sample t-tests were carried out, comparing the scores on the follow-up (T2) with those at baseline (T0). Also, paired-sample t-tests were carried out for the control group, to measure the effect of the MBCT intervention after the waiting time period, comparing scores at post-treatment (T2 for the control group) with those at pre-treatment (T1 for the control group).

Effect sizes at post-treatment (T0-T1) were calculated with Cohen's d using the means and the pooled standard deviations of the measurements in the conditions. For the effect sizes at follow-up (T0-T2) the Cohen's d was corrected for dependence among means by using the correlation between the two means [35]. To interpret Cohen's d an effect size of less than 0.33 is considered small, while 0.33 to 0.55 is considered moderate and effect sizes of 0.56 to 1.2 are considered large [36]. Comparisons were two-tailed and interpreted with a significance value of $p<0.05$.

With the Jacobson and Truax methodology, the proportion of participants was determined who made a clinically significant change on the CES-D from baseline to post-treatment [37]. First, the reliable change was calculated with the reliable change index (RCI). Jacobson and Truax suggest that subjects can be considered to have improved when they shift from a dysfunctional distribution to a functional one, and the reliable change scores exceed measurement error (calculated by dividing the difference between the pretest and posttest scores by the standard error of the measurement). Second, the recovery criterion was defined as a post-treatment score below the cut-off value of 16 for clinically relevant depressive symptoms [38,39]. Because we studied a population with a mild to moderate symptomatology, the mean score at baseline was already at the recovery criterion (M = 16.04; range 1–43; S.D. = 8.08). A clinically significant change on the CES-D is thus defined as having a reliable change between the measurements, which required a post-treatment score below the cut-off of 16. Participants that had a clinically significant change were either coded 1 (implying a favorable treatment response, 'success') or 0 ('failure'). The binary outcome was used to calculate the odds ratio (OR) using logistic regression. Based on the clinically significant change proportions, the number needed to treat (NNT) was calculated [40]. To provide a more complete representation of the effects of the intervention, the outcomes were also analyzed for intervention completers only (somewhat arbitrarily defined as participants that attended at least 9 sessions).

The process measures were expected to be mediators between the MBCT intervention and post-treatment levels of depressive symptomatology (CES-D). Mediation was performed for all process measures that were significantly different between the intervention and control condition in the ANOVA. Then, all steps outlined by Baron and Kenny [41] were used. In the first step linear regression analysis was performed, with treatment group as independent variable and depressive symptoms post-treatment as the dependent variable. In the second step we tested the effect of the independent variable on the proposed mediators with linear regression analyses, with treatment group as independent variable and the residual change scores of the proposed mediators as the dependent variables. The third step tested the effect of the proposed mediator on the dependent variable. The indirect effect of the mediator on the outcome was assessed to examine whether an increase in psychological flexibility and mindfulness during the intervention would mediate the effects of the intervention on depressive symptomatology at post-intervention. Simple mediational analyses with bootstrapping procedures (n = 5000 bootstrap resamples) were used to assess the indirect effect of the mediator on the outcome [42]. An indirect effect was considered significant in the case zero was not contained in the 95% confidence interval.

Results

Enrollment, treatment adherence, satisfaction and drop-out

Figure 1 provides an overview of the flow of participants. A total of 251 persons were interested in the training. During telephone screening, 43 persons presented other psychiatric symptoms or practical restraints that precluded them from participation in the trial. The remaining 208 applicants were assessed for eligibility. Through interviewing, a further 57 were excluded. After signing the informed consent form, the included 151 participants were randomly assigned to the MBCT intervention (n = 76) and the waiting list condition (n = 75).

After randomization, two participants decided not to start with the intervention due to time constraints (n = 1) and health problems (n = 1). Four other participants in the MBCT (8%) group did not complete the intervention (attendance of at least 9 sessions). The reasons given for non-completion were that the intervention was too time consuming (n = 1), practicality reasons (n = 1), insufficient concentration (n = 1), and an unknown reason (n = 1). Two of the four community mental health centers evaluated the course resulting in anonymous evaluation forms of all participants, including those who did not participate in the study. Based on these results overall the intervention was evaluated as positive on a scale from 1 to 10 (m = 7.98, sd = 0.72, n = 130).

At T1 (post-treatment for the MBCT group and pre-treatment for the waiting list group), data was available for 143 participants (drop-out rate 5.3%) and at T2 (follow-up for the MBCT group and post-treatment for the waiting list group), data was available for 139 participants (drop-out rate 7.9%). There were no significant differences at baseline on all the measurements between participants who completed the assessments and those who did not complete all measures.

Baseline characteristics

Table 1 shows an overview of the participants' characteristics. Participants had a mean age of 48 years (SD = 11.29, range 20–81) and were predominantly female (78.1%). The majority was of Dutch origin (96%), had a paid job (66.9%), and were living with a partner (75.5%). The level of education was high for 65.5% of the participants and intermediate for 30.5%. At the entry of the study, 2.6% met the criteria of mild MDE and 4% were diagnosed with moderate MDE. There were no significant differences at baseline between the MBCT group and the control group for any of the demographic variables or outcome measurements. Also, there were no significant changes in the waiting time period for the control group, comparing scores at baseline (T0) with pre-treatment measurement (T1), on any of the outcome measures.

Treatment effects

Primary outcome

The means and standard deviations for the primary outcome measure, the results of the ANCOVA and the effect sizes are presented in Table 2. Compared to the control condition, participants in the intervention condition reported significantly decreased depressive symptoms at post-treatment (Table 2). The effects of the intervention condition on depressive symptoms were maintained at follow-up compared to baseline measurement [$t(75) = -3.46$, $p<0.01$]. Moderate effect sizes were found at post-treatment ($d = 0.50$) and follow-up ($d = 0.40$). The control group also showed significant reductions in depression after they received the intervention at T2 [$t(74) = -3.03$, $p<0.01$].

Clinically significant change

The reliable change on the CES-D appeared to be a pre-post difference of at least 7 scale points. Clinically significant change was thus defined as a recovery condition of a score ≤16 points on the CES-D (n = 138) and a RCI of 7 points. The proportion of participants with a score of ≥7 at T0 that reached a clinically significant change was 24/70 (34%) in the intervention group, versus 10/68 (15%) in the control condition [OR 3.026, 95% confidence interval (CI) 1.316–6.961, p<0.01, NNT = 5.10, under an intention-to-treat analysis]. These results compare well with completers-only findings: OR 2.916, 95% CI 1.252–6.795, p< 0.01, NNT = 5.26.

Secondary outcome measures

The means and standard deviations for the secondary outcome measures, the results of the ANCOVA and the effect sizes are presented in Table 2. Compared to the control condition, participants in the intervention condition reported significantly decreased anxiety symptoms after the intervention. At follow-up, the effects of the intervention condition on anxiety symptoms were maintained compared to baseline measurement [$t(75) = -8.40$,

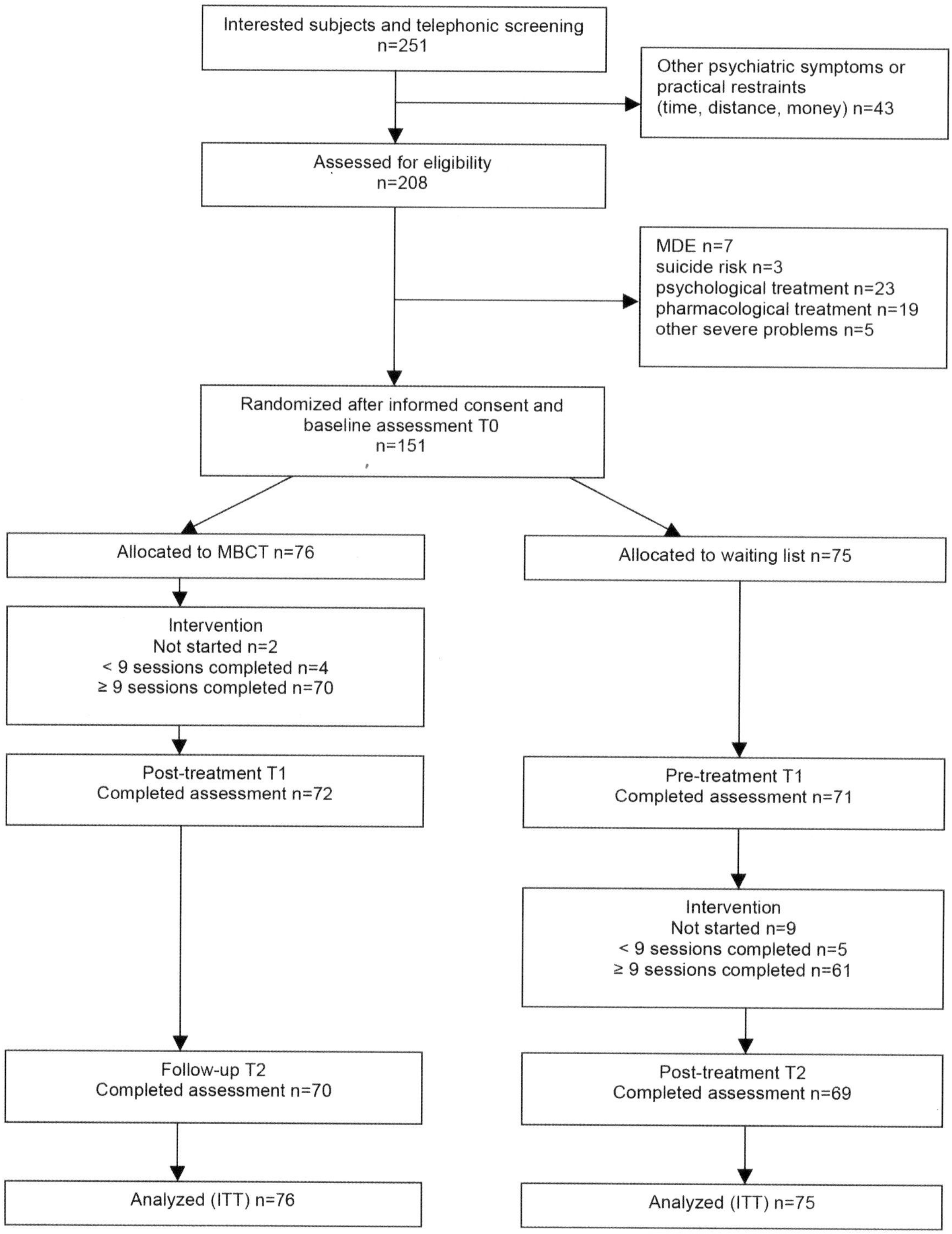

Figure 1. Participant flow. MDE = major depressive episode.

$p<0.001$]. The effect sizes for anxiety symptoms at post-treatment ($d = 0.56$) and at follow-up ($d = 0.97$) were large. The control group also showed significant reductions in anxiety after they received the intervention at T2 [$t(74) = -5.15$, $p<0.001$].

At post treatment, significant improvements in emotional well-being and psychological well-being were found. The effects of the intervention condition on emotional and psychological well-being were maintained at follow-up compared to baseline measurement [emotional well-being $t(75) = 4.13$, $p<0.001$; psychological well-being $t(75) = 5.20$, $p<0.001$]. Effect sizes at post-treatment were small (emotional well-being, $d = 0.31$) to moderate (psychological well-being, $d = 0.34$). The effect sizes at follow-up were moderate (emotional well-being, $d = 0.50$) to large (psychological well-being, $d = 0.56$). No significant effects were found at post-treatment for social well-being, with a small effect size ($d = 0.22$). At follow-up, there was a significant increase in social well-being compared to

Table 1. Baseline characteristics of the total sample, MBCT intervention and waiting list control condition.

		MBCT (n = 76)		**Waiting list (n = 75)**		**Total (n = 151)**	
		n	**%**	**n**	**%**	**n**	**%**
Age[a]	Mean (SD)	47.99 (10.59)		47.88 (12.02)		47.93 (11.29)	
	Range	24–74		20–81		20–81	
Gender[b]	Female	59	77,6	59	78,7	118	78,1
	Male	17	22,4	16	21,3	33	21,9
Marital status[b]	Single	17	22,4	20	26,7	37	24,5
	Living with partner	59	77,6	55	73,3	114	75,5
Race[b]	Dutch	71	93,4	74	98,7	145	96,0
	Other	5	6,6	1	1,3	6	4,0
Education[b]	Low	2	2,6	4	5,3	6	4,0
	Middle	21	27,6	25	33,3	46	30,5
	High	53	69,7	46	61,3	99	65,5
Employment[b]	Paid	53	69,7	48	64,0	101	66,9
	No paid	23	30,3	27	36,0	50	33,1
Diagnosis[b]	Mild MDE	3	3,9	1	1,3	4	2,6
	Moderate MDE	0	0,0	6	8,0	6	4,0

Note. MDE, major depressive episode.
[a] No significant differences between intervention and control condition (t-test with $P<0.05$).
[b] No significant differences between intervention and control condition (chi-square-test with $P<0.05$).

Table 2. Means and standard deviations for outcome measures and results of ANCOVA for intervention effects, and Cohen's d.

Measures	MBCT		Waiting list				
	(n = 76)		(n = 75)				
	M[a]	SD[a]	M[a]	SD[a]	F(df)[b]	*P*	*d*
Primary outcome							
CES-D baseline	15.62	7.86	16.46	8.32			
CES-D post-treatment	11.79	8.76	16.43	9.94	10.91(1)	0.001	0.50
CES-D follow-up[c]	11.77	8.25	13.60	8.88			
Secondary outcomes							
HADS-A baseline	7.96	3.40	8.57	3.58			
HADS-A post-treatment	6.14	3.52	8.22	3.89	12.42(1)	0.001	0.56
HADS-A follow-up[c]	4.88	2.88	6.54	3.84			
MHC-SF-EM baseline	3.15	0.95	3.15	0.78			
MHC-SF-EM post-treatment	3.46	0.85	3.19	0.88	5.32(1)	0.023	0.31
MHC-SF-EM follow-up[c]	3.54	0.95	3.61	0.78			
MHC-SF-SOC baseline	2.38	1.04	2.28	0.96			
MHC-SF-SOC post-treatment	2.72	1.08	2.49	1.05	1.62(1)	0.206	0.22
MHC-SF-SOC follow-up[c]	2.91	1.12	2.85	0.86			
MHC-SF-PSY baseline	2.92	0.89	2.96	1.00			
MHC-SF-PSY post-treatment	3.26	0.98	2.90	1.11	8.60(1)	0.004	0.34
MHC-SF-PSY follow-up[c]	3.37	0.93	3.41	0.89			

Note. ANCOVA, Analysis of covariance; CES-D, Center for Epidemiologic Studies - Depression.
Scale; HADS-A, Hospital Anxiety and Depression Scale - Anxiety subscale; MHC-SF, Mental Health Continuum - Short form; EM, emotional; SOC, social; PSY, psychological.
[a] Unadjusted condition means and standard deviations (SD).
[b] F-value, corrected for baseline values.
[c] Follow-up for intervention group and post-treatment for waiting list group.

baseline measurement [$t(75) = 5.58$, $p<0.001$], with a large effect size ($d = 0.63$).

The control group showed significant reductions on positive mental health after they received the intervention at T2 [social well-being $t(74) = 4.79$, $p<0.001$; emotional well-being $t(74) = 5.47$, $p<0.001$; psychological well-being $t(74) = 6.21$, $p< 0.001$].

Process measures

Table 3 shows all process measurements, the results of the ANOVA, and the effect-sizes. Compared to the control condition, participants in the intervention condition showed significant improvement in psychological flexibility and all mindfulness facets (except for FFMQ-Describe). The effects of the intervention condition on all process measures were maintained at follow-up compared to baseline measurement [psychological flexibility, $t(75) = 6.17$, $p<0.001$; FFMQ observing, $t(75) = 7.67$, $p<0.001$; FFMQ describing, $t(75) = 6.82$, $p<0.001$; FFMQ acting with awareness, $t(75) = 6.20$, $p<0.001$; FFMQ non-judging of inner experience, $t(75) = 6.46$, $p<0.001$; FFMQ non-reactivity to inner experience, $t(75) = 8.97$, $p<0.001$]. The effect sizes post-treatment were small to large ($d = 0.13$–0.84) and large at follow-up ($d = 0.71$–1.03).

Mediational analyses

Figure 2 shows the results of the first three steps of mediation. The FFMQ-Describe was excluded from the mediational analyses, having no significantly different effect in the ANOVA. The first step shows that the intervention condition had significantly decreased depressive symptoms at post-treatment, compared to the control condition. Step two shows that the intervention condition was significantly improved in psychological flexibility and mindfulness compared to the control condition. In step 3, all change scores of the process measures were significantly associated with the scores on the CES-D at post-treatment. In the last step of the mediational analysis, following Preacher & Hayes [42], results showed that the effect of the intervention on depressive symptoms was mediated by all process measures. Full mediation was found for improvement of psychological flexibility (direct effect $\beta = .145$, $p = 0.057$; indirect effect $\beta = -.387$, 95% CI 0.89–3.45), and mindfulness facets Observing (direct effect $\beta = 0.132$, $p = 0.106$; indirect effect $\beta = -.308$, 95% CI 0.98–3.60), and Non-reactivity to inner experience (direct effect $\beta = .135$, $p = 0.108$; indirect effect $\beta = -.275$, 95% CI 0.83–3.73). Partial mediation was found for improvement of mindfulness facets Acting with awareness (direct effect $\beta = .176$, $p = 0.044$; indirect effect $\beta = -.160$, 95% CI 0.18–2.84), and Non-judging of inner experience (direct effect $\beta = .208$, $p = .011$; indirect effect $\beta = -.158$, 95% CI 0.06–1.74).

Discussion

Main findings

To our best knowledge, this is the first study that evaluated MBCT as a public mental health intervention for adults with mild to moderate depressive symptomatology within a large pragmatic multi-site trial. The potential of offering MBCT to the community as a public mental health intervention is of importance, as the idea that MBCT is only effective in patients suffering from recurrent depression is superseded. In the present study the participants suffered from mild to moderate depressive symptoms but differed from severe clinical samples, as indicated by the substantially lower mean degree of severity of depressive symptoms as measured by the CES-D and the MINI. This corresponds to the nature and structure of the community-based MBCT, offered in our study. The results from this study indicate that MBCT as a public mental health intervention is effective in reducing depressive symptoms. We found a moderate effect size for depressive symptoms at post-treatment in comparison with the control group ($d = 0.50$). This effect size is comparable to the effect size of 0.42 that was found for psychological treatments on subthreshold depression [43]. The only studies of MBCT in community-based samples to our knowledge are from Kaviani et al. [20] and Cavanagh et al. [21]. Both conducted a randomized controlled trial in a sample of students comparing MBCT to a waiting list control group. They showed significant reductions of depressive and anxiety symptoms over time, with effect limited by low generalizability. Our study corroborates with these findings, further showing that MBCT seems to be effective in a population of adults with mild to moderate depressive symptomatology, and that MBCT can be used as a public mental health intervention in the community. Our finding that the results are maintained at 3 months follow-up is promising, but needs to be substantiated by longer follow-up measurements under controlled conditions. Offering a public mental health intervention in a positive framework might be less stigmatizing for participants with depressive symptomatology or minor depression [5]. MBCT focuses on the enhancement of promoting positive skills and therefore has the potential to offer an alternative to stigmatization.

The likelihood of a clinically significant change in depressive symptomatology in our study was substantially higher in the intervention condition compared to the waiting-list control group. As the presence of clinically relevant depressive symptoms is known to be an important risk factor for clinical depression [44], this outcome suggests that MBCT implemented as a public mental health intervention for adults with mild to moderate depressive symptomatology may decrease the risk of developing a MDE. It is shown that the effects on clinical cases of interventions for people with sub-clinical symptomatology are most prominently found after longer periods of time [45]. However this result needs to be corroborated with longer follow-up measurement and the use of diagnostic instruments as outcome measures.

Moreover, the MBCT intervention resulted in significant reductions in anxiety symptoms with large effect sizes post-treatment and at the 3-month follow-up. The effect of MBCT on anxiety symptoms are consistent with the meta-analysis by Vøllestad et al. [46], which found a large effect size ($g = 0.83$) for controlled studies of mindfulness and acceptance-based interventions for patients with anxiety symptoms. Strauss et al. [14] found no effects on anxiety symptom severity in their meta-analysis, applying a more stringent definition and excluding trials with interventions based on Acceptance and Commitment Therapy. Our study supports the findings of Vøllestad et al. [46], indicating that MBCT as a public mental health intervention could be effective in not only reducing depressive symptoms, but also in significantly reducing anxiety symptoms post-treatment and, even more substantially, at the 3-month follow-up. As anxiety symptoms often coexist with depression and may precipitate depression [47], these findings could indicate that the application of MBCT has the potential to further decrease the incidence of depression. However, this needs to be substantiated by further research.

The results also show a significant effect on positive mental health. It thus seems that MBCT has the potential not only to reduce psychological distress, but also to improve emotional, psychological, and social (only at follow-up) well-being as well. This finding confirms earlier studies that show that MBCT can promote well-being in patients with anxiety or depression [20,48]. The effects of MBCT on positive mental health are of importance.

Table 3. Means and standard deviations for process measures, results of ANOVA and Cohen's d for intervention effects.

Measures	MBCT		Waiting list				
	(n = 76)		(n = 75)				
Process outcomes	M	SD	M	SD	F(df)	*P*	*d*
AAQ-II baseline	44.28	8.42	43.03	7.86			
AAQ-II post-treatment	49.59	8.80	44.36	10.01	11.62(1)	0.001	0.56
AAQ-II follow-up[a]	50.93	9.04	48.91	8.89			
FFMQ - Observe baseline	24.77	5.58	25.21	5.77			
FFMQ - Observe post-treatment	27.98	5.15	25.28	6.29	8.34(1)	0.004	0.47
FFMQ - Observe follow-up[a]	28.46	4.54	29.07	4.74			
FFMQ - Describe baseline	26.39	6.14	27.43	6.89			
FFMQ - Describe post-treatment	28.60	5.56	27.80	6.35	0.68(1)	0.410	0.13
FFMQ - Describe follow-up[a]	29.24	6.03	29.77	6.76			
FFMQ - ActAware baseline	20.92	5.45	22.61	5.48			
FFMQ - ActAware post-treatment	25.31	5.53	22.67	6.05	7.86(1)	0.006	0.46
FFMQ - ActAware follow-up[a]	25.08	5.51	26.31	5.30			
FFMQ - NonJudge baseline	23.64	6.04	22.87	5.48			
FFMQ - NonJudge post-treatment	27.68	5.16	24.72	5.66	11.28(1)	0.001	0.55
FFMQ - NonJudge follow-up[a]	28.16	5.57	28.05	5.52			
FFMQ - NonReact baseline	19.73	4.29	19.31	4.29			
FFMQ - NonReact post-treatment	23.86	4.27	20.24	4.32	26.82(1)	0.000	0.84
FFMQ - NonReact follow-up[a]	24.24	4.04	23.54	4.22			

Note. AAQ-II, Acceptance and Action Questionnaire-II; ANOVA, Analysis of variance; FFMQ, Five Facet Mindfulness Questionnaire; Observe, observing; Describe, describing; ActAware, acting with awareness; NonJudge, non-judging of inner experience; NonReact, non-reactivity to inner experience.

[a] Follow-up for intervention group and post-treatment for waiting list group.

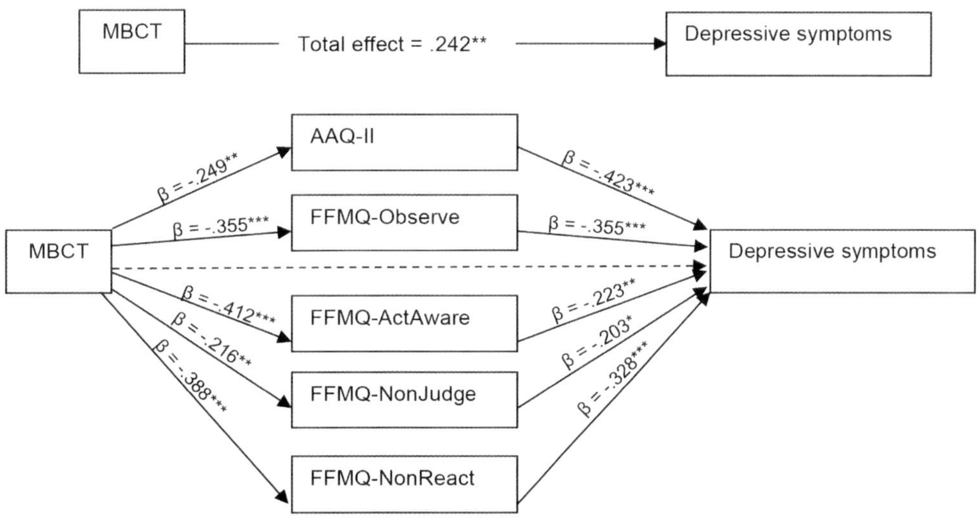

Figure 2. Mediation model of psychological flexibility and mindfulness as mediators. *Note.* AAQ-II, Acceptance and Action Questionnaire-II; FFMQ, Five Facet Mindfulness Questionnaire; Observe, observing; ActAware, acting with awareness; NonJudge, non-judging of inner experience; NonReact, non-reactivity to inner experience. $^{*}P<0.05$; $^{**}P<0.01$; $^{***}P<0.001$.

There is growing evidence that positive mental health and psychopathology are related but different dimensions of mental health [49], and that positive mental health is a protective factor against mental illnesses [6,7]. Several researchers suggest that aspects of psychological well-being (e.g. meaning, mastery, autonomy, goals) increase personal resilience [50–52]. The findings of this study suggest that adults with mild to moderate depressive symptomatology that participated in this public mental health intervention will be able to better cope with life adversity in the future. Moreover, offering a public mental health intervention in a positive framework might be less stigmatizing for participants with depressive symptomatology [5].

Mediational analyses show that the efficacy of MBCT compared to the control group on reducing post-treatment depressive symptoms is mediated by an increase in psychological flexibility and all mindfulness skills, except for the subscale 'describe'. Our results are in line with Kuyken et al. [53], which showed that 15-month follow-up level of depression were mediated by mindfulness skills and self-compassion. Developing a compassionate attitude toward one's own negative thoughts and feelings mediated the effect of MBCT on depressive symptoms and relapse. These findings are also in line with earlier studies that demonstrated the association between low psychological flexibility (i.e. experiential avoidance) and mindfulness and psychopathology [15,54,55]. The increase of psychological flexibility and mindfulness that mediated the effects of MBCT on depressive symptomatology suggests that participants have gained additional adaptive emotion regulation skills in response to negative affect-producing stressors [19,54].

The original MBCT training was designed for people with a history of depression and requires participants to commit to a 2.5-hour group session and to 45 to 60 minutes of mindfulness practice each day for 8 weeks [9]. The current study suggests that mindfulness exercises of a total of 15 minutes a day may be effective for adults with mild to moderate depressive symptomatology. Much of the research on the effects of MBCT is conducted based on a clinical population. For the non-clinical population, mostly still working and active socially, the required time commitment on a weekly and daily basis may be a barrier to effectively integrate exercises into daily life. Carmody and Baer [56] concluded in their review that the correlation between mean effect size and number of in-class hours was non-significant for both clinical and non-clinical samples. They suggested that adaptations that include less class time may be worthwhile for populations for whom reduction of psychological distress is an important goal and for whom longer time commitment may be a barrier to their ability or willingness to participate. Our findings are in line with a number of studies which have shown that short-term meditation can lead to more tolerance, and a lower distress of pain and perceived stress (e.g. [57,58]). For example, Klatt et al. [57] showed that a 60-minute training together with 20 minutes of daily practice of meditation can have a significant positive effect on levels of perceived stress in healthy working adults ($p = .0025$). Also, Cavanagh et al. [21] effectively adapted their online MBCT to a brief intervention with daily mindfulness meditation practices of 10 minutes. Our finding that an 11-week MBCT training with 15 minutes of daily mindfulness meditation practice can sufficiently and significantly reduce depressive symptomatology seems promising from a public mental health perspective and is in line with Carmody and Baer [56]. The finding that the community-based MBCT intervention was very positively evaluated by the participants (scoring 7.98 out of 10), and that very few people dropped out of the intervention or dropped out of the study, underscores the feasibility and the attractiveness of the intervention.

Limitations

Some limitations must also be acknowledged. First, for the design of the study as a waiting-list compared RCT, controlling for the influence of possible non-specific factors, such as attention and social interaction, was unlikely. Future research should use an active control intervention or an attention placebo controlled design to overcome this limitation. Secondly, the study used a short follow-up period of 3 months for which the follow-up was limited to a within group analysis. For ethical reasons, the time until the control group could receive the intervention was limited to 3 months. For future research, a longer follow-up (e.g. 1-year follow-up) is recommended to study the impact of MBCT on the incidence of depression. Third, the design was a pragmatic randomized controlled trial with self-referred participants, so the results of the study may have been influenced by a selection bias. All measures were self-report: no psychiatric diagnoses were available because participants were recruited from the general public. Generalizability of the findings to patients seeking treatment cannot be assumed. On the other hand, no restrictions were made to the level of depressive symptoms, as is customary to the procedures applied in community mental health centers. In this regard, the study was representative for standard general practice.

Conclusion

This study shows that MBCT as a public mental health intervention for adults with mild to moderate depressive symptomatology is effective by not only reducing depressive symptoms and anxiety symptoms, but also enhancing positive mental health and psychological flexibility. Furthermore, this study shows that the intervention is applicable and effective in a natural setting.

Supporting Information

Checklist S1 CONSORT Checklist.

File S1 Metadata file.

Protocol S1 Trial protocol English translation.

Protocol S2 Trial protocol original Dutch language.

Acknowledgments

The authors wish to thank the therapists and participants that took part in this study.

Author Contributions

Conceived and designed the experiments: WTP PAM MMV JJK ETB. Performed the experiments: JJK. Analyzed the data: WTP PAM MMV. Contributed reagents/materials/analysis tools: WTP PAM MMV JJK ETB. Wrote the paper: WTP PAM MMV JJK ETB.

References

1. Cuijpers P, Smit F, Oostenbrink J, De Graaf R, Ten Have M, et al. (2007) Economic costs of minor depression: A population-based study. Acta Psychiatr Scand 115: 229–236.
2. Muñoz RF, Cuijpers P, Smit F, Barrera AZ, Leykin Y (2010) Prevention of major depression. Annu Rev Clin Psychol 6: 181–212.
3. Jané-Llopis E, Barry M, Hosman C, Patel V (2005) Mental health promotion works: a review. Promot Educ Suppl 2: 9–25, 61, 67.
4. Cuijpers P, Beekman ATF, Reynolds CF (2012) Preventing depression: A global priority. JAMA 307: 1033–1034.
5. Cuijpers P, Van Straten A, Warmerdam L, Van Rooy MJ (2010) Recruiting participants for interventions to prevent the onset of depressive disorders: Possibile ways to increase participation rates. BMC Health Serv Res 10: 181.
6. Keyes CLM, Dhingra SS, Simoes EJ (2010) Change in level of positive mental health as a predictor of future risk of mental Illness. Am J Public Health 100: 2366–2371.
7. Wood AM, Joseph S (2010) The absence of positive psychological (eudemonic) well-being as a risk factor for depression: A ten year cohort study. J Affect Disord 122: 213–217.
8. Fledderus M, Bohlmeijer ET, Smit F, Westerhof GJ (2010) Mental health promotion as a new goal in public mental health care: A randomized controlled trial of an intervention enhancing psychological flexibility. Am J Public Health 100: 2372–2378.
9. Segal ZV, Williams JMG, Teasdale JD (2002) Mindfulness-based Cognitive Therapy for Depression: A New Approach to Preventing Relapse. New York: The Guilford Press.
10. Ma SH, Teasdale JD (2004) Mindfulness-Based Cognitive Therapy for Depression: Replication and Exploration of Differential Relapse Prevention Effects. J Consult Clin Psychol 72: 31–40.
11. Teasdale JD, Segal ZV, Williams JMG, Ridgewaya VA, Soulsby JM, et al. (2000) Prevention of relapse/recurrence in major depression by mindfulness-based cognitive therapy. J Consult Clin Psychol 68: 615–623.
12. Piet J & Hougaard E (2011) The effect of mindfulness-based cognitive therapy for prevention of relapse in recurrent major depressive disorder: A systematic review and meta-analysis. Clin Psychol Rev, 31: 1032–1040.
13. Williams JMG, Crane C, Barnhofer T, Brennan K, Duggan DS, et al. (2014) Mindfulness-based cognitive therapy for preventing relapse in recurrent depression: A randomized dismantling trial. J Consult Clin Psychol 82: 275–286.
14. Strauss C, Cavanagh K, Oliver A, Pettman D (2014) Mindfulness-based interventions for people diagnosed with a current episode of an anxiety or depressive disorder: A meta-analysis of randomised controlled trails. PLOS ONE 9:e96110. doi: 10.1371/journal.pone.0096110
15. Hayes SC, Luoma JB, Bond FW, Masuda A, Lillis J (2006) Acceptance and Commitment Therapy: Model, processes and outcomes. Behav Res Ther 44: 1–25.
16. Aldao A, Nolen-Hoeksema S (2010) Specificity of cognitive emotion regulation strategies: A transdiagnostic examination. Behav Res Ther 48: 974–983.
17. Kabat-Zinn J (1990) Full catastrophe living: Using the wisdom of your body and mind to face stress, pain and illness. New York: Delacorte.
18. Chiesa A, Serretti A (2011) Mindfulness based cognitive therapy for psychiatric disorders: A systematic review and meta-analysis. Psychiatry Res 187: 441–453.
19. Chiesa A, Anselmi R, Serretti A (2014) Psychological mechanisms of mindfulness-based interventions: What do we know? Holist Nurs Pract 28: 124–148.
20. Kaviani H, Hatami N, Javaheri F (2012) The impact of Mindfulness-based Cognitive Therapy (MBCT) on mental health and quality of life in a sub-clinically depressed population. Arch Gen Psychiatry 14: 21–28.
21. Cavanagh K, Strauss C, Cicconi F, Griffiths N, Wyper A, et al. (2012) A randomised controlled trial of a brief online mindfulness-based intervention. Behav Res Ther 51: 573–578.
22. Sheehan DV, Lecrubier Y, Sheehan KH, Amorim P, Janavs J, et al. (1998) The Mini-International Neuropsychiatric Interview (M.I.N.I.): the development and validation of a structured diagnostic psychiatric interview for DSM-IV and ICD-10. J Clin Psychiatry 59: 22–33.
23. Van Vliet IM, De Beurs E (2007) The MINI-International Neuropsychiatric Interview (M.I.N.I.). A brief structured diagnostic psychiatric interview for DSM-IV and ICD-10 psychiatric disorders [in Dutch]. Tijdschr Psychiatr 49: 393–397.
24. Radloff LS (1977) The CES-D scale, a self report depression scale for research in the general population. Appl Psychol Meas 1: 385–401.
25. Haringsma R, Engels GI, Beekman ATF, Spinhoven P (2004) The criterion validity of the Center for Epidemiological Studies Depression Scale (CES-D) in a sample of self-referred elders with depressive symptomatology. Int J Geriatr Psychiatry 19: 558–563.
26. Zigmond AS, Snaith RP (1983) The hospital anxiety and depression scale. Acta Psychiatr Scand 67: 361–370.
27. Spinhoven P, Ormel J, Sloekers PPA, Kempen GIJM, Speckens AEM, et al. (1997) A validation study of the hospital anxiety and depression scale (HADS) in different groups of Dutch subjects. Psychol Med 27: 363–370.
28. Keyes CLM, Wissing M, Potgieter JP, Temane M, Kruger A, et al. (2008) Evaluation of the mental health continuum-short form (MHC-SF) in Setswana-speaking South Africans. Clin Psychol Psychother 15: 181–192.
29. Lamers SMA, Westerhof GJ, Bohlmeijer ET, Ten Klooster PM, Keyes CLM (2011) Evaluating the psychometric properties of the mental health Continuum-Short Form (MHC-SF). J Clin Psychol 67: 99–110.
30. Bond FW, Hayes SC, Baer RA, Carpenter KM, Guenole N, et al. (2011) Preliminary Psychometric Properties of the Acceptance and Action Questionnaire-II: A Revised Measure of Psychological Inflexibility and Experiential Avoidance. Behav Ther 42: 676–688.
31. Fledderus M, Oude Voshaar MAH, ten Klooster PM, Bohlmeijer ET (2012) Further evaluation of the psychometric properties of the acceptance and action questionnaire-II. Psychol Assess 24: 925–936.
32. Baer RA, Smith GT, Hopkins J, Krietemeyer J, Toney L (2006) Using self-report assessment methods to explore facets of mindfulness. Assessment 13: 27–45.
33. Bohlmeijer E, Klooster PM, Fledderus M, Veehof M, Baer R (2011) Psychometric properties of the five facet mindfulness questionnaire in depressed adults and development of a short form. Assessment 18: 308–320.
34. Dempster AP, Laird NM, Rubin DB (1977) Maximum likelihood from incomplete data via the EM algorithm. J R Stat Soc Series B Stat Methodol 39: 1–38.

35. Morris SB, DeShon RP (2002) Combining effect size estimates in meta-analysis with repeated measures and independent-groups designs. Psychol Methods 7: 105–125.
36. Lipsey MW, Wilson DB (1993) The efficacy of psychological, educational, and behavioral treatment: Confirmation from meta-analysis. Am Psychol 48: 1181–1209.
37. Jacobson NS, Truax P (1991) Clinical significance: A statistical approach to defining meaningful change in psychotherapy research. J Consult Clin Psychol 59: 12–19.
38. Beekman ATF, Deeg DJH, Van Limbeek J, Braam AW, De Vries MZ, et al. (1997) Criterion validity of the Center for Epidemiologic Studies Depression scale (CES-D): Results from a community-based sample of older subjects in the Netherlands. Psychol Med 27: 231–235.
39. Smit F, Ederveen A, Cuijpers P, Deeg D, Beekman A (2006) Opportunities for cost-effective prevention of late-life depression: An epidemiological approach. Arch Gen Psychiatry 63: 290–296.
40. Cook RJ, Sackett DL (1995) The number needed to treat: A clinically useful measure of treatment effect. Br Med J 310: 452–454.
41. Baron RM, Kenny DA (1986) The moderator-mediator variable distinction in social psychological research: conceptual, strategic, and statistical considerations. J Pers Soc Psychol 51: 1173–1182.
42. Preacher KJ, Hayes AF (2008) Asymptotic and resampling strategies for assessing and comparing indirect effects in multiple mediator models. Behav Res Methods 40: 879–891.
43. Cuijpers P, Smit F, Van Straten A (2007) Psychological treatments of subthreshold depression: A meta-analytic review. Acta Psychiatr Scand 115: 434–441.
44. Cuijpers P, Smit F (2004) Subthreshold depression as a risk indicator for major depressive disorder: A systematic review of prospective studies. Acta Psychiatr Scand 109: 325–331.
45. Cuijpers P, Van Straten A, Smit F, Mihalopoulos C, Beekman A (2008) Preventing the onset of depressive disorders: A meta-analytic review of psychological interventions. Am J Psychiatry 165: 1272–1280.
46. Vollestad J, Nielsen MB, Nielsen GH (2012) Mindfulness- and acceptance-based interventions for anxiety disorders: A systematic review and meta-analysis. Br J Clin Psychol 51: 239–260.
47. Horn PJ, Wuyek LA (2010) Anxiety disorders as a risk factor for subsequent depression. Int J Psychiatry Clin Pract 14: 244–247.
48. Kuyken W, Byford S, Taylor RS, Watkins E, Holden E, et al. (2008) Mindfulness-Based Cognitive Therapy to Prevent Relapse in Recurrent Depression. J Consult Clin Psychol 76: 966–978.
49. Lamers SMA, Westerhof GJ, Kovács V, Bohlmeijer ET (2012) Differential relationships in the association of the Big Five personality traits with positive mental health and psychopathology. J Res Pers 46: 517–524.
50. Fava GA, Tomba E (2009) Increasing psychological well-being and resilience by psychotherapeutic methods. J Pers 77: 1903–1934.
51. Ruini C, Fava GA (2012) Role of Well-Being Therapy in Achieving a Balanced and Individualized Path to Optimal Functioning. Clin Psychol Psychother 19: 291–304.
52. Ryff CD, Friedman EM, Morozink JA, Tsenkova V (2012) Psychological resilience in adulthood and later life: Implications for health. Annu Rev Gerontol Geriatr 32: 73–92.
53. Kuyken W, Watkins E, Holden E, White K, Taylor RS, et al. (2010) How does mindfulness-based cognitive therapy work? Behav Res Ther 48: 1105–1112.
54. Kashdan TB, Rottenberg J (2010) Psychological flexibility as a fundamental aspect of health. Clin Psychol Rev 30: 865–878.
55. McCarney RW, Schulz J, Grey AR (2012) Effectiveness of mindfulness-based therapies in reducing symptoms of depression: A meta-analysis. European Journal of Psychotherapy and Counselling 14: 279–299.
56. Carmody J, Baer RA (2009) How long does a mindfulness-based stress reduction program need to be? A review of class contact hours and effect sizes for psychological distress. J Clin Psychol 65: 627–638.
57. Klatt MD, Buckworth J, Malarkey WB (2009) Effects of low-dose mindfulness-based stress reduction (MBSR-ld) on working adults. Health Educ Behav 36: 601–614.
58. Liu X, Wang S, Chang S, Chen W, Si M (2012) Effect of Brief Mindfulness Intervention on Tolerance and Distress of Pain Induced by Cold-Pressor Task. Stress Health 29: 199–204.

3

Modeling the Dynamics of Disease States in Depression

Selver Demic[1,2,3], Sen Cheng[1,2,3]*

1 International Graduate School of Neuroscience, Bochum, Germany, **2** Mercator Research Group "Structure of Memory", Bochum, Germany, **3** Faculty of Psychology, Ruhr University Bochum, Bochum, Germany

Abstract

Major depressive disorder (MDD) is a common and costly disorder associated with considerable morbidity, disability, and risk for suicide. The disorder is clinically and etiologically heterogeneous. Despite intense research efforts, the response rates of antidepressant treatments are relatively low and the etiology and progression of MDD remain poorly understood. Here we use computational modeling to advance our understanding of MDD. First, we propose a systematic and comprehensive definition of disease states, which is based on a type of mathematical model called a finite-state machine. Second, we propose a dynamical systems model for the progression, or dynamics, of MDD. The model is abstract and combines several major factors (mechanisms) that influence the dynamics of MDD. We study under what conditions the model can account for the occurrence and recurrence of depressive episodes and how we can model the effects of antidepressant treatments and cognitive behavioral therapy within the same dynamical systems model through changing a small subset of parameters. Our computational modeling suggests several predictions about MDD. Patients who suffer from depression can be divided into two sub-populations: a high-risk sub-population that has a high risk of developing chronic depression and a low-risk sub-population, in which patients develop depression stochastically with low probability. The success of antidepressant treatment is stochastic, leading to widely different times-to-remission in otherwise identical patients. While the specific details of our model might be subjected to criticism and revisions, our approach shows the potential power of computationally modeling depression and the need for different type of quantitative data for understanding depression.

Editor: H. Sunny Sun, National Cheng Kung University Medical College, Taiwan

Funding: S.C. was supported by a grant from the Stiftung Mercator. S.D. was supported by the International Graduate School of Neuroscience. The funders had no role in study design, data collection and analysis, decision to publish, or preparation of the manuscript.

Competing Interests: The authors have declared that no competing interests exist.

* Email: sen.cheng@rub.de

Introduction

Major depressive disorder (MDD) affects around 20% of the population at some point during the life time of an individual [1–4]. Depression is a common and costly disorder that is usually associated with severe and persistent symptoms leading to important social role impairment, increased medical co-morbidity and mortality [5–7]. Depression can strike anyone regardless of age, ethnic background, socioeconomic status or gender [8,9]. According to the World Health Organization, MDD is currently the leading cause of disease burden in North America and the 4th leading cause worldwide [5,10–12]. The onset of MDD is usually between the ages of 20 and 30 years and peaks between 30 and 40 years [13,14].

The understanding of the nature and causes of depression has evolved over the centuries, though this understanding is incomplete and has left many aspects of depression as a subject of discussion and research. The heterogeneity of depression implies that multiple neural substrates and mechanisms contribute to its etiology [15]. Proposed causes include psychological, psychosocial, hereditary, evolutionary and biological factors. Family, twin, and adoption studies provide evidence that genetic factors might account for some risk of developing MDD [16–18]. According to diathesis-stress theories of depression, genetic liability (diathesis) interacts with negative life experiences (stress) to cause depressive symptoms and disorders [19,20]. Indeed, there is some evidence for the involvement of specific genes and gene-by-environment interactions in the pathogenesis of MDD, even though they cannot account for all occurrences of MDD [5].

One major theory about the biological etiology of depression suggests that the underlying pathophysiological basis of depression is a depletion of the neurotransmitters serotonin, nor-epinephrine or dopamine in the central nervous system [21–23]. Although most antidepressants drugs (ADs) produce a rapid increase in extracellular level of the monoamines, the onset of an appreciable clinical effect usually takes at least 3–4 weeks [24–29]. This delayed onset of action, or response, which is usually defined as a 50% reduction in depression rating scale score compared to baseline [30], suggests that dysfunctions of monoaminergic neurotransmitter systems found in MDD represent the down-stream effects of other, more primary abnormalities. In addition, success of AD treatment is relatively low. Selective serotonin re-uptake inhibitors (SSRIs) are frequently used as a first medication for MDD, but have response rates of 50% to 60% in daily practice [31–35]. In some studies, ADs even fail to show superiority over placebo [36–38]. More precisely, the response to inert placebos is approximately 75% of the response to active AD medication [36,39]. The high rate of inadequate treatment of the disorder remains a serious concern. Research comparing AD medication to cognitive behavioral therapy (CBT) has found that both are equally effective for non-psychotic forms of depression [40].

Indeed, in some theories of depression, cognitive aspects are dominant factors in the etiology and maintenance of the disorder [41–43]. These models postulate that depressed patients process depression-congruent information selectively, which seems to form part of a vulnerability factor.

In addition to the heterogeneous etiology of MDD, the disorder shows complex transitions between several disease states. According to the Diagnostic and Statistical Manual of Mental Disorder, 4th edition, text revision (DSM-IV-TR), the standard for the diagnosis of mental disorders, a depressive episode (DE) is characterized as a period lasting at least 14 days, during which the patient is consistently within the symptomatic range of a sufficient number of symptoms [1,44]. A DE can be interrupted by remission, which is defined as an asymptomatic period of at least 14 days [45]. A remission and recovery are accompanied by the same behavioral symptoms and, at the behavioral level, distinguished only by their duration. A remission that lasts for 6 months or longer is called recovery [45]. This term refers to recovery from the episode, not from MDD per se. The appearance of a new DE after recovery is called a recurrence [45]. A relapse is a return of the symptoms satisfying the full syndrome criteria for an DE during the period of remission, but before recovery [1,45]. According to a population-based study among depressive patients, about 15% of first lifetime onsets have unremitting course, and 35% recover but have one or more future episodes [46,47]. These cases may represent chronic and more severe forms of MDD [46,48]. About 50% of first lifetime onsets recover and have no future episodes [46]. However, the disease states in depression are not defined consistently by different investigators, thus making it difficult to interpret the results and precluding comparisons between different studies.

All hypotheses that try to explain the dynamics of depression have certain limitations, so our understanding what causes depression is still incomplete. Existing hypotheses are not exclusive, but rather complementary. The question is how to integrate the different hypotheses. Mathematical models are well-suited for this problem. Here, we aim to systematically define the states in the course of MDD and to study the dynamics of MDD. We developed a single abstract model that is consistent with many existing theories about depression. Although our model is not mechanistic, it helps us to understand and analyze the etiology and dynamics of MDD. Finally, we modeled the influence of three types of therapies (antidepressant treatment, cognitive behavioral therapy, and life style changes) on the occurrence and duration of depressive episode.

Methods

Dynamical systems model of major depressive disorder

To model the dynamics of depression, we first need a way to describe the state of a person, i.e., whether a person is suffering from MDD or not. We adopted the simplest approach possible, which is to describe the state of a person by a single variable. We call this variable M, loosely for mood. $M<0$ indicates that the person suffers from symptoms associated with MDD; the person is in the symptomatic state. In our simple model with only one variable, we do not model which precise symptoms patients suffer from. A negative value of the state variable indicates that the person satisfies a sufficient number of symptoms (Table 1) to meet the syndromal criterion for a depressive episode according to DSM-IV-TR [1]. If this state persists for fourteen days or more, the person is considered to suffer from MDD [1,45]. $M>0$ indicates that the person does not meet the syndromal criterion for a depressive episode; the person is in the asymptomatic state.

The variable M changes across time to account for changes in the symptoms and progression of MDD. We model the time evolution of M in discrete time steps according to this simple equation

$$M(t+\Delta t)=M(t)+\frac{dM}{dt}\Delta t \qquad (1)$$

.

In each time step Δt, the mood changes by the amount $\frac{dM}{dt}\Delta t$. The crucial issue is how to model the dynamics of the mood given by $\frac{dM}{dt}$. The dynamics fully determines the behavior of the system and should account for the major empirical observations in MDD as outlined in the Introduction. We were looking for a simple model that can capture many of the important clinical observations related to MDD. The simplest model is a linear one with a single stable point. Preliminary work showed that linear dynamics does not account for many important observations. It was too easy to switch from positive to negative mood and vice versa, which is in contradiction with the phenomenology of MDD. Thus it was evident that we needed a model that has two stable states, one corresponding to a depressive state and the other to a non-depressive state. We therefore chose to model the dynamics with a polynomial of third degree (Fig. 1A).

$$\frac{dM}{dt}=-0.01a(M-b)(M-c)(M-d)+I+\varepsilon \qquad (2)$$

,where $a>0$; b, c, d are parameters to be studied, I is an external input, and ε is a Gaussian noise term with zero mean and a standard deviation of one to set the scale. In our model, the system is driven both by deterministic intrinsic dynamics (cf. Fig. 1B) and a stochastic noise process (cf. Fig. 1C, D). The intrinsic dynamics is an abstract model of the changes in the mood of a person driven by deterministic physiological processes, processes which we do not attempt to model mechanistically here. The dynamical system in Eq. (2) has two stable fix points, separated by an unstable fix point. The parameters b, c, and d are ordered such that $b \leq c \leq d$ (Fig. 1A). The parameters of the model specify the unique dynamics of a system, which represents a person. Depending on how the parameters affect the dynamics of MDD, we assign them to possible physiological correlates (Table 2). Within a subpopulation in our model, all individuals share identical parameters. By contrast, the noise process captures stochastic physiological processes as well as external environmental factors. Fluctuations in the mood can be caused, for instance, by random hormonal changes or by changes due to the circadian rhythm. Also, external changes might cause fluctuation in the mood of a person during the day, i.e., stressful situations at work or rapid weather changes. The name "noise" does not imply that the noise process is irrelevant or unimportant. On the contrary, the noise term is crucial in our model since it introduces unpredictable changes to the mood. This stochasticity is what makes the time-course of the mood of one modeled person (cf. Fig. 1D) different from that of another person.

Relating occurrence and recurrence rates to the distribution of the number of depressive episodes

We use empirical occurrence and recurrence rates to compute the distribution of the number of depressive episodes during an individual's lifetime (NDE) since the latter is rarely reported by

Table 1. DSM-IV-TR Criteria for Major Depressive Disorder [1].

Five or more of the following symptoms should be present daily for most of the day for at least 2 weeks
At least one symptom is either depressed mood or anhedonia
Changes in appetite or weight
Insomnia or hypersomnia
Psychomotor agitation or retardation
Fatigue or loss of energy
Feelings of guilty or worthlessness
Difficulty with thinking, concentrating, or making decisions
Suicidal ideation or suicidal attempts

epidemiological studies but quite informative. The occurrence rate (OR) is the fraction of the population that suffers from at least one DE during their life time. The OR thus equals the probability of having one or more depressive episodes, i.e.,

$$OR = p[NDE \geq 1] \tag{3}$$

The rate of first recurrence RR(1) is the fraction of patients who suffer from depression a second time out of those patients who suffered from one previous depressive episode. The rates of second recurrence RR(2), third recurrence RR(3), etc. are defined similarly. In general, RR(i) can be calculated using the following equation

$$RR(i) = \frac{p[NDE \geq i+1]}{p[NDE \geq i]} \tag{4}$$

The probability of having no depressive episode is

$$p[NDE = 0] = 1 - OR \tag{5}$$

The probability of having exactly one depressive episode is

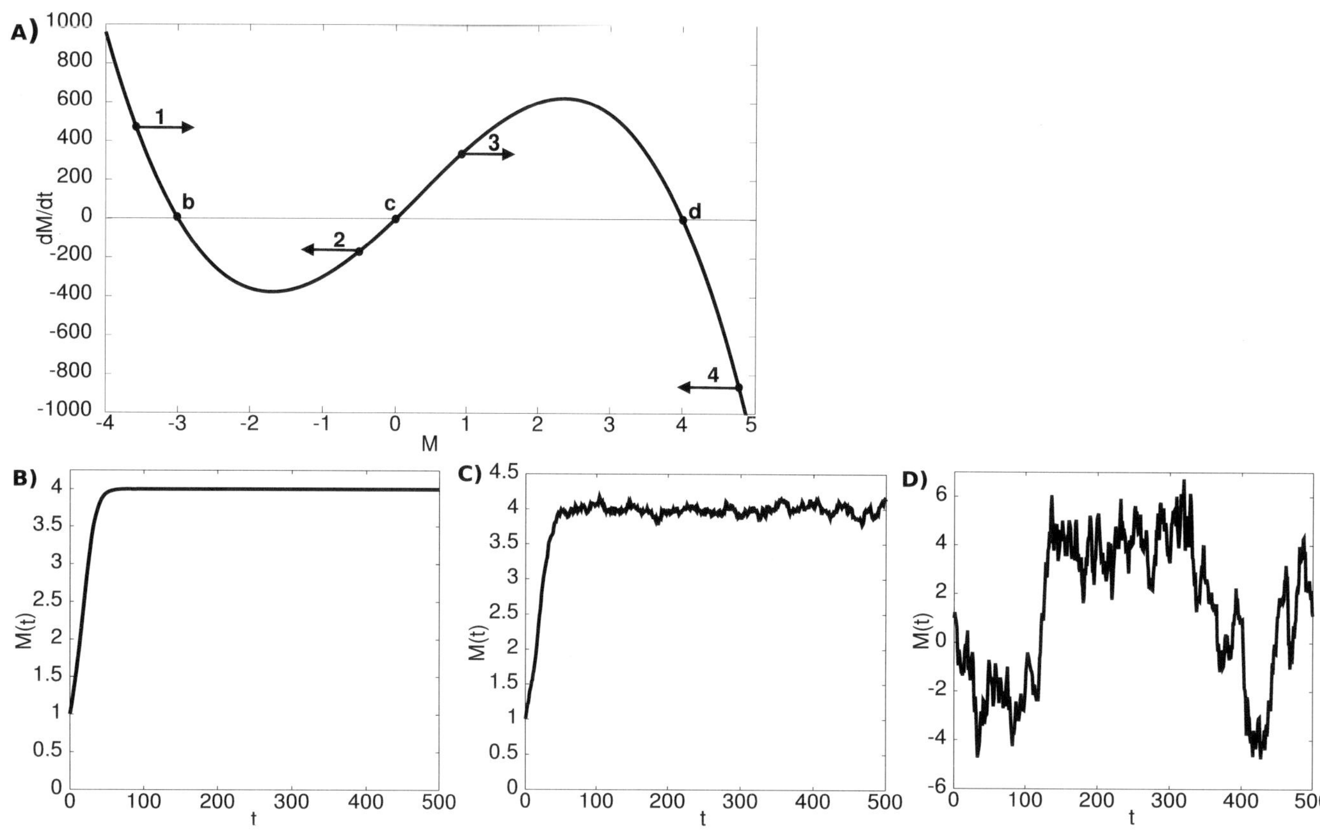

Figure 1. Dynamical systems model for the dynamics of mood. A) A schematic showing the mood change as a function of the state variable M without external inputs and noise ($I = \varepsilon = 0$). The arrows at 1, 2, 3, 4 indicate the direction of change in those states. The points labeled with b, c, and d are fix points. At these points, the value of the change is zero (dM/dt = 0). Therefore, when there is no noise, the state will not change once it has reached a fix point. The fix points b and d are stable, meaning that the system will return to these states if slightly perturbed. The fix point c is unstable and has different properties, the system will move further away from point c even if the system is only slightly perturbed. In that case, the system will evolve until it reaches one of the stable fixed points. If $M > c$, the system will move towards the fix point d. The system will evolve towards the other fix point b, if $M < c$. Therefore, the fix point c separates the basins of attraction of the two stable fix points. Samples of the evolution of M over time **B**) without noise, **C**) with a moderate level of noise and **D**) with high level of noise. Note, that with high level of noise the system exhibits stochastic transition between positive and negative values.

Table 2. Potential physiological correlates of the model parameters.

Symbol	Parameter	Potential physiological correlates
a	Decay rate	Hippocampal volume and rate of adult neurogenesis
b	Negative stable fix point	Level of monoamines (i.e. serotonin)
c	Instable fix point	Pessimistic attitude c>0, optimistic attitude c<0
d	Positive stable fix point	Amygdala activity (higher activity is represented by a smaller d)
I	External input	Environmental influence
ε	Noise	Unpredictable internal or external changes that cause fluctuation in the mood

$$p[\mathrm{NDE}=1]=(1-\mathrm{RR}(1))\mathrm{OR} \quad (6)$$

The probability of having two or more depressive episode is computed according to this equation

$$p[\mathrm{NDE}=i]=(1-RR(i))\mathrm{OR}\prod_{j=1}^{i-1}RR(j) \quad (7)$$

for $i \geq 1$.

To study the OR and RR, we initialized the system in a positive state $M(0)=1.75$ and simulated the dynamics of MDD for a period of 70 years using a time-step $\Delta t=0.1$d. For both the single population and the two sub-populations model, the analyses are based on simulations of 10000 individuals. In the two sub-populations model, *93%* of individuals belong to the low-risk sub-population while the remaining *7%* belong to the high-risk sub-population.

Studying treatment effects

To study the time-to-remission and time-to-response in our model, we initialized the system in a negative state $b \leq M(0) < 0$. The initial value was drawn from a uniform distribution. We simulated the dynamics of MDD for a period of 20 years using a time-step $\Delta t=0.1$d. To study the effects of different treatments, we used only simulations of the two-subpopulations model in which a DE occurred. Hence, *63%* of the simulations belong to the low-risk sub-population while the remaining 37% belong to the high-risk sub-population. We initialized the finite-state machine in the rebound depressive episode state and considered the time when M increases above 50% as time-to-response, and the time at which the first remission or recovery occurred as the time-to-remission. Fourteen days were added to the time-to-remission to account for the fact that symptoms have to be present for at least fourteen days to qualify as an DE. In the control group, parameters were identical to those used for the simulation of the occurrence rate. In the experimental group, we changed certain parameters in order to simulate the effect of various treatments such as AD treatment (change in parameter a, and d or b), CBT (change in parameter c) and life style changes (change in parameter I).

All simulations and analyses were performed in Matlab R2012a (MathWorks; Natick, Massachusetts, USA) using custom-written software. The code is freely available online at http://cns.mrg1.rub.de/index.php/software

Results

Finite state machine: systematic definition of disease states

We developed a finite state machine (Fig. 2) to systematically define the disease states of MDD: *depressive episode, remission, recovery*, and *relapse*, which were described above. This mathematical model analyzes the transitions of M from the asymptomatic to the symptomatic state, and vice versa, and assigns a disease state to each time interval. The disease state changes depending on the length of periods for which M remains positive (T_p) or negative (T_n) (see Fig. 3 for an example). In addition to the disease states of clinical relevance, we had to introduce auxiliary disease states to account for short interruptions of a disease state that are clinically irrelevant. For instance, if a one-month-long depressive episode is interrupted by a 2-day-long period in the asymptomatic state, there is little reason to assume that the short interruption has any relevance. Clinicians frequently make such intuitive judgments without making them explicit [45], but such discounting has to be build in explicitly in a mathematical model.

In the following, we describe the auxiliary disease states in more detail. The *null state* is the initial state, before any data is available to make a more specific determination of the disease state. Short periods in the symptomatic state, $T_n < 14$, and any duration in the asymptomatic state, $T_p > 0$, will not change this state (Fig. 2&3). The only possible transition out of the null state is to a DE, if the syndromal criterion is met for at least 14 consecutive days, i.e., $T_n \geq 14$. A *rebound depressive episode* is an interruption of a DE that is shorter than two weeks (Fig. 2&3). The duration in the positive state is added to the duration of the DE (boxes connected to rebound depressive episode in Fig. 2). Similarly, *rebound relapse, interrupted remission*, and *interrupted recovery* are interruptions of the relapse, remission and recovery states of MDD, respectively. The auxiliary disease states are necessary to discount short interruptions of the disease states in our model and have little clinical relevance. We therefore focus our attention on the clinically relevant disease states in the following.

One point requires special attention. Recovery occurs after an asymptomatic period of 6 months or more, even if that period is interrupted by short periods (<14 days) in the negative state. If the first period in the positive state lasts for longer than 14 days and less than 6 month, then the finite-state machine will initially label this period as remission. Short interruptions in the negative state and the following periods in the positive state are added to duration of remission. If the total duration of the "remission" period exceeds 6 months, then the period becomes recovery. To correct the initial classification, we included an action "change

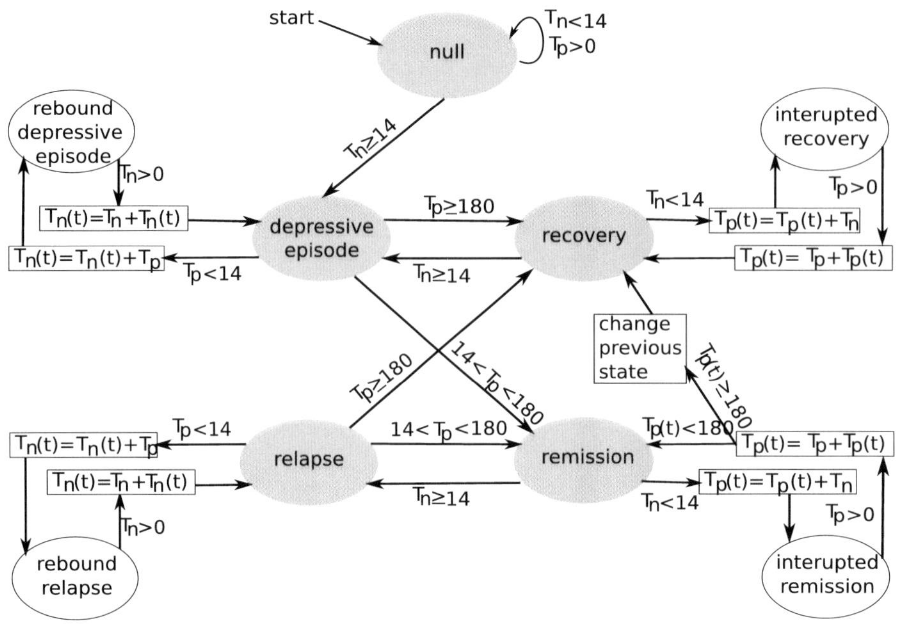

Figure 2. Finite state machine modeling the transitions between the disease states in depression. State diagram for the finite state machine. Ellipses represent the disease states in depression. Grey filled ellipses are clinically relevant disease states; unfilled ellipses are auxiliary disease states that are needed to discount short interruptions of clinically relevant disease states. The arrows indicate transitions between disease states. Transitions only occur when the state variable *M* changes sign, i.e., either from positive to negative, or vice versa. Each arrow is labeled by the criteria that trigger the transition. T_n represents the length (in days) of the period during *M*<*0* before transition to a positive value occurred. In other words, T_n is the duration that a person meets the syndromal criterion for a depressive episode according to DSM-IV-TR [1]. Accordingly, T_p represents the length (in days) of the period during *M*>*0*, i.e., the duration in which a person does not meet the syndromal criterion for a depressive episode. The rectangles indicate a change to previously identified states. Short interruptions of disease states are added to the duration of disease states.

previous state" (Fig. 2). This finite-state machine unambiguously defines the disease states and can be used to track their evolution over the lifespan of patients as well as in our theoretical simulations.

Dynamical systems model for the dynamics of major depressive disorder

We developed a simple dynamical systems model (see Methods) to simulate and study the progression of disease states over 70

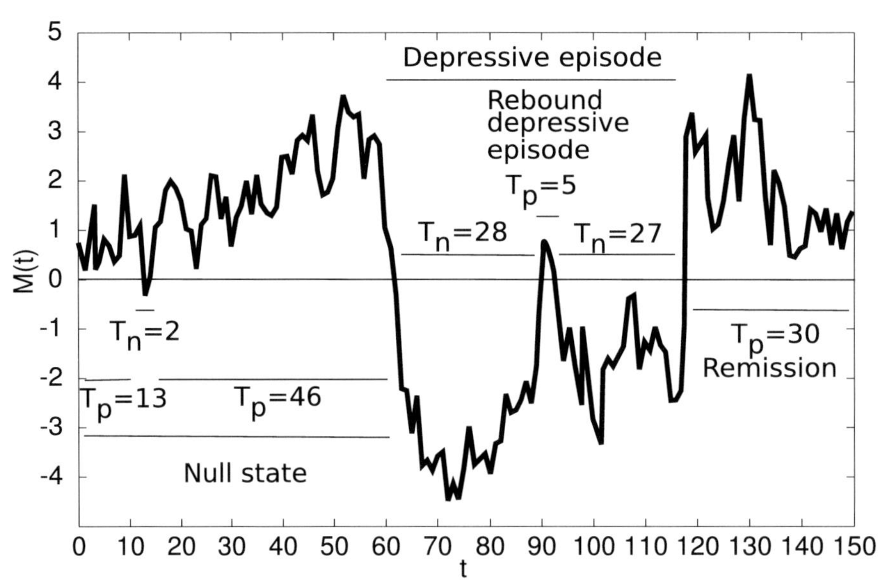

Figure 3. Example of the time course of the state variable *M* and the disease states identified by the finite state machine. In this example, a symptomatic period lasting 28d is interrupted by an asymptomatic period of 5d and followed by another symptomatic period of 27d. Therefire, our model identifies the three periods together as a single depressive episode of length 60d. T_n and T_p represent the length (in days) of the period when *M*<0 and *M*>0, respectively.

years. In a first attempt, we speculated that perhaps all people share the same dynamics parameters, and thus similar physiological parameters, and that depressive episodes occur stochastically.

If our model captures some aspect of the dynamics of MDD, it should be able to account for the epidemiological data on occurrence and recurrence rates of MDD (see Methods). According to DSM-IV-TR, $OR = 20\%$, $RR(1) = 50\%$, $RR(2) = 70\%$, and $RR(3) = 90\%$ [1]. In our first modeling attempt, we chose a single set of parameters representing a homogeneous population to match the epidemiological occurrence rate. The parameters of the single population model were: $a = 4.65$; $b = -3$; $c = 0.175$; $d = 5$; $I = 0.02$. However, this model does not match any of the epidemiological recurrence rates (Fig. 4A). The mismatch is not simply a numerical issue, the model yields qualitatively different data. Rather than having rates that increase with the number of DE as in epidemiological studies, in our single-population model, the rates decrease.

This is not surprising. Since a one-dimensional model has no memory other than the current state, the probability of the second DE (the first recurrence) occurring within a certain time period is the same as the probability of the first DE. However, the first DE can occur anytime within the full 70 years of simulated time whereas the second DE can only occur after the first DE had already occurred. Since the number of DE are proportional to the length of the observation period, the first recurrence rate is lower than the occurrence rate. The same logic applies to the second and third recurrence rates, which are successively lower (Fig. 4A). Our argument implies that this property is not specific to the particular parameters that we chose. Indeed, additional simulations show for a range of the parameters a and b that, in the single population model, the rate of first recurrence is lower than the occurrence rate, and the rate of second recurrence is lower than the rate of first recurrence (Fig. 5). To further investigate how the single population model deviates from the true dynamics of MDD, we calculated the distribution of NDE (Fig. 4B). In the simulated data, the likelihood monotonically decreases such that four or more DE are absent from our simulated data. In contrast, the epidemiological data show that four or more DE occur with a substantial probability of around 7% and is even higher than the probability of two or three DE. Since the epidemiological data follows a bimodal distribution, we hypothesized that two subpopulations might be required to account for empirical occurrence and recurrence rates of MDD.

We therefore simulated data for two sub-populations. In this model, ninety-three percent of the population shares low-risk parameters and develops depression with low probability. The parameters of this sub-population were chosen ($a = 5$; $b = -2.85$; $c = 0.175$; $d = 5$; $I = 0.02$) such that $OR = 13\%$. The remaining seven percent of the population belongs to the high-risk sub-population and develops depression with very high probability ($\sim 100\%$). The parameters for this sub-population were: $a = 4.4$; $b = -3.75$; $c = 0.175$; $d = 4.25$; $I = 0$. At this point, we would like to stress that the two sub-populations together represent the entire population, which implies that no one is absolutely immune to depression. By design, the two sub-population model yields a bimodal distribution of NDE (Fig. 6B). With this two sub-population model, we were able to match the empirical occurrence and recurrence rates of MDD (Fig. 6A).

Modeling the effect of antidepressant treatment

The most commonly used antidepressants are those that regulate the metabolism of monoamines in the brain, in particular serotonin. Our initial hypothesis was that the parameter d correlates with monoamine levels. Furthermore, it was shown that treatment with AD increases the rate of adult neurogenesis in the dentate gyrus [49] and it has been suggested that adult neurogenesis is important for memory [50]. Since the parameter a determines how quickly the current state is forgotten, we hypothesized that AD treatment increases parameter a. Since the intended effect of AD treatment is to reduce the time that patients suffer from the symptoms of MDD, we decided to use the time-to-remission as the target parameter for AD treatment. Our simulation results contradict our initial hypothesis, increasing the parameters a and d increases, rather than decreases, the time-to-remission (Fig. 7B&C). One potential resolution could be to assume that we correctly guessed the physiological correlates of the parameters a and d, but the relationship is inverse to our expectation. However, this interpretation is inconsistent with the OR in our simulations. Decreasing parameters a and/or d, increases the OR. Thus if we modeled the effect of AD treatment as a decrease in parameters a and/or d, it would imply paradoxically that AD treatment of healthy patients increases the OR of MDD (Fig. 7A, C). An extensive parameter search did not yield any parameter changes in a and d that have the desired change time-to-remission and OR simultaneously. We therefore turned to model the increase in the level of monoamines as an increase in parameter b (Fig. 8). In this scenario, the time-to-remission is reduced by an increase in b, but elevated by an increase in a (Fig. 8B, E). While the latter outcome is an undesirable property, there are combinations of simultaneous increases in parameters a and b that yield a lower time-to-remission. This is possible because the contour lines are not parallel to the axes or, in other words, the parameters are inter-dependent. Similarly, the OR is reduced by an increase in a, as desired, but elevated by an increase in b (Fig. 8A, C). Again, there are combinations of simultaneous increases in parameters a and b that yield a lower occurrence rate. Importantly for the change of parameters indicated by the black and white points, representing pre- and post-treatment parameters, the change in both the time-to-remission and occurrence rate are in the desired directions. We therefore suggest that parameter a correlates with the rate of adult neurogenesis and parameter b with monoamine levels (Table 2). It is worthwhile to note that AD treatment in our model does not work like a deterministic switch. Even though AD treatment in our model alters the physiological parameters immediately, remission remains a stochastic process driven by the intrinsic dynamics and the noise term. The results of our model demonstrate that the time required to see a significant effect of antidepressants is about three weeks, which is highly similar to the epidemiological data (see Table 3). Figure 9 shows the distribution of the duration of DEs. Both the treated (Fig, 9D, E, F) and control groups (Fig. 9A, B, C) exhibit distributions with large variances and long tails. This result is somewhat surprising given that within each subpopulation all individuals share the same parameters and it underlines the difficulty in understanding the physiological mechanisms of AD treatment. These highly skewed distributions might explain why the median duration of depressive episodes reported in the literature varies widely from three to twelve months, even if most studies suggest that the median duration of depressive episode is about three months [51–56]. Overall, we find that our model reproduces rather well other variables which are often used in a clinical and epidemiological studies to examine the efficacy of AD treatment (Table 3).

Modeling the effects of cognitive behavioral therapy and life style changes

CBT instructs patients with MDD to develop a more optimistic approach to life and to detect and transform negative thoughts

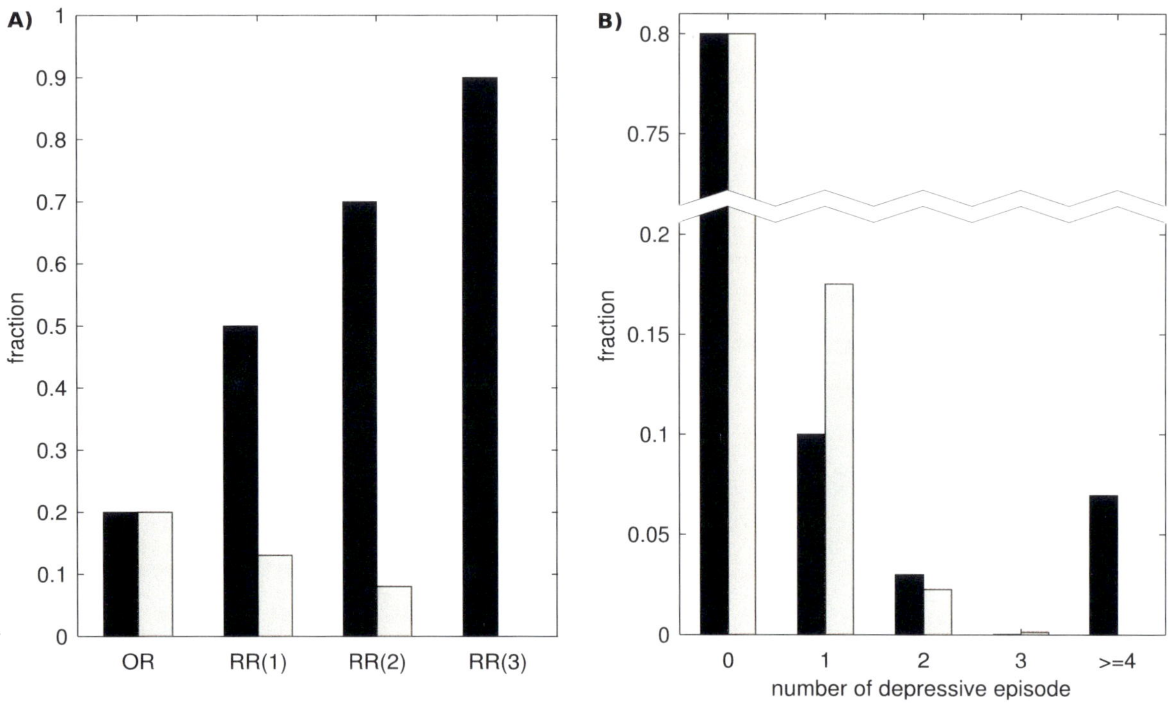

Figure 4. Single population model can account for empirical occurrence rate but not for recurrence rates. A) The occurrence rate (OR) from our simulation (grey bars) was fit to the result from epidemiological studies (black bars). The parameters of the model are: $a = 4.65$; $b = -3$; $c = 0.175$; $d = 5$; $I = 0.02$. However, in our simulation, the recurrence rates, RR(i), decrease with the number of prior depressive episodes, which is contrary to epidemiological data. **B**) The distribution of the number of depressive episodes (DE). The probability of zero DE is 0.8. The bars were cut off to show more clearly the smaller probabilities for the higher numbers of DE. The epidemiological distribution is clearly bimodal (black bars), whereas the simulated distribution is unimodal (grey bars).

into positive thinking [40,57,58]. The effect of CBT is an improved ability to deal with difficult circumstances and shorter durations of DEs [59,60]. A similar effect occurs in our simulations when we decrease parameter c: both the OR and the time-to-remission decrease (Fig. 10, the black and white points represent pre- and post-treatment value of parameter c, respectively). Moreover, the results of our model show that about half of the patients treated with CBT will be in remission after three months of treatment and that the number of patients in remission increases with elapsed time, in line with the epidemiological data (see Table 3). Hence, we hypothesize that smaller c correspond to optimistic attitude and larger c to pessimistic attitude (Table 2).

Life style changes such as, for instance, exercise, social support, and stress reduction lead to a lower probability of having another DE and to shorter duration of DEs, if they do occur [61–63]. Indeed, a recent study compared exercise, antidepressant medication and combined medication and exercise in adults and found that all treatments were effective [61,62]. Since external factors enter our model through the parameter I, we suggest that the parameter I correlates with environmental influence, where larger I corresponds to positive environmental influence and smaller I to negative influence (Table 2). Our simulations confirm that increasing I indeed decreases the time-to-remission and the OR (Fig. 10). In addition, our results suggest that the combination of

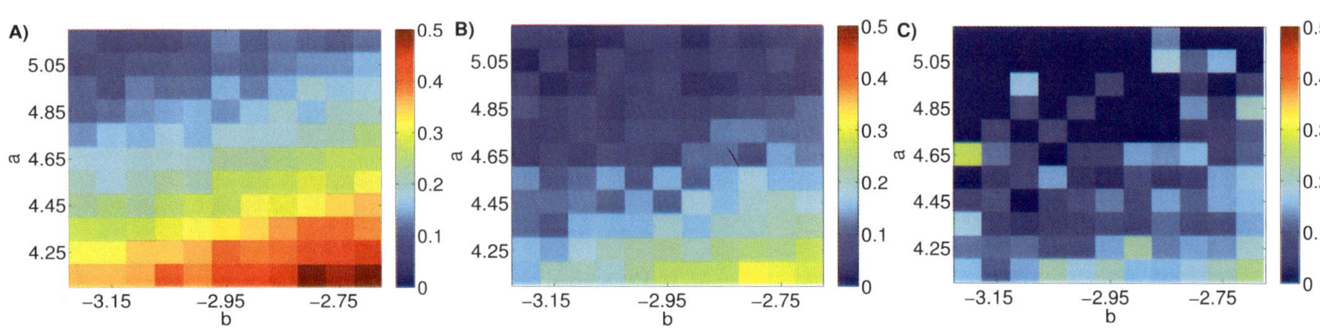

Figure 5. Influence of parameters a and b on the occurrence and recurrence rate in the single population model. A) Occurrence rate, **B**) first recurrence rate, and **C**) second recurrence rate, each represented by color scales, for a range of the parameters a and b. The remaining parameters are: $c = 0.175$; $d = 5$; $I = 0.02$. Note, that for all combinations of the parameters a and b, the rate of first recurrence is lower than the occurrence rate, and the rate of second recurrence is lower than the rate of first recurrence.

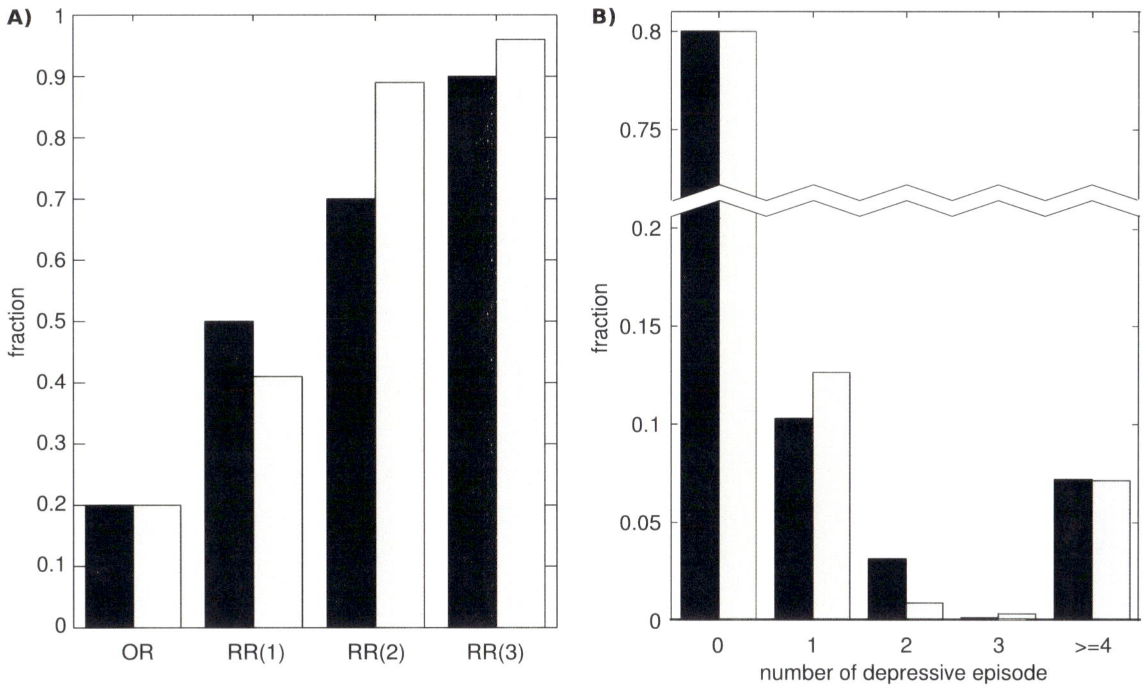

Figure 6. Two sub-population model can account for empirical occurrence and recurrence rate. A) The parameters of the two sub-population model are: $a = 5$; $b = -2.85$; $c = 0.175$; $d = 5$; $I = 0.02$ for the low-risk sub-population and $a = 4.4$; $b = -3.75$; $c = 0.175$; $d = 4.25$; $I = 0$ for the high-risk sub-population. Our simulation data (grey bars) closely matches the empirical (black bars) occurrence and recurrence rates and **B**) the distribution of the number of depressive episodes.

the two interventions, CBT and life style changes, will yield better results in the treatment of depression and the prevention of relapses and recurrence than their individual application.

Discussion

In this article, we have developed a finite-state machine to systematically define the states in the course of MDD together with operational criteria for the terms remission, recovery, relapse, and recurrence. We used a simple dynamical systems model to simulate the day-to-day fluctuations in the mood that might correlate with depression. While this model is not a physiological model, it incorporates several parameters that can be associated with physiological mechanisms. The advantage of this model is that it can incorporate several biological and psychological factors that are thought to affect MDD, and describe their potential interactions. Combining the finite-state machine and dynamical systems model, we studied the dynamics of disease states in depression and found that two sub-populations, one high-risk and one low-risk, are required in our model to account for the empirical data. The two sub-populations model is able to reproduce many, though not all, observations quite well.

One parameter, *d*, we have not associated with a physiological or cognitive roles, yet. The influence that parameter *d* has on the

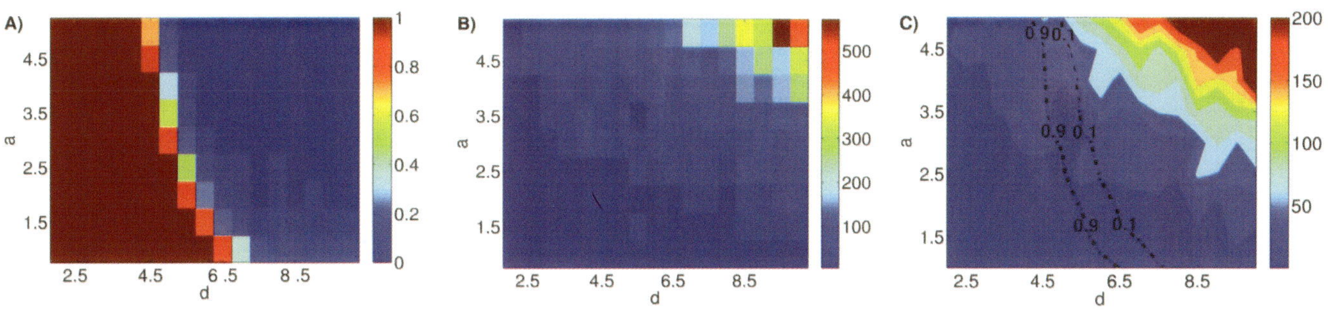

Figure 7. Modification of parameters a and d cannot account for the effect of antidepressant treatment. Shown in the color scales are the occurrence rate (**A**), the median time-to-remission (**B**) and the contours of the median time-to-remission (**C**) in simulated data. Consistent with the assumption that monoamine levels correlate with parameter *d* and the rate of adult neurogenesis with parameter *a*, the occurrence rate decreases with increasing parameters *a* and *d* (A). However, modeling the effect of antidepressant treatment as increases in parameters *a* and *d* would make the paradoxical prediction that antidepressant treatment increases the time-to-remission (B). **C**) To show this conflict more explicitly we plot both the occurrence rate and the time-to-remission in the same panel. The dashed lines represents contours in the occurrence rate at the indicated values, while the color scale represents median time-to-remission. It is highly unlikely to find parameter combinations of *a* and *d* which reduces the time-to-remission while keeping the occurrence rate constant or lowering it.

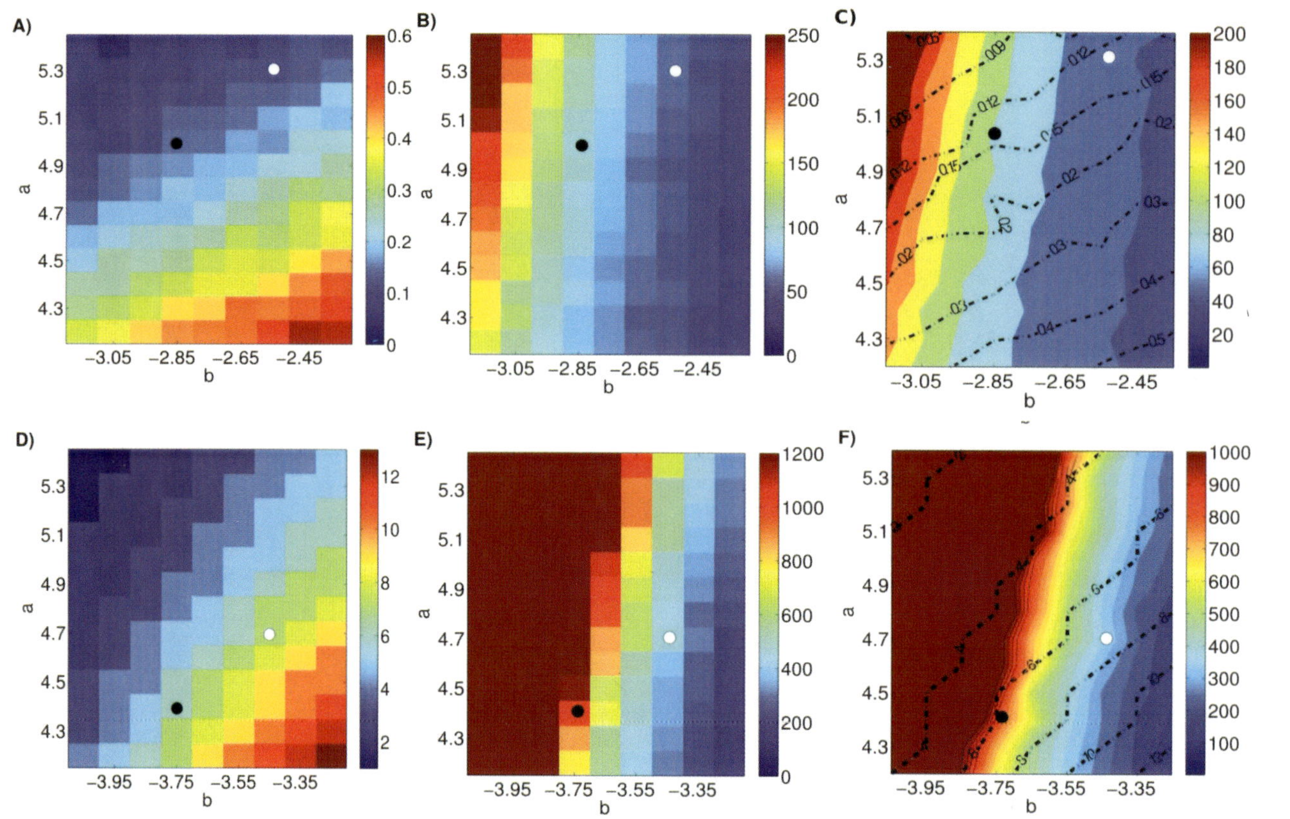

Figure 8. Increases in parameters a and b are consistent with the effect of antidepressant treatment. The first row of panels shows the results of simulations for the low-risk sub-population where the color scales in **A**) and **B**) represent the occurrence rate and median time-to-remission, respectively. Panel **C**) displays the same data using contour lines (occurrence rate) and color scale (media time-to-remission). The second row of panels shows the results for the high-risk sub-population where the color scale represents **D**) the median number of depressive episodes and **E**) median time-to-remission. Panel **F**) displays the same data using contour lines (median number of depressive episodes) and color scheme (median time-to-remission). The black and white points mark pre- and post-treatment parameters, respectively. For certain parameter combinations an increase in the parameters *a* and *b* reduces the median time-to-remission while keeping the occurrence rate (the median number of depressive episodes for the high risk sub-population) constant or lowering it.

occurrence rate and time-to-remission suggests that *d* might correlate partly with amygdala activity. Indeed, other authors before us have tied the amygdala to depression [64,65]. Hyperactivity in the amygdala is a common finding during baseline conditions in MDD [66] and has been interpreted as a valence-specific effect that causes a negative memory bias [67,68].

Dimensionality of the model and history-dependence

DSM-IV-TR, used worldwide as a diagnostic tool, does not define absolute boundaries between mental disorder and no mental disorder. However, the use of a categorical classification is fundamental in everyday clinical practice and research, as well as for health services and insurance purposes. The categories are prototypes, which define certain criteria related to symptoms, i.e., we say that a patient with a close approximation of the ill-prototype is ill. However, it has been argued that MDD should not be treated as a categorical condition and instead be viewed along a continuum [69]. Instead of categorizing subjects as ill or healthy, they should be scored on a graded scale according to how may symptoms the subject expressed and/or how severe the symptoms are. Some authors go even further to suggest that a one-dimensional approach is not sufficient and that multiple dimensions have to be used to capture the multiple facets of depression. In this study, we reject the view that depression is a categorical condition, and model the dynamics of MDD with a continuous state variable (*M*). However, since virtually all existing observations on MDD have been based on categorical classification and clinical practice depends on it, we developed the finite-state model to translate between the dynamics of a continuous one-dimensional system and the categorical classification of disease states. Since we are at an early stage of the modeling process, it appeared prudent to start with a single state variable to model the dynamics of MDD, especially given the paucity of data that could constrain higher-order systems. In addition, the general approach in modeling is to start with a parsimonious model and to include more complexity only if and when additional mechanisms are required. So far, the simple model we studied has been able to account for a surprisingly wide range of observations.

A consequence of the choice of a one-dimensional model is that, at a given point in time, the system's behavior is fully determined by the one state variable. As a result, the system does not depend on the previous history of the system. For instance, the probability of developing a DE does not depend on whether the patient has previously experienced a DE or not. To allow the history to affect the behavior of the system, we would have to include additional state variables which would imply more complex higher-order systems. We are aware that to fully understand depression, it eventually will be necessary to incorporate such history-depen-

Table 3. Comparison of quantitative measures of disease progression between model and clinical observation.

Variable	Observations	Model
Occurrence rate, OR	20% [1,82,85]	20%
1st recurrence, RR(1)	50% [1,85]	40%
2nd recurrence, RR(2)	70% [1]	90%
3rd recurrence, RR(3)	90% [1]	96%
Mean time-to-response	2 to 3 we [26], 3 to 4 we [24], 20 to 31 we [87]	20d
DE duration in patients treated with AD (from onset of DE to remission/recovery)		
Mean	8.4 mo [51]	267d
Median	3 mo [51], 16 we [82], 22 we (1st DE) [55], 19 we (4th DE) [55]	96d
p(TDE< = 90 d)	50% [51], 53% [60]	48%
p(TDE< = 180 d)	63% [51]	68%
p(TDE< = 360 d)	76% [51]	80%
p(TDE< = 630 d)	80% [51]	87%
p(TDE>720 d)	12% [84],15% [46], 20% [51], 20% [54], 22% [83]	11%
DE duration in patients treated with AD (from onset of AD treatment to remission/recovery)		
Mean	5.6 mo [81]	252 d
Median	3 mo [81]	85 d
p(TDE< = 30 d)	26% [81]	24.5%
p(TDE< = 90 d)	63% [81]	52%
p(TDE< = 180 d)	77% [81]	69%
p(TDE< = 360 d)	85% [81]	80%
p(TDE< = 720 d)	88% [81]	87%
Median age of onset of 1st DE	early-to-mid twenties [84]	25 y
DE duration in patients treated with CBT		
p(TDE< = 3 m)	50% [60]	49%
p(TDE< = 16 week)	52% [86]	57%

AD: antidepressant; **DE**: depressive episode; **TDE**: duration of depressive episode

dence. For instance, epidemiological studies have found evidence that adverse experience during childhood, such as sexual or physical abuse, neglect or loss of parents, is associated with substantial increase in the risk of developing depression [70–73]. Additionally, childhood trauma can change symptom patterns and the clinical course of MDD. For example, childhood trauma has been consistently associated with an early onset of depression [74,75], as well as larger numbers of depressive episodes or more chronic depression [76,77]. Moreover, childhood adverse experience has been associated with a decreased responsiveness to pharmacological treatment in patients with dysthymia and depression [78,79]. However, not all forms of depression are associated with childhood adversity, and we may speculate that the high-risk sub-population in our model may partly include the group of depressive patients with a history of childhood trauma. Indeed, patients within the high-risk sub-population in our model tend to have more episodes, longer duration of episodes as well as more chronic episodes than those in the low-risk sub-population.

Comparison between observations and model outputs

Our model offers an account for why AD treatment has only low rates of success and in some studies did not show superiority over placebo [36–38]. In our model, the distribution of DE durations in the treated patients is very broad with a peak at about 3 months and a long tail including episodes longer than 9 years. The properties of this distribution suggests two things. First, many studies were not able to see an effect of the AD treatment because the time window of observation was not long enough. Second, any effect of AD treatment is highly variable. Note that the parameters are identical for each simulation, so the widely different durations of depressive episodes did not emerge as a result of differences in the parameters. Furthermore, the risk of relapse seemed similar across heterogeneous groups of patients including those who had recently responded to treatment of an acute episode and those who had been successfully taking maintenance treatment for several months or even years [80]. Similarly, our modeling results indicate that AD treatment does not decrease the probability of developing another DE in the future.

Practical implications

Our results imply that people who suffer from depression can be assigned to two sub-populations. The low-risk sub-population develops depression by chance, and those from this sub-population who suffer from MDD do not otherwise differ from those who never develop depression. The high-risk sub-population has an increased likelihood of developing depression, and tends to have more DEs during their life time, and longer DE durations. This prediction of our model may have relevance for clinicians, because

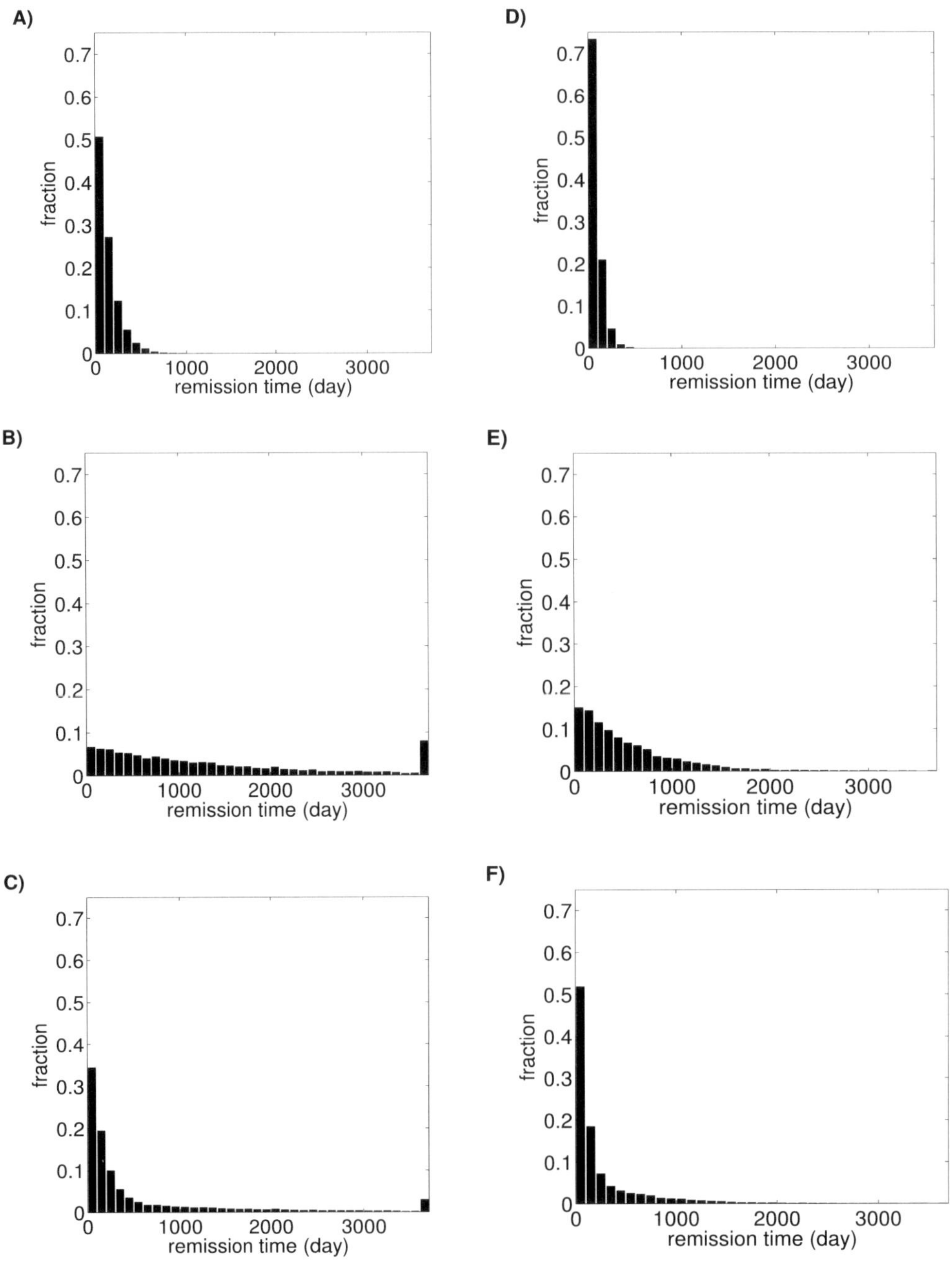

Figure 9. Distribution of the duration of depressive episodes. A), B), and C) show data for control group with pre-treatment parameters. D), E), and F) show data for treatment group with post-treatment parameters. The first row (A, D) of panels shows the duration of depressive episodes for the low-risk subpopulation, the second row (B, E) for the high-risk subpopulation, and the third row (C, F) for the joint distribution. Note that the distributions have long tails, indicating that some patients take much longer to improve than others, even though they all share the same parameters.

it suggests that the patients who belong to the high-risk subpopulation are at high risk of developing a chronic course of the disease. Moreover, this group of patients demands long-term treatment and regular check-ups after recovery.

We do not claim that our model is the final word on modeling the dynamics of depression. On the contrary, it has several apparent limitations some of which we have discussed above. The main goal of our article is to show the potential power of computationally modeling depression and the need for different quantitative data for understanding depression. We therefore hope that our modeling work will promote new empirical studies and/or reexaminations of existing data. In particular, we believe that it is important to monitor the disease progression in MDD on a day-to-day basis. The finite-state machine model that we developed here could be used to define the disease state of MDD more consistently and the operational criteria we suggested here might lead to improved design, interpretation, and comparison of studies of the natural course and clinical therapeutic trials. Ultimately, we hope

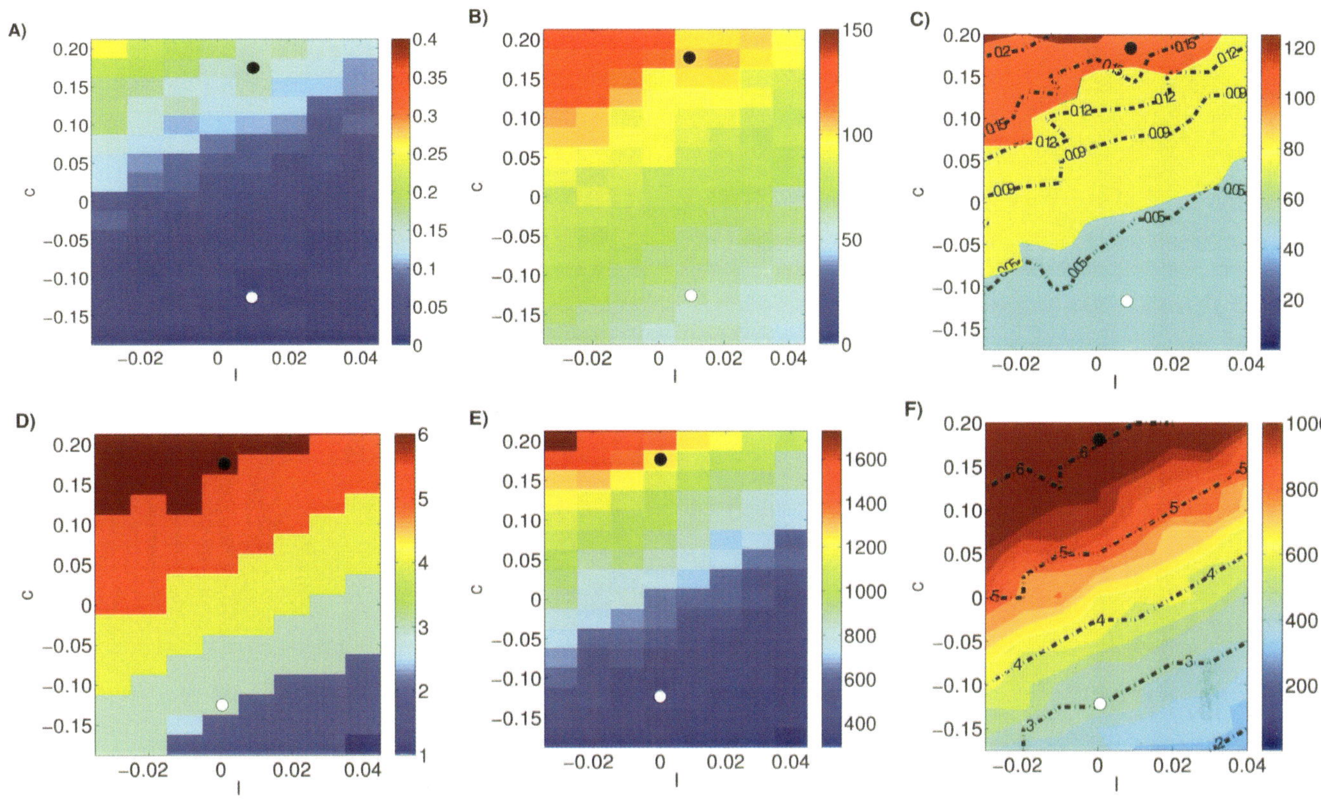

Figure 10. Modeling the effect of cognitive behavioral therapy and life style changes on MDD. Plotting convention as in Figure 8. An increase in the parameter *I* and/or decrease in *c* reduces the occurrence rate (A) (the median number of depressive episodes for the high-risk sub-population, D) and the median time-to-remission (B and E). These results suggests that smaller values of parameter *c* correlates with more positive attitude and larger values of *I* correlate with more positive environmental influences.

that such efforts will lead to a clearer understanding of the nature of MDD.

Acknowledgments

We thank Martin Brüne for helpful comments on an earlier version of the manuscript.

Author Contributions

Conceived and designed the experiments: SD SC. Performed the experiments: SD SC. Analyzed the data: SD SC. Contributed reagents/materials/analysis tools: SD SC. Wrote the paper: SD SC.

References

1. American Psychiatric Association (2000) Diagnostic and Statistical Manual of Mental Disorders IV Edition Text Revision (DSM IV TR). Washington DC, USA: APA.
2. Blazer DG, Kessler RC, McGonagle KA, Swartz MS (1994) The prevalence and distribution of major depression in a national community sample: the National Comorbidity Survey. The American journal of psychiatry 151: 979–986.
3. Hasin DS, Goodwin RD, Stinson FS, Grant BF (2005) Epidemiology of major depressive disorder: results from the National Epidemiologic Survey on Alcoholism and Related Conditions. Archives of general psychiatry 62: 1097–1106. doi:10.1001/archpsyc.62.10.1097.
4. Kessler RC, Berglund P, Demler O, Jin R, Merikangas KR, et al. (2005) Lifetime prevalence and age-of-onset distributions of DSM-IV disorders in the National Comorbidity Survey Replication. Archives of general psychiatry 62: 593–602. doi:10.1001/archpsyc.62.6.593.
5. Hasler G (2010) Pathophysiology of depression: do we have any solid evidence of interest to clinicians? World psychiatry: official journal of the World Psychiatric Association (WPA) 9: 155–161.
6. Angst F, Stassen HH, Clayton PJ, Angst J (2002) Mortality of patients with mood disorders: follow-up over 34–38 years. Journal of affective disorders 68: 167–181.
7. Murray CJ, Lopez AD (1997) Global mortality, disability, and the contribution of risk factors: Global Burden of Disease Study. Lancet 349: 1436–1442. doi:10.1016/S0140-6736(96)07495-8.
8. Weissman MM (1996) Cross-National Epidemiology of Major Depression and Bipolar Disorder. JAMA: The Journal of the American Medical Association 276: 293. doi:10.1001/jama.1996.03540040037030.
9. Nolen-Hoeksema S (2001) Gender Differences in Depression. Current Directions in Psychological Science 10: 173–176. doi:10.1111/1467-8721.00142.
10. Kessler R, Berglund P, Demler O, Jin R, Koretz D, et al. (2003) The epidemiology of major depressive disorder: results from the National Comorbidity Survey Replication (NCS-R). JAMA: the journal of the American Medical Association 289: 3095–3105. doi: doi: 10.1001/jama.289.23.3095.
11. Greenberg PE, Kessler RC, Birnbaum HG, Leong SA, Lowe SW, et al. (2003) The economic burden of depression in the United States: how did it change between 1990 and 2000? The Journal of clinical psychiatry 64: 1465–1475.
12. Murray CJ, Lopez AD (1996) Evidence-based health policy—lessons from the Global Burden of Disease Study. Science (New York, NY) 274: 740–743.
13. Kessler RC, McGonagle KA, Zhao S, Nelson CB, Hughes M, et al. (1994) Lifetime and 12-month prevalence of DSM-III-R psychiatric disorders in the United States. Results from the National Comorbidity Survey. Archives of general psychiatry 51: 8–19. doi: 10.1001/archpsyc.1994.03950010008002.
14. Kessler RC, Bromet EJ (2013) The epidemiology of depression across cultures. Annual review of public health 34: 119–138. doi:10.1146/annurev-publhealth-031912-114409.
15. Nestler E, Barrot M, DiLeone R, Eisch A, Gold S, et al. (2002) Neurobiology of depression. Neuron 34: 13–25.
16. Sullivan PF, Neale MC, Kendler KS (2000) Genetic epidemiology of major depression: review and meta-analysis. The American journal of psychiatry 157: 1552–1562.
17. Flint J, Kendler KS (2014) The Genetics of Major Depression. Neuron 81: 484–503. doi:10.1016/j.neuron.2014.01.027.

18. Kendler KS, Gatz M, Gardner CO, Pedersen NL (2006) A Swedish national twin study of lifetime major depression. The American journal of psychiatry 163: 109–114. doi:10.1176/appi.ajp.163.1.109.
19. Monroe SM, Simons AD (1991) Diathesis-stress theories in the context of life stress research: implications for the depressive disorders. Psychological bulletin 110: 406–425.
20. Hornung OP, Heim CM (2014) Gene-Environment Interactions and Intermediate Phenotypes: Early Trauma and Depression. Frontiers in endocrinology 5: 14. doi:10.3389/fendo.2014.00014.
21. Belmaker RH, Agam G (2008) Major depressive disorder. The New England journal of medicine 358: 55–68. doi: 10.1056/nejmra073096.
22. Lopez-Munoz F, Alamo C (2009) Monoaminergic Neurotransmission: The History of the Discovery of Antidepressants from 1950s Until Today. Current Pharmaceutical Design 15: 1563–1586. doi:10.2174/138161209788168001.
23. Morilak DA, Frazer A (2004) Antidepressants and brain monoaminergic systems: a dimensional approach to understanding their behavioural effects in depression and anxiety disorders. The international journal of neuropsychopharmacology/official scientific journal of the Collegium Internationale Neuropsychopharmacologicum (CINP) 7: 193–218. doi:10.1017/S1461145704004080.
24. Santarelli L, Saxe M, Gross C, Surget A, Battaglia F, et al. (2003) Requirement of hippocampal neurogenesis for the behavioral effects of antidepressants. Science (New York, NY) 301: 805–809. doi: 10.1126/science.1083328.
25. Thompson C (2002) Onset of action of antidepressants: results of different analyses. Human psychopharmacology 17 Suppl 1: S27–32. doi:10.1002/hup.386.
26. Stassen HH, Delini-Stula A, Angst J (1993) Time course of improvement under antidepressant treatment: A survival-analytical approach. European Neuropsychopharmacology 3: 127–135. doi:10.1016/0924-977X(93)90264-M.
27. Segman RH, Gorfine M, Lerer B, Shapira B (1995) Onset and time course of antidepressant action: psychopharmacological implications of a controlled trial of electroconvulsive therapy. Psychopharmacology 119: 440–448. doi:10.1007/BF02245860.
28. Quitkin FM, Stewart JW, McGrath PJ, Nunes E, Ocepek-Welikson K, et al. (1993) Further evidence that a placebo response to antidepressants can be identified. The American journal of psychiatry 150: 566–570.
29. Machado-Vieira R, Salvadore G, Luckenbaugh DA, Manji HK, Zarate CA (2008) Rapid onset of antidepressant action: a new paradigm in the research and treatment of major depressive disorder. The Journal of clinical psychiatry 69: 946–958.
30. Macedo-Soares MB de, Moreno RA, Rigonatti SP, Lafer B (2005) Efficacy of electroconvulsive therapy in treatment-resistant bipolar disorder: a case series. The journal of ECT 21: 31–34.
31. Ruhé H, Huyser J, Swinkels J, Schene A (2006) Switching antidepressants after a first selective serotonin reuptake inhibitor in major depressive disorder: a systematic review. The Journal of clinical psychiatry 67: 1836–1855.
32. Walsh BT, Seidman SN, Sysko R, Gould M (2002) Placebo Response in Studies of Major Depression. JAMA 287: 1840. doi:10.1001/jama.287.14.1840.
33. Anderson IM, Tomenson BM (1994) The efficacy of selective serotonin reuptake inhibitors in depression: a meta-analysis of studies against tricyclic antidepressants. Journal of psychopharmacology (Oxford, England) 8: 238–249. doi:10.1177/026988119400800407.
34. Fava M (2000) New approaches to the treatment of refractory depression. The Journal of clinical psychiatry 61 Suppl 1: 26–32.
35. Nelson JC (1998) Treatment of antidepressant nonresponders: augmentation or switch? The Journal of clinical psychiatry 59 Suppl 1: 35–41.
36. Kirsch I, SG (1998) Listening to prozac but hearing placebo: a meta-analysis of antidepressant medicatione. Prevention and treatment article 0002a I, article.
37. Ellis HC, Ottaway SA, Varner LJ, Becker AS, Moore BA (1997) Emotion, motivation, and text comprehension: the detection of contradictions in passages. Journal of experimental psychology General 126: 131–146.
38. Thase ME (1999) How should efficacy be evaluated in randomized clinical trials of treatments for depression? The Journal of clinical psychiatry 60 Suppl 4: 23–31; discussion 32.
39. Perry R, Cassagnol M (2009) Desvenlafaxine: a new serotonin-norepinephrine reuptake inhibitor for the treatment of adults with major depressive disorder. Clinical therapeutics 31 Pt 1: 1374–1404. doi:10.1016/j.clinthera.2009.07.012.
40. Nemeroff CB, Heim CM, Thase ME, Klein DN, Rush a J, et al. (2003) Differential responses to psychotherapy versus pharmacotherapy in patients with chronic forms of major depression and childhood trauma. Proceedings of the National Academy of Sciences of the United States of America 100: 14293–14296. doi:10.1073/pnas.2336126100.
41. Beck AT (1976) Cognitive therapy and the emotional disorders.
42. Moore MT, Fresco DM (2012) Depressive realism: a meta-analytic review. Clinical psychology review 32: 496–509. doi:10.1016/j.cpr.2012.05.004.
43. DeRubeis RJ, Crits-Christoph P (1998) Empirically supported individual and group psychological treatments for adult mental disorders. Journal of consulting and clinical psychology 66: 37–52.
44. Kennedy SH (2008) Core symptoms of major depressive disorder: relevance to diagnosis and treatment. Dialogues in clinical neuroscience 10: 271–277.
45. Frank E, Prien RF, Jarrett RB, Keller MB, Kupfer DJ, et al. (1991) Conceptualization and rationale for consensus definitions of terms in major depressive disorder. Remission, recovery, relapse, and recurrence. Archives of general psychiatry 48: 851–855.
46. Eaton W, Shao H, Nestadt G, Lee HB, Lee BH, et al. (2008) Population-based study of first onset and chronicity in major depressive disorder. Archives of general psychiatry 65: 513–520. doi: 10.1001/archpsyc.65.5.513.
47. Hardeveld F, Spijker J, De Graaf R, Nolen WA, Beekman ATF (2010) Prevalence and predictors of recurrence of major depressive disorder in the adult population. Acta psychiatrica Scandinavica 122: 184–191. doi:10.1111/j.1600-0447.2009.01519.x.
48. Torpey DC, Klein DN (2008) Chronic depression: update on classification and treatment. Current psychiatry reports 10: 458–464.
49. Sahay A, Hen R (2007) Adult hippocampal neurogenesis in depression. Nature neuroscience 10: 1110–1115. doi:10.1038/nn1969.
50. Cheng S (2013) The CRISP theory of hippocampal function in episodic memory. Frontiers in neural circuits 7: 88. doi:10.3389/fncir.2013.00088.
51. Spijker J, de Graaf R, Bijl R, Beekman A, Ormel J, et al. (2002) Duration of major depressive episodes in the general population: results from The Netherlands Mental Health Survey and Incidence Study (NEMESIS). The British journal of psychiatry: the journal of mental science 181: 208–213. doi: 10.1192/bjp.181.3.208.
52. Furukawa TA, Kitamura T, Takahashi K (2000) Time to recovery of an inception cohort with hitherto untreated unipolar major depressive episodes. The British journal of psychiatry: the journal of mental science 177: 331–335.
53. Angst J, Preisig M (1995) Course of a clinical cohort of unipolar, bipolar and schizoaffective patients. Results of a prospective study from 1959 to 1985. Schweizer Archiv für Neurologie und Psychiatrie (Zurich, Switzerland: 1985) 146: 5–16.
54. Keller MB, Shapiro RW, Lavori PW, Wolfe N (1982) Recovery in major depressive disorder: analysis with the life table and regression models. Archives of general psychiatry 39: 905–910.
55. Solomon DA, Keller MB, Leon AC, Mueller TI, Shea MT, et al. (1997) Recovery from major depression. A 10-year prospective follow-up across multiple episodes. Archives of general psychiatry 54: 1001–1006.
56. Mueller TI, Keller MB, Leon AC, Solomon DA, Shea MT, et al. (1996) Recovery after 5 years of unremitting major depressive disorder. Archives of general psychiatry 53: 794–799.
57. Beck JS (1995) Cognitive therapy: Basics and Beyond. New York: Guilford Press.
58. Hollon SD, Thase ME, Markowitz JC (2002) Treatment and Prevention of Depression. Psychological Science in the Public Interest 3: 39–77. doi:10.1111/1529-1006.00008.
59. Jarrett RB, Schaffer M, McIntire D, Witt-Browder A, Kraft D, et al. (1999) Treatment of atypical depression with cognitive therapy or phenelzine: a double-blind, placebo-controlled trial. Archives of general psychiatry 56: 431–437.
60. Hollon SD, DeRubeis RJ, Evans MD, Wiemer MJ, Garvey MJ, et al. (1992) Cognitive therapy and pharmacotherapy for depression. Singly and in combination. Archives of general psychiatry 49: 774–781.
61. Dunn AL, Trivedi MH, Kampert JB, Clark CG, Chambliss HO (2005) Exercise treatment for depression: efficacy and dose response. American journal of preventive medicine 28: 1–8. doi:10.1016/j.amepre.2004.09.003.
62. Blumenthal JA, Babyak MA, Doraiswamy PM, Watkins L, Hoffman BM, et al. (2007) Exercise and pharmacotherapy in the treatment of major depressive disorder. Psychosomatic medicine 69: 587–596. doi:10.1097/PSY.0b013e318148c19a.
63. Martinsen EW (2008) Physical activity in the prevention and treatment of anxiety and depression. Nordic journal of psychiatry 62 Suppl 4: 25–29. doi:10.1080/08039480802315640.
64. Siegle G, Thompson W, Carter C, Steinhauer S, Thase M (2007) Increased amygdala and decreased dorsolateral prefrontal BOLD responses in unipolar depression: related and independent features. Biological psychiatry 61: 198–209. doi: doi: 10.1016/j.biopsych.2006.05.048.
65. Surguladze S, Brammer M, Keedwell P, Giampietro V, Young A, et al. (2005) A differential pattern of neural response toward sad versus happy facial expressions in major depressive disorder. Biological psychiatry 57: 201–209. doi: 10.1016/j.biopsych.2004.10.028.
66. Drevets W, Bogers W, Raichle M (2002) Functional anatomical correlates of antidepressant drug treatment assessed using PET measures of regional glucose metabolism. European neuropsychopharmacology: the journal of the European College of Neuropsychopharmacology 12: 527–544.
67. Hamilton P, Gotlib I (2008) Neural substrates of increased memory sensitivity for negative stimuli in major depression. Biological psychiatry 63: 1155–1162. doi: 10.1016/j.biopsych.2007.12.015.
68. Ramel W, Goldin P, Eyler L, Brown G, Gotlib I, et al. (2007) Amygdala reactivity and mood-congruent memory in individuals at risk for depressive relapse. Biological psychiatry 61: 231–239. doi: 10.1016/j.biopsych.2006.05.004.
69. Widiger TA, Samuel DB (2005) Diagnostic categories or dimensions? A question for the Diagnostic And Statistical Manual Of Mental Disorders–fifth edition. Journal of abnormal psychology 114: 494–504. doi:10.1037/0021-843X.114.4.494.
70. Edwards VJ, Holden GW, Felitti VJ, Anda RF (2003) Relationship between multiple forms of childhood maltreatment and adult mental health in community respondents: results from the adverse childhood experiences study. The American journal of psychiatry 160: 1453–1460.
71. Chapman DP, Whitfield CL, Felitti VJ, Dube SR, Edwards VJ, et al. (2004) Adverse childhood experiences and the risk of depressive disorders in adulthood. Journal of affective disorders 82: 217–225. doi:10.1016/j.jad.2003.12.013.

72. Heim C, Newport DJ, Mletzko T, Miller AH, Nemeroff CB (2008) The link between childhood trauma and depression: insights from HPA axis studies in humans. Psychoneuroendocrinology 33: 693–710. doi:10.1016/j.psyneuen.2008.03.008.
73. Felitti VJ, Anda RF, Nordenberg D, Williamson DF, Spitz AM, et al. (1998) Relationship of childhood abuse and household dysfunction to many of the leading causes of death in adults. The Adverse Childhood Experiences (ACE) Study. American journal of preventive medicine 14: 245–258.
74. Gladstone GL, Parker GB, Mitchell PB, Malhi GS, Wilhelm K, et al. (2004) Implications of childhood trauma for depressed women: an analysis of pathways from childhood sexual abuse to deliberate self-harm and revictimization. The American journal of psychiatry 161: 1417–1425. doi:10.1176/appi.ajp.161.8.1417.
75. Bernet CZ, Stein MB (1999) Relationship of childhood maltreatment to the onset and course of major depression in adulthood. Depression and anxiety 9: 169–174.
76. Zlotnick C, Mattia J, Zimmerman M (2001) Clinical features of survivors of sexual abuse with major depression. Child abuse & neglect 25: 357–367.
77. Zlotnick C, Ryan CE, Miller IW, Keitner GI (1995) Childhood abuse and recovery from major depression. Child abuse & neglect 19: 1513–1516.
78. Hayden EP, Klein DN (2001) Outcome of dysthymic disorder at 5-year follow-up: the effect of familial psychopathology, early adversity, personality, comorbidity, and chronic stress. The American journal of psychiatry 158: 1864–1870.
79. Kaplan MJ, Klinetob NA (2000) Childhood emotional trauma and chronic posttraumatic stress disorder in adult outpatients with treatment-resistant depression. The Journal of nervous and mental disease 188: 596–601.
80. Geddes JR, Carney SM, Davies C, Furukawa T a, Kupfer DJ, et al. (2003) Relapse prevention with antidepressant drug treatment in depressive disorders: a systematic review. Lancet 361: 653–661. doi:10.1016/S0140-6736(03)12599-8.
81. Furukawa T a (2000) Time to recovery of an inception cohort with hitherto untreated unipolar major depressive episodes. The British Journal of Psychiatry 177: 331–335. doi:10.1192/bjp.177.4.331.
82. Mueller TI, Leon a C, Keller MB, Solomon D a, Endicott J, et al. (1999) Recurrence after recovery from major depressive disorder during 15 years of observational follow-up. The American journal of psychiatry 156: 1000–1006.
83. Keller MB, Lavori PW, Rice J, Coryell W, Hirschfeld RM (1986) The persistent risk of chronicity in recurrent episodes of nonbipolar major depressive disorder: a prospective follow-up. The American journal of psychiatry 143: 24–28.
84. Andrade L, Caraveo-Anduaga JJ, Berglund P, Bijl RV, De Graaf R, et al. (2003) The epidemiology of major depressive episodes: results from the International Consortium of Psychiatric Epidemiology (ICPE) Surveys. International journal of methods in psychiatric research 12: 3–21.
85. Consensus Development Panel (1985) NIMH/NIH Consensus Development Conference statement. Mood disorders: pharmacologic prevention of recurrences. Consensus Development Panel. American Journal of Psychiatry 142: 469–476.
86. Luty SE, Carter JD, McKenzie JM, Rae AM, Frampton CMA, et al. (2007) Randomised controlled trial of interpersonal psychotherapy and cognitive-behavioural therapy for depression. The British journal of psychiatry: the journal of mental science 190: 496–502. doi:10.1192/bjp.bp.106.024729.
87. Möller HJ, Müller H, Volz HP (1996) How to assess the onset of antidepressant effect: comparison of global ratings and findings based on depression scales. Pharmacopsychiatry 29: 57–62. doi:10.1055/s-2007-979545.

Diagnostic Criteria for Depression in Type 2 Diabetes: A Data-Driven Approach

Sergio E. Starkstein[2]*, Wendy A. Davis[1], Milan Dragovic[2], Violetta Cetrullo[1], Timothy M. E. Davis[1], David G. Bruce[1]

1 School of Medicine & Pharmacology, University of Western Australia, Crawley, Western Australia, Australia, **2** School of Psychiatry & Clinical Neuroscience, University of Western Australia, Crawley, Western Australia, Australia

Abstract

Background: While depression is a frequent psychiatric comorbid condition in diabetes and has significant clinical impact, the syndromal profile of depression and anxiety symptoms has not been examined in detail.

Aims: To determine the syndromal pattern of the depression and anxiety spectrum in a large series of patients with type 2 diabetes, as determined using a data-driven approach based on latent class analysis (LCA).

Method: Type 2 diabetes participants from the observational community-based Fremantle Diabetes Study Phase II underwent assessment of lifetime depression using the Brief Lifetime Depression Scale, the Patient Health Questionnaire 9-item version (PHQ-9) for current depression symptoms, and the Generalized Anxiety Disorder Scale that was specifically developed and validated for this study. The main outcome measure was classes of patients with a specific syndromal profile of depression and anxiety symptoms based on LCA.

Results: LCA identified four classes that were interpreted as "major anxious depression", "minor anxious depression", "subclinical anxiety", and "no anxious depression". All nine DSM-IV/5 diagnostic criteria for major depression identified a class with a high frequency of major depression. All symptoms of anxiety had similar high probabilities as symptoms of depression for the "major depression-anxiety" class. There were significant differences between classes in terms of history of depression and anxiety, use of psychoactive medication, and diabetes-related variables.

Conclusions: Patients with type 2 diabetes show specific profiles of depression and anxiety. Anxiety symptoms are an integral part of major depression in type 2 diabetes. The different classes identified here provide empirically validated phenotypes for future research.

Editor: Kenji Hashimoto, Chiba University Center for Forensic Mental Health, Japan

Funding: Funding was provided by National Health and Medical Research Council (Project Grant 513781). The funders had no role in study design, data collection and analysis, decision to publish, or preparation of the manuscript.

Competing Interests: The authors have declared that no competing interests exist.

* Email: ses@cyllene.uwa.edu.au

Introduction

Depression is one of the most frequent psychiatric disorders in patients with type 2 diabetes, with a lifetime prevalence of 24%–29% and a point prevalence of 10%-15% [1]. Depression in type 2 diabetes is significantly associated with poor glycaemic control [2], chronic complications [2], increased mortality [3], reduced physical and mental functioning [4], higher health costs and decreased adherence to diet and hypoglycaemic medications [5]. A recent epidemiological study demonstrated that individuals with diabetes and comorbid depression have a worse health-related quality of life and higher health service usage [6]. Collaborative care models for depression in diabetes demonstrated to significantly improve outcomes for depression and glycaemic control [7].

Depression may be underdiagnosed in diabetes. The limitations in diagnosing depression in diabetes include the lack of specific diagnostic criteria and the overlap of symptoms. Egede and Ellis [8] noted that poor management of diabetes is a barrier for early recognition of depressive symptoms, such as fatigue, changes in weight and appetite, sleep disturbances, and motor retardation. Furthermore, increased appetite is a cardinal diagnostic criterion for both major depression and diabetes, anhedonia may result from changes in lifestyle due to diabetes, loss of interest may be secondary to limitations to pursue usual free-time activities due to diabetes complications (e.g., visual problems, neuropathy), and loss of libido and reduced self-esteem may result from sexual dysfunction. Campayo and co-workers [9] suggested that depression in diabetic patients may be qualitatively different from depression observed among individuals without diabetes who have 'primary' (i.e. no organic cause) depression, but no supporting data were provided. A recent large prospective study showed that individuals with current depressive and/or anxiety disorders fad a 10-fold increased odds of diabetes incidence at two years, and the

Table 1. Generalized Anxiety Disorder Scale.

Over the last 6 months, how often have you been bothered by any of the following problems?	**Not at all**	**Several days**	**More than half the days**	**Nearly every day**
1. worrying excessively or being anxious about several things?	0	1	2	3
2. difficulty controlling the worries or found the worries interfering with your ability to focus on what you were doing?	0	1	2	3
3. feeling restless, keyed up or on edge?	0	1	2	3
4. feeling tense?	0	1	2	3
5. feeling tired, weak or exhausted easily?	0	1	2	3
6. difficulty concentrating or finding your mind going blank?	0	1	2	3
7. feeling irritable?	0	1	2	3
8. difficulty sleeping (falling asleep, waking in the middle of the night, early morning wakening, or sleeping excessively)?	0	1	2	3
9. the symptoms of anxiety caused you significant distress or impaired your ability to function at work, socially, or in some other important way?	0	1	2	3
10. Were you taking any drugs or medicines just before the symptoms began?				
☐ No ☐ Yes	If YES, which drugs/medicines? ____________			
11. 10b. Did you have any medical illness just before these symptoms began?				
☐ No ☐ Yes	If YES, what was the illness? ____________			

incidence was highest for those with comorbid depression and anxiety [10]. A valid and timely diagnosis of depression is of clinical relevance especially given that detection and treatment of depression improves glycaemic control [9].

Another potential confounder for a valid diagnosis of depression in diabetes is the potential comorbidity with anxiety. This is substantial in the general population, with 57% of individuals with major depression also meeting diagnostic criteria for an anxiety disorder [11]. Generalized anxiety disorder (GAD) is more frequent in diabetes than in age-comparable healthy controls [12], and is associated with poor health behaviours [13]. In the general population, comorbid depression and anxiety is highly prevalent [14]. Several studies examined the comorbidity between depression and anxiety in diabetes, but they were limited by important methodological shortcomings, such as a diagnosis of diabetes based only on self-report [13].

The aim of the present study was to examine the syndromal pattern of depression and anxiety in type 2 diabetes using a data-driven approach, as well as to examine the overlap with anxiety. We used baseline data from community-based participants of the Fremantle Diabetes Study Phase II (FDS2) [15], and used latent class analysis (LCA) to examine the homogeneity of depressive symptoms and the comorbidity between depression and anxiety. LCA assesses the symptom profile of individual patients and produces classes of patients in terms of their pattern of symptoms. Given that the classes thus identified do not overlap, individual patients can belong to only one group. Based on our experience with LCA in medical conditions, we expected to find three classes characterized by high, moderate and low probabilities for symptoms of depression, as well as a high comorbidity between depression and anxiety.

Methods

Patients

The FDS2 is a longitudinal observational study of known diabetes conducted in a postcode-defined geographical area surrounding the city of Fremantle (Western Australia) [15].

Details of FDS2 recruitment procedures, sample characteristics including classification of diabetes type and non-recruited patients have been published elsewhere [15]. Briefly, between 2008 and 2011, 4,667 diabetic patients were identified in the local population of 153,000 (crude diabetes prevalence 3%), of whom 1,668 (36%) were recruited to FDS2, in addition to 64 surviving FDS phase I participants who had moved out of the study area (1,732 participants altogether).

Ethics Statement

The Human Research Ethics Committee of the Southern Metropolitan Area Health Service specifically approved the study, and all subjects gave written informed consent.

Clinical and psychiatric assessment

Each participant underwent a baseline assessment that included a comprehensive clinical questionnaire, physical examination and fasting biochemical tests [15]. Diabetes type was assessed from treatment history, BMI, age at diagnosis, and nature of first presentation and/or self-identification. Non-insulin treated patients and those ≥60 years of age at diagnosis were usually considered to have type 2 diabetes, as were patients <60 years of age at diagnosis and taking insulin at the time of the study entry but whose first treatment was not insulin. In these cases, case records were consulted for evidence of ketonemia, as well as islet cell antibody, GAD antibodies, serum insulin and C-peptide levels, if available. Complications were ascertained using standard criteria [15,16].

All participants were assessed with the PHQ-9 [17], a brief and accurate assessment of depression that has been validated in patients with diabetes [16]. The PHQ-9 is a dual-purpose instrument that can establish depressive disorder diagnoses as well as ratings of depressive symptom severity [17]. Patients with type 2 diabetes have significant physical complaints that may artificially increase PHQ-9 scores on items that are not necessary symptoms of major depression. Using a PHQ-9 cut point rather than the diagnostic algorithm may increase the frequency of false-positive cases of depression [18]. Therefore, as suggested by the PHQ-9 authors [18], we used the instrument's diagnostic algorithm for making diagnoses of major and minor depression. Major depression was diagnosed when the first or second symptoms (i.e. depressed mood or loss of interest/anhedonia) were present more than half the days, and at least 5 of the 9 symptoms were present during the same period [19]. Minor depression was diagnosed whenever 2 to 4 symptoms (including depressed mood or loss of interest/anhedonia) were present for more than half the days. Lifetime history of depression was assessed with the Brief Lifetime Depression Scale (BLDS). This instrument was developed and validated by our group for use in diabetes [20]. The BLDS was modelled on the PHQ-9 and included similar items, general format and language, but the participants were asked whether they had ever had a period during their lives lasting for two weeks or more when they experienced any of the nine symptoms of depression listed in the DSM-IV/5.

For the study of anxiety in the FDS2, a specific questionnaire (the Generalized Anxiety Disorder Scale (GADS)) was devised by one of the authors (SES) with experience in developing psychiatric instruments to rate the severity of anxiety (Table 1). The GADS includes 9 items that correspond to all 9 DSM-IV criteria for GAD. Based on the PHQ-9, GADS items were rated as "not at all present", "present several days", "present more than half of the days", and "present nearly every day". As with the PHQ-9, a symptom was rated positive whenever the patient rated "more than half of the days" or "nearly every day". To make the instrument comparable to the DSM-IV criteria for GAD, the time criterion was the past 6 months. The validity of the GADS was examined by having a psychiatrist (SES) assess a convenience sample of 23 patients with the Structured Clinical Interview for the DSM-IV-Research Version (SCID)-Anxiety Disorders Module, blind to the GADS results. Kappa statistics showed a high diagnostic concordance for DSM-IV GAD diagnosis (kappa $= 0.88$). Six of the 23 patients received a diagnosis of GAD based on the SCID, as compared to 4 based on the GADS (McNemar's test, $P = 0.50$). Test-retest reliability was assessed in 25 patients, who completed the GADS twice, with an interval of (mean ± SD) 9±6 days. The intra-class correlation (ICC) was high (ICC $= 0.88$). The presence of cognitive deficits was based on the following algorithm (Bruce et al., 2008): patients scoring ≤26 on the MMSE were further assessed with the Clinical Dementia Rating (CDR) (Hughes et al., 1982) to establish the presence of dementia. This instrument generates ratings ranging from normal cognition (CDR 0) to severity levels of dementia (CDR 1–3) and

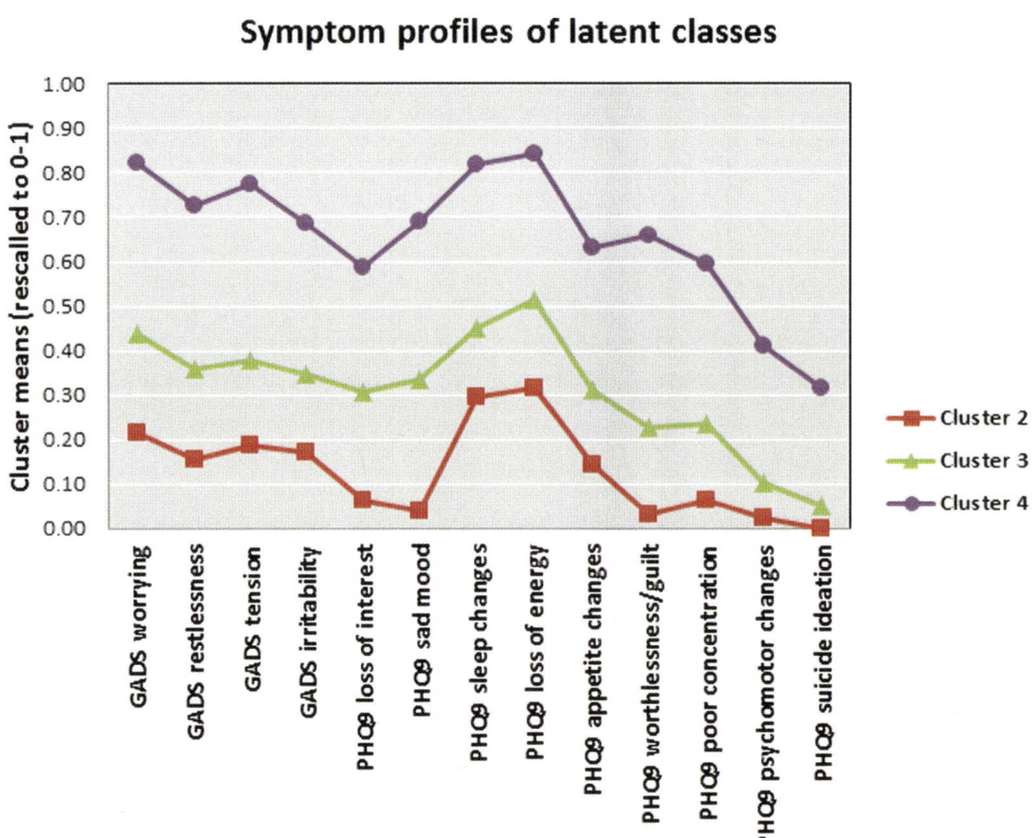

Figure 1. Symptom profile of the 4 (ordered) latent class model graph showing partial conditional probabilities for the 4-class model (LCA response profiles).

Table 2. Testing Six Subsequent Latent Class Analysis Models.

Number of classes	L^2	Reduction from baseline	Gain (%)	Classification error	BIC*	AWE*	CAIC
One class	17470.9	-		0.00	33396.3	33797.7	33435.3
Two classes	12744.7	27.1	27.1	0.04	28772.2	29555.7	28825.3
Three classes	11449.9	34.5	7.4	0.06	27579.6	28733.8	27646.6
Four classes	10988.6	37.8	2.6	0.10	27222.3	28785.1	27301.2
Five classes	10720.2	38.6	1.5	0.13	27053.9	28964.8	27148.9

* Information criteria evaluating the quality of latent class solution: L2 - The likelihood-ratio goodness-of-fit, BIC (Bayes Information Criterion), AWE (Approximate Weight of Evidence, similar to BIC but also takes classification performance into account), CAIC (Corrected Akaike Information Criterion).

an intermediate category defines very mild cognitive impairment or questionable dementia (CDR 0.5).

Statistical Analysis

To test for group differences, generalised linear modelling (GLM) was used. LCA (cluster procedure) was used to determine the latent structure of patients with diabetes and to categorize individuals based on their responses to the PHQ-9 and GADS. LCA was calculated using the software LatentGold version 4.0.4 [21]. LCA assumes that a 'class' explains the association among a set of symptoms. LCA computes latent class probabilities or prevalence, and conditional probabilities. The basic assumption of LCA is that a (presumably homogeneous) population of individuals is a mixture of distinct, but internally homogeneous subgroups [22]. LCA assesses the symptom profile of individual patients and produces classes of patients as suggested by their pattern of symptoms. Since the clusters do not overlap, individual patients can belong to only one group. For this analysis, we included the nine DSM-IV symptoms for major depression and the four DSM-IV symptoms for generalized anxiety disorder that do not overlap with major depression as latent class indicators. Models with one to five classes were estimated. Each patient was assigned to the latent class to which the largest posterior probability was calculated. The best-fitting model was chosen based on having the lowest values for the following goodness of fit indices: Bayes Information Criterion (BIC), Approximate Weight of Evidence (AWE) (which takes into account classification performance), and the Corrected Akaike Information Criterion (CAIC). The level of contribution of each indicator to the final latent class structure is assessed by the information content statistic (R^2), which can be interpreted similarly to the commonalities in traditional factor analysis. For the clinical interpretation, the mean level and frequency of responses for each psychiatric symptom within each class were examined. After determining the best class solution, we used latent class membership as a between-subject variable in a one-way analysis of variance (ANOVA) followed by post-hoc comparisons using Tukey's HSD, and X^2 analyses to examine demographic and clinical differences among the latent classes. The computer package IBM SPSS Statistics 20 (IBM Corporation, Somers, NY, USA) was used to compare baseline characteristics across the four LCA classes. Data are presented as proportions, mean ± SD, geometric mean (SD range), or, in the case of variables which did not conform to a normal or log-normal distribution, median [inter-quartile range, IQR]. For independent samples, two-way comparisons for proportions were by Fisher's exact test, for normally distributed variables by Student's t-test, and for non-normally distributed variables by Mann-Whitney U-test. Multiple comparisons for proportions were by Fisher's exact test or Chi-squared test, for normally distributed variables by one-way ANOVA, and for non-normally distributed variables by Kruskal-Wallis H-test, adjusted using the Bonferroni correction. A two-tailed significance level of $P<0.05$ was used throughout.

Results

Demographic and clinical findings

FDS2 recruited 1,551 participants (90%) with clinically defined type 2 diabetes. Complete data for our study was obtained from 1,337 patients (86%). When compared with the 214 patients with missing data, the latter were more likely to be female (46% vs. 57%, $P=0.005$), and had worse glycaemic control (HbA_{1c} (median [IQR]) 6.8% median [IQR] [6.2%–7.6%] vs. 7.0% [6.4%–8.5%], respectively, $P=0.001$). On the other hand, there were no significant between-group differences in age (mean years

Table 3. Scores for anxiety and depression items for the four LCA classes.

Symptom	No anxious – depression	Subsyndromal anxiety	Minor anxious depression	Major anxious depression	F	*P*
Worrying	0.06 (0.23)	0.65 (0.63)	1.33 (0.87)	2.49 (0.73)	548.6	0.0001
Restlessness	0.01 (0.09)	0.47 (0.53)	1.09 (0.70)	2.17 (0.83)	597.3	0.0001
Tension	0.01 (0.10)	0.57 (0.55)	1.15 (0.72)	2.33 (0.74)	654.6	0.0001
Irritability	0.06 (0.24)	0.52 (0.58)	1.04 (0.69)	2.06 (0.89)	430.5	0.0001
Loss of interest	0.02 (0.17)	0.18 (0.45)	0.96 (0.84)	1.75 (0.91)	398.3	0.0001
Sad mood	0.02 (0.13)	0.12 (0.33)	1.03 (0.74)	2.06 (0.81)	754.3	0.0001
Sleep changes	0.28 (0.66)	0.90 (1.00)	1.35 (1.06)	2.47 (0.85)	162.7	0.0001
Loss of energy	0.20 (0.43)	0.96 (0.83)	1.55 (0.97)	2.55 (0.68)	204.8	0.0001
Appetite changes	0.09 (0.33)	0.44 (0.78)	0.94 (1.03)	1.88 (1.17)	179.0	0.0001
Worthlessness/guilt	0.01 (0.48)	0.09 (0.30)	0.70 (0.77)	1.96 (1.08)	131.1	0.0001
Poor concentration	0.01 (0.08)	0.19 (0.47)	0.72 (0.87)	1.76 (1.04)	104.0	0.0001
Psychomotor changes	0.01 (0.04)	0.08 (0.34)	0.30 (0.59)	1.25 (1.17)	207.7	0.0001
Suicide ideation	0.00 (0.00)	0.01 (0.04)	0.17 (0.50)	0.91 (1.09)	57.7	0.0001

± SD) (65.8±11.1 vs. 64.9±14.4 years, respectively, $P = 0.41$), diabetes duration (8.8 years [2.8–15.6] vs. 10.0 years [3.0–17.8], respectively, $P = 0.12$), or cognition (8.0% vs. 7.1% cognitively impaired (P = 1.00).

Latent class analysis

Items selected for the LCA included all 9 items from the PHQ-9, and the items of worrying/anxiety, feeling restless, feeling tense, and feeling irritable from the GADS (the remaining items were not included due to overlap with PHQ-9 items). The modelling started with probing the presence of conventional latent classes (i.e., cluster modelling), running cluster models of up to 5 latent clusters. Inspection of conditional probabilities showed a reduction in BIC and CAIC values from the 2- to the 5-cluster model, but at the cost of increasing number of parameters (NPar) (Table 2). From the 4-class model onwards, decreased accuracy was unacceptably high (i.e., >10%) and the AWE index has started to ascend. The 4-cluster model showed a pattern of probabilities extending from one extreme (low probabilities for all symptoms) to the other (high probabilities for all symptoms), with the exception of two intermediate classes showing a mixed pattern of probabilities. This finding suggests that a single discrete factor (anxious depression) with 4 ordered levels or classes (e.g., no anxious depression, subclinical anxiety, minor anxious depression and major anxious depression) provides the best explanatory model. Thus, an inter-factorial effect and orderliness of latent classes was obtained, as opposed to random and/or pseudonominal composition of latent classes. Class-specific endorsement profiles for depression and anxiety symptoms are shown in Figure 1.

Latent class 4 included 104 patients (8%) and showed high partial conditional probabilities (>0.60) for all the anxiety and depression symptoms, except for psychomotor changes (>0.40) and suicidal ideation (>0.30). This class was labelled "major anxious depression". Latent class 1 included 439 patients (33%) and showed low partial conditional probabilities (<0.10) for all symptoms of depression and anxiety. This class was labelled "no anxious depression". Latent class 3 included 293 patients (22%) with partial conditional probabilities intermediate between classes 1 and 4, and was labelled "minor anxious depression". Finally, latent class 2 included 501 patients (38%) and showed higher conditional probabilities than class 4 on the anxiety items, sleep changes and loss of energy. This class was labelled "subclinical anxiety". We used final class membership as a between-subject variable to evaluate differences in depressive and anxiety symptoms as a function of latent class membership. The ANOVAs evaluating mean symptom severity differences on each item as a function of latent class membership were all significant at the $P < 0.001$ level. Follow-up pairwise comparisons using Tukey's HSD tests demonstrated the following differences: For GAD worry the ANOVA was significant (Table 3), and all four groups were significantly different to each other (Tukey HSD $P = 0.0001$). Similar results were obtained for GADS restlessness, GADS tension, GADS irritability, loss of interest, sad mood, sleep changes, loss of energy, appetite changes, worthlessness/guilt, and poor concentration. For the items of psychomotor changes and suicide ideation there were significant differences on post-hoc tests between all classes except between classes 1 and 2.

There were significant demographic and clinical differences between classes (Table 4). The *major anxious depression class* was significantly younger than the other classes, whilst the *minor anxious depression class* was significantly younger than the subclinical anxiety class. Depression (major or minor) was significantly more frequent in the *major anxious depression class* as compared to the other classes, and in the *minor anxious depression class* as compared to the remaining two classes. Depression before the onset of diabetes was significantly higher in the *major anxious depression class* as compared to the other classes, and in the *minor anxious depression class* as compared to the remaining two classes. Patients in the *major anxious depression class* had a significantly higher frequency of GAD as compared to the other classes, whilst patients in the *minor anxious depression class* had a significantly higher frequency of GAD than the remaining two classes. Depression (minor or major) and/or GAD were present in 89% of patients in the *major anxious depression class*, 29% in the *minor anxious depression class*, 2% in the *subclinical anxiety class*, and none in the *no anxious depression class*.

Finally, the *major anxious depression class* showed a significantly younger age at onset of diabetes, higher HbA_{1c} levels, higher serum triglycerides levels and a higher frequency of insulin use

Table 4. FDS2 baseline associates of four LCA groups in participants with type-2 diabetes.

	LCA group				
FDS2 baseline variable	**No anxious depression (Cluster 1)**	**Subsyndromal anxiety (Cluster 2)**	**Minor anxious depression (Cluster 3)**	**Major anxious depression (Cluster 4)**	***P*-value**
N (%)	439 (32.8)	501 (37.5)	293 (21.9)	104 (7.8)	
Age (years)	67.4±10.8	66.1±10.8	64.7±11.1††	60.6±12.3***,†††,‡‡	**<0.001**
Any depressive syndrome (%)	0	1.0	26.3***,†††	77.9***,†††,‡‡‡	**<0.001**
Major depressive syndrome (%)	0	0	4.1***,†††	67.3***,†††,‡‡‡	**<0.001**
Taking antidepressant medication (%)	6.6	13.6**	23.5***,†††	35.6***,†††	**<0.001**
No depression/ depression before diabetes/concomitant diagnoses/depression after diabetes (%)	88.2/7.7/1.2/3.0	64.0/19.6/5.4/11.0***	29.8/32.4/10.2/27.6***,†††	2.1/43.3/16.5/38.1***,†††,‡‡‡	**<0.001**
Current GAD (%)	0	0	3.8***,†††	51.0***,†††,‡‡‡	**<0.001**
Lifetime GAD (%):	5.1	14.7***	35.6***,†††	70.3***,†††,‡‡‡	**<0.001**
Any depressive syndrome and/or current GAD (DSMIV) (%)	0	1.6	29.4***,†††	89.4***,†††,‡‡‡	**<0.001**
Male (%)	58.5	52.3	50.2	45.2	**0.030**
Educated beyond primary level (%)	88.2	88.1	88.5	80.4	0.17
Currently married	65.1	65.9	63.1	63.5	0.87
Alcohol consumption (standard drinks/day)	0.1 [0–1.5]	0.1 [0–1.2]	0.1 [0–1.5]	0 [0–0.3]***,†,‡‡	**0.003**
Age at diagnosis of diabetes (years)	57.4±11.7	56.2±11.5	54.7±11.5†	49.9±11.6***,†††,‡‡	**<0.001**
Diabetes duration (years)	8.5 [3.0–15.8]	8.0 [2.3–15.4]	9.0 [2.0–15.5]	10.0 [4.0–15.5]	0.57
Fasting serum glucose (mmol/L)	7.1 [6.2–8.7]	7.1 [6.2–8.5]	7.1 [6.1–8.9]	8.1 [6.2–10.3]*,†	**0.021**
HbA_{1c} (%)	6.8 [6.3–7.5]	6.7 [6.2–7.5]	6.8 [6.2–7.6]	7.5 [6.3–8.9]***,†††,‡‡‡	**0.001**
Diabetes treatment (% diet/OGLMs/insulin/ insulin + OGLMs)	23.9/57.2/3.2/15.7	27.1/52.3/3.4/17.2	24.9/51.2/6.8/17.1	18.3/43.3/9.6/28.8***,††	**0.001**
BMI (kg/m^2)	30.9±5.9	30.9±5.8	32.0±6.6	33.5±7.0**,††	**<0.001**
Central adiposity (% obese by waist circumference)	68.6	70.9	74.4	83.5*,†	**0.013**
Total serum cholesterol (mmol/L)	4.3±1.0	4.4±1.0	4.4±1.2	4.5±1.3	0.09
HDL-cholesterol (mmol/L)	1.26±0.35	1.24±0.34	1.24±0.34	1.15±0.27	**0.033**
Serum triglycerides (mmol/L)	1.4 (0.9–2.4)	1.5 (0.9–2.5)	1.5 (0.9–2.5)	2.0 (1.0–3.8)***,†††,‡‡‡	**<0.001**
eGFR <60 ml/min/ 1.73 m^2 (%)	16.5	18.8	18.2	22.3	0.52
Peripheral sensory neuropathy (%)	57.6	59.7	61.6	56.3	0.67
Any retinopathy (%)	20.6	21.9	22.9	24.5	0.83
Self-reported MI/angina (%)	15.5	14.8	22.5†	25.0	**0.005**
Self-reported stroke (%)	2.5	4.0	6.5	7.7	**0.018**

Table 4. Cont.

FDS2 baseline variable	LCA group				P-value
	No anxious depression (Cluster 1)	Subsyndromal anxiety (Cluster 2)	Minor anxious depression (Cluster 3)	Major anxious depression (Cluster 4)	
Peripheral arterial disease (%)	23.5	20.2	21.8	24.3	0.59

*$P<0.05$,
**$P<0.01$,
***$P<0.001$ vs no depression-anxiety;
†$P<0.05$,
††$P<0.01$,
†††$P<0.001$ vs minor depression-anxiety;
‡$P<0.05$,
‡‡$P<0.01$,
‡‡‡$P<0.001$ vs subsyndromal anxiety after Bonferroni adjustment for multiple comparisons.

than the other three classes. This class also showed a higher BMI than the *subclinical anxiety* and the *no anxious depression classes*. When the class with major anxious-depression was compared with patients meeting DSM-IV criteria for major depression, there were no differences on demographic, diabetes-related or psychiatric variables (Table 5).

Discussion

To our knowledge, this is the first study to examine the validity of diagnostic criteria for depression in diabetes using LCA in a large community sample of patients with type 2 diabetes, and there were several important findings. First, LCA of depressive and anxiety symptoms from our sample produced evidence for a 4-class solution: a *major depression-anxiety class*, a *minor depression-anxiety class*, a *subsyndromal anxiety class*, and a class with *no depression or anxiety*. Second, all nine DSM-IV diagnostic criteria for major depression identified a class of patients with a high frequency of major depression, and further changes to these criteria are not necessary. Third, all symptoms of anxiety had similar high probabilities as symptoms of depression for the *major depression-anxiety class*, suggesting that anxiety symptoms should be added to the DSM-IV/5 diagnostic criteria for major depression to identify a class with more severe psychopathology. Therefore, our findings do not support separating anxiety from depressive symptoms for patients with type 2 diabetes. Fourth, the *major depression-anxiety class* had worse diabetes-related parameters than the class without anxiety or depression, suggesting that anxious depression is a marker of more malignant diabetes. Finally, we also identified a class that included anxiety and depression symptoms of a lesser severity, which we termed *minor depression-anxiety*. About one third of this group had clinically relevant anxiety and/or depression, but there were no demographic or clinical differences when compared to the class without anxiety or depression.

These findings should be considered in the light of some limitations of our study. First, given the large sample of individuals to be assessed and the comprehensive quantity of clinical assessments, we were unable to interview patients with more appropriate structured psychiatric interviews. Nevertheless, we assessed depression using the PHQ-9, a valid and reliable instrument to diagnose depression based on DSM-IV criteria and to measure the severity of depression. Second, anxiety symptoms were assessed with the GADS, a new instrument specifically developed and validated for the present study. As with the PHQ-9, the GADS allows a diagnosis of GAD based on DSM-IV criteria and measures the severity of anxiety. We did not use the Generalized Anxiety Disorder 7-item scale (GAD-7) given that this instrument was not available when our study was designed. However, we believe that the GADS is an improvement over the GAD-7 given that the GADS assesses all the DSM-IV/5 criteria for GAD over the past 6 months, whilst the GAD-7 assesses a partial list of symptoms during the past 2 weeks. This was a cross-sectional study, and the clinical progression of the classes identified in this study will need to be examined in our ongoing biennial follow-up study. Finally, we did not assess for the category of 'diabetes distress' in our study. The syndrome of major depression was criticized for not differentiating an expected emotional reaction to a significant stressor from a pathological reaction, whereas 'diabetes distress' may better capture the worries and fears of a chronic illness [23]. However, the construct of 'diabetes distress' is in need of further validation, and it is not included into the major psychiatric nomenclatures. Our study provides empirical support for a class that includes the symptoms of major depression in diabetes, and demonstrates this class to be significantly related to worse diabetes outcomes.

While depression is recognized as one of the most frequent psychiatric disorders in type 2 diabetes, questions remain regarding the validity of using DSM-IV/5 diagnostic criteria when the symptoms of depression and diabetes can overlap. Given the impact of depression on the management and prognosis of diabetes, it is critical to validate diagnostic criteria for depression for use in clinical practice. Using LCA, we found for the first time that all nine- DSM-IV criteria for major depression identify a class of patients with a high chance of having major depression. Moreover, this group also showed significantly worse clinical parameters, such as higher fasting plasma glucose, higher HbA1c, greater use of insulin, higher BMI, increased central adiposity and increased serum triglycerides than the class without anxious depression, which provides partial validation of the classes obtained.

The classes with high probability of depressive symptoms also included a high probability of anxiety symptoms (worrying, restlessness, tension and irritability) and had a high frequency of GAD. This finding demonstrates the high comorbidity of depression and anxiety in diabetes, and suggests that a new diagnostic category of "major anxious depression" should be used in type 2 diabetes. In the general population, this comorbidity is

Table 5. FDS2 baseline associates of major anxious depression class vs major depression (DSM-IV criteria) in participants with type-2 diabetes.

FDS2 baseline variable	Major depression (DSM-IV)	Major anxious-depression (Cluster 4)
N (%)	82 (6.1)	104 (7.8)
Age (years)	60.6±12.5	60.6±12.3
Any depressive syndrome (%)	100.0	77.9
Major depressive syndrome (%)	100.0	67.3
Taking antidepressant medication (%)	42.7	35.6
No depression/depression before diabetes/concomitant diagnoses/ depression after diabetes (%)	0/38.2/19.7/42.1	2.1/43.3/16.5/38.1
Current GAD (%)	43.9	51.0
Lifetime GAD (%):	67.1	70.3
Any depressive syndrome and/or current GAD (DSMIV) (%)	100.0	89.4
Male (%)	46.3	45.2
Educated beyond primary level (%)	79.0	80.4
Currently married	59.8	63.5
Alcohol consumption (standard drinks/day)	0 [0–0.4]	0 [0–0.3]
Age at diagnosis of diabetes (years)	49.3±11.3	49.9±11.6
Diabetes duration (years)	11.0 [4.0–16.1]	10.0 [4.0–15.5]
HbA_{1c} (%)	7.5 [6.2–9.0]	7.5 [6.3–8.9]
Diabetes treatment (% diet/OGLMs/insulin/insulin + OGLMs)	22.0/41.5/9.8/26.8	18.3/43.3/9.6/28.8
BMI (kg/m^2)	33.5±6.1	33.5±7.0
Central adiposity (% obese by waist circumference)	85.4	83.5
Total serum cholesterol (mmol/L)	4.5±1.4	4.5±1.3
HDL-cholesterol (mmol/L)	1.14±0.29	1.15±0.27
Serum triglycerides (mmol/L)	2.0 (1.0–3.8)	2.0 (1.0–3.8)
eGFR <60 ml/min/1.73 m^2 (%)	18.5	22.3
Peripheral sensory neuropathy (%)	53.7	56.3
Any retinopathy (%)	21.8	24.5
History of ischaemic heart disease (%)	36.6	25.0
History of cerebrovascular disease (%)	12.2	7.7
Peripheral arterial disease (%)	23.2	24.3

associated with a poor prognosis, recurrent depression, worse treatment outcomes of depression, more frequent suicide attempts, greater symptom severity, diminished social supports, and more past-year distressing life events [24]. Starr and Davila [25] proposed a model of depression-anxiety comorbidity in which anxiety symptoms lead to depressive symptoms via maladaptive anxiety response styles.

Another relevant finding from our study was a class with intermediate symptoms of anxiety and depression, which we labelled *minor depression-anxiety*. This class included a relatively large proportion of our sample (22%), and future studies may determine whether this class may evolve into a more severe depression with significant impact upon diabetes variables. Cyranowsky et al [24] recently demonstrated that anxiety commonly emerges alongside subthreshold depressive symptoms. The finding that 29% of this class had depression and/or anxiety suggests that this class is clinically relevant. It has been demonstrated that subclinical depression has a significant negative impact on diabetes control [26] and the relationship between depressive symptoms and poor self-care appears to be linear [1]. A third class, which included 38% of the sample, had minor symptoms of anxiety but no depression. Only 2% of this group had clinical depression and/or anxiety, but had a significantly higher lifetime prevalence of GAD and depression as compared to the class with no anxiety or depression. The clinical relevance of this class should be further examined in longitudinal studies.

In conclusion, we demonstrated that the DSM-IV criteria for major depression may be used unmodified to diagnose depression in diabetes. We also found a high comorbidity between depression and anxiety, suggesting that symptoms of anxiety may be included into a new set of diagnostic criteria for major depression or mixed anxiety-depression in type 2 diabetes. Future longitudinal studies will validate this construct and examine the clinical relevance of minor anxious depression and subclinical anxiety in type 2 diabetes.

Author Contributions

Conceived and designed the experiments: SES WAD MD. Performed the experiments: SES WAD VC. Analyzed the data: MD WAD. Contributed reagents/materials/analysis tools: WAD MD. Wrote the paper: SES DB TMED.

References

1. Blay SL, Fillenbaum GG, Marinho V, Andreoli SB, Gastal FL (2011) Increased health burden associated with comorbid depression in older Brazilians with diabetes. J Affect Disord. 134(1–3): 77–84.
2. Gonzalez JS, Peyrot M, McCarl LA, Collins EM, Serpa L, et al (2008) Depression and diabetes treatment nonadherence: a meta-analysis. Diabetes Care. 31(12): 2398–403.
3. de Groot M, Anderson R, Freedland KE, Clouse RE, Lustman PJ (2001) Association of depression and diabetes complications: a meta-analysis. Psychosom Med. 63(4): 619–30.
4. Bruce DG, Davis WA, Starkstein SE, Davis TM (2005) A prospective study of depression and mortality in patients with type 2 diabetes: the Fremantle Diabetes Study. Diabetologia 48(12): 2532–9.
5. Markowitz SM, Gonzalez JS, Wilkinson JL, Safren SA (2011) A review of treating depression in diabetes: emerging findings. Psychosomatics 1; 52(1): 1–18.
6. Atlantis E, Goldney RD, Eckert KA, Taylor AW, Phillips P (2012) Trends in health-related quality of life and health service use associated with comorbid diabetes and major depression in South Australia, 1998–2008. Social psychiatry and psychiatric epidemiology 47(6): 871–7.
7. Atlantis E, Fahey P, Foster J (2014) Collaborative care for comorbid depression and diabetes: a systematic review and meta-analysis. BMJ open 4(4): e004706.
8. Egede LE, Ellis C (2010) Diabetes and depression: global perspectives. Diabetes research and clinical practice 87(3): 302–12.
9. Campayo A, Gomez-Biel CH, Lobo A (2011) Diabetes and depression. Current psychiatry reports 13(1): 26–30.
10. Atlantis E, Vogelzangs N, Cashman K, Penninx BJ (2012) Common mental disorders associated with 2-year diabetes incidence: the Netherlands Study of Depression and Anxiety (NESDA). J Affect Disord 142 Suppl: S30–5.
11. Kessler RC, Merikangas KR, Wang PS (2007) Prevalence, comorbidity, and service utilization for mood disorders in the United States at the beginning of the twenty-first century. Annual review of clinical psychology 3: 137–58.
12. Collins MM, Corcoran P, Perry IJ (2009) Anxiety and depression symptoms in patients with diabetes. Diabet Med 26(2): 153–61.
13. Edwards LE, Mezuk B (2012) Anxiety and risk of type 2 diabetes: evidence from the Baltimore Epidemiologic Catchment Area Study. J Psychosom Res 73(6): 418–23.
14. Nutt D, Argyropoulos S, Hood S, Potokar J (2006) Generalized anxiety disorder: A comorbid disease. European neuropsychopharmacology: the journal of the European College of Neuropsychopharmacology 16 Suppl 2: S109–18.
15. Davis TM, Bruce DG, Davis WA (2013) Cohort profile: the Fremantle Diabetes Study. Int J Epidemiol 42(2): 412–21.
16. Roy T, Lloyd CE, Pouwer F, Holt RI, Sartorius N (2012) Screening tools used for measuring depression among people with Type 1 and Type 2 diabetes: a systematic review. Diabet Med 29(2): 164–75.
17. Kroenke K, Spitzer RL, Williams JB (2001) The PHQ-9: validity of a brief depression severity measure. J Gen Intern Med 16(9): 606–13.
18. Kroenke K, Strine TW, Spitzer RL, Williams JB, Berry JT (2009) The PHQ-8 as a measure of current depression in the general population. J Affect Disord 114(1–3): 163–73.
19. Kroenke K, Spitzer RL, Williams JB, Lowe B (2010) The Patient Health Questionnaire Somatic, Anxiety, and Depressive Symptom Scales: a systematic review. Gen Hosp Psychiatry 32(4): 345–59.
20. Bruce DG, Davis WA, Cetrullo V, Starkstein SE, Davis TM (2013) Clinical Impact of the Temporal Relationship between Depression and Type 2 Diabetes: The Fremantle Diabetes Study Phase II. PLoS One 8(12): e81254.
21. Vermunt JK, Magidson J (2005) Technical Guide for Latent GOLD Choice 4.0: Basic and Advanced. Belmont, Massachussetts.
22. Ruscio J, Brown TA, Meron Ruscio A (2009) A taxometric investigation of DSM-IV major depression in a large outpatient sample: interpretable structural results depend on the mode of assessment. Assessment 16(2): 127–44.
23. Fisher L, Gonzalez JS, Polonsky WH (2014) The confusing tale of depression and distress in patients with diabetes: a call for greater clarity and precision. Diabet Med 31(7): 764–72.
24. Cyranowski JM, Schott LL, Kravitz HM, Brown C, Thurston RC, et al (2012) Psychosocial features associated with lifetime comorbidity of major depression and anxiety disorders among a community sample of mid-life women: the SWAN mental health study. Depress Anxiety 29(12): 1050–7.
25. Starr LR, Davila J (2012) Responding to Anxiety with Rumination and Hopelessness: Mechanism of Anxiety-Depression Symptom Co-Occurrence? Cognitive therapy and research 36(4): 321–37.
26. Fisher L, Skaff MM, Mullan JT, Arean P, Mohr D, et al. (2007) Clinical depression versus distress among patients with type 2 diabetes: not just a question of semantics. Diabetes Care 30(3): 542–8.

5

Waist-to-Hip Ratio, Dyslipidemia, Glycemic Levels, Blood Pressure and Depressive Symptoms among Diabetic and Non-Diabetic Chinese Women

Yu Zheng[1,2], Qihong Sun[1,3], Kang Chen[1], Wenhua Yan[1], Changyu Pan[1], Juming Lu[1], Jingtao Dou[1], Zhaohui Lu[1], JianmingBa[1], Baoan Wang[1], Yiming Mu[1]*

1 Department of Endocrinology, Chinese PLA General Hospital, Beijing, China, **2** School of Medicine, Nankai University, Tianjin, China, **3** Internal Medicine, Fushun Hospital of TCM, Liaoning, China

Abstract

Objectives: To explore the relationship between depressive symptoms and waist-to-hip ratio, dyslipidemia, glycemic levels or blood pressure among diabetic and non-diabetic Chinese women.

Methods: 11,908 women aged ≥40 years were enrolled in this cross-sectional study, including 2,511 with type 2 diabetes and 9,397 without. Depressive symptoms (defined as having mild-to-severe depressive symptoms) were assessed by the Patient Health Questionnaire-9 (PHQ-9) diagnostic algorithm. The prevalence and the odds ratios (ORs) with 95% confidence intervals (CIs) for having depressive symptoms were estimated using logistic regression analysis.

Results: The age-adjusted prevalence of depressive symptoms was significantly higher in non-diabetic subjects with waist-to-hip ratio (WHR) ≥0.9 (8.6%, age-adjusted OR 1.51 [95% CI 1.17, 1.95]), total cholesterol (TC)>6.22 mmol/L (8.8%, 1.58 [1.16, 2.15]), and Hemoglobin A1c (HbA1c) ≥6.00 mmol/L (7.7%, 1.69 [1.34, 2.14]), while it was significantly lower in non-diabetic subjects with diastolic blood pressure (DBP) between 80 to 89 mmHg (6.2%, 0.78 [0.64, 0.95]). These relationships remained significant even after controlling for multiple factors (WHR ≥0.9: multivariable-adjusted OR 1.39 [95% CI 1.07, 1.80]; TC>6.22 mmol/L: 1.56 [1.14, 2.12]; HbA1c ≥6.00 mmol/L: 1.64 [1.30, 2.08]; DBP 80-89 mmHg: 0.78 [0.64, 0.95]). However, no significant trend between depressive symptoms and WHC, TC, HbA1c, DBP was observed in diabetic women, and no significant trend relationship between depressive symptoms and BMI, WC, TG, or SBP was observed in both non-diabetic and diabetic women. Moreover, the prevalence of depressive symptoms was significantly higher in previously-diagnosed diabetes, compared with non-diabetic subjects, while no significant differences were observed between newly-diagnosed diabetes and non-diabetic subjects.

Conclusion: The present study showed a relationship between WHR, TC, HbA1c, DBP and depressive symptoms among non-diabetic women, while no significant relationship between them was observed among diabetic women, even after controlling for multiple confounding factors.

Editor: David Meyre, McMaster University, Canada

Funding: This work was supported by National Science and Technology Major Project (2011ZX09307-001-08). The funder had no role in study design, data collection and analysis, decision to publish, or preparation of the manuscript.

Competing Interests: The authors have declared that no competing interests exist.

* Email: muyiming@yeah.net

Introduction

Depression is a mental health illness responsible for 11.8% of YLDs (years lived with disability), with a point prevalence of approximately 6% in the Chinese population [1],[2]. Women are more prone to depression and this could be explained by gender roles and norms attached to those roles [3]. Better knowledge of its risk factors is required for effective prevention of this disorder. Recently, there is an increasing interest in the relationship between depression and metabolic syndrome or its components, including abdominal obesity, dyslipidemia, hypertension and hyperglycemia. However, researches on the relationship between them have generated controversial findings. Several studies reported a positive link between depression and metabolic syndrome or its components [4–6], while some negative findings have been reported as well [7–9]. In addition, it is estimated that 20% of patients with diabetes suffer from clinically relevant depressive symptoms [10]. There are substantive data to suggest that depression is a risk factor for type 2 diabetes, while diabetes is also a risk factor for depression, and a bidirectional relationship is formed between depression and type 2 diabetes over time [11]. The present cross-sectional study examined the relationship between depressive symptoms and type 2 diabetes. As type 2 diabetes has a marked impact on depression, the present study then divided the subjects into diabetic and non-diabetic groups, and evaluated the relationship between depression and metabolic syndrome components—abdominal obesity, dyslipidemia, and glycemic control, blood pressure–in both diabetic and non-diabetic Chinese women. Moreover, in most prior studies, the estimation of obesity only used Body mass index (BMI) or waist circumference (WC), which is easily distorted by muscle mass and bone structure or takes no account of body composition. In the present study, we examined the relationships between BMI, WC vis-a-vis waist-hip ratio (WHR), and depressive symptoms in Chinese women, as WHR is a measure of body shape and to some extent of lower trunk adiposity since it does not account for the differing ratios of adipose to lean tissue, nor does it distinguish between general or central obesity.

Materials and Methods

Participants and measures

The present study was nested in an ongoing longitudinal (REACTION) study that was designed to investigate the relationship between type 2 diabetes, pre-diabetes and the risk of cancer in the Chinese population, described previously [12]. All permanent residents of Jingding, Laoshan and Gucheng communities of Beijing, China, aged ≥40 years, were invited to participate in a screening examination for diabetes. These research centers are all urban areas, with upper-middle degree of urbanization and economic development status, and the subjects represent the general middle-aged and elderly population of Beijing. Recruitment was performed by local resident associations, and was conducted in the primary health care centers located at these communities. During the recruitment period, the opportunity to participate in the study was offered daily to all residents. A total of 19,314 persons were registered between March and December, 2012. Participants meeting the following criteria were excluded: 1) those who were type 1 or other types of diabetes (n = 205); 2) those without complete data to define depressive symptoms or diabetes (n = 689); 3) males (n = 6,512). A total of 11,908 females (2,511 with type 2 diabetes, 9,397 without) were included in the final analysis. We tested fasting plasma glucose (FPG) and 2 h post-load plasma glucose (PPG), and classified the participants: non-diabetic subjects, defined as an FPG level less than 7.0 mmol/L (126 mg/dL), a PPG level less than 11.1 mmol/L (200 mg/dL) and no history of diabetes; diabetes subjects, defined as an FPG level of 7.0 mmol/L or greater or a PPG level 11.1 mmol/L or greater or a history of diabetes. The two groups were then divided into two subgroups respectively according to their depressive symptoms (defined as having mild-to-severe depressive symptoms): 756 subjects with depressive symptoms, 8,705 subjects without in the non-diabetic group; 228 subjects with depressive symptoms, 2,283 subjects without in the diabetic group.

All participants received comprehensive examinations that included a detailed questionnaire, anthropometric measurement, a standard 75 g oral glucose tolerance test, and blood collection.

The self-administered questionnaire covered history of diabetes, alcohol intake, smoking habits, vocation, educational status, physical activity level, and depressive symptoms. Alcohol intake was classified as either consumption nearly/more than once a week currently or not. Smoking habits was defined as either smoking more than once a day or not. Vocation was classified as farmer or worker, official or soldier or technician, businessman, unemployed, retired and others. Educational status was classified as <high school diploma, high school graduate, and> high school diploma. Regular exercise was defined as engaging in sports more than once a week. Depressive symptoms were assessed by using the Patient Health Questionnaire-9 (PHQ-9) diagnostic algorithm, which has been described in detail elsewhere [13]. Specifically, participants were asked about how often over the last 2 weeks they had experienced each of the following symptoms: 1) little interest or pleasure in doing things; 2) feeling down, depressed, or hopeless; 3) trouble falling or staying asleep or sleeping too much; 4) feeling tired or having little energy; 5) having a poor appetite or overeating; 6) feeling bad as a failure or having let themselves or their family down; 7) having trouble concentrating on things such as reading newspaper or watching TV; 8) moving or speaking so slowly that other people could have noticed, or being so fidgety or restless that they had been moving around a lot more than usual; and 9) thinking of suicide or self-injury in some way. The responses to each item were scored as 0 point for "not at all", 1 point for "having the symptoms for several days", 2 points for "having the symptoms for more than half the days", and 3 points for "having the symptoms for nearly every day". The total score for each item produced a total depression severity score, and subjects who scored 5 or more points were defined as having mild-to-severe depressive symptoms [13]. The PHQ-9 was developed in 1999 and was derived from the Primary Care Evaluation of Mental Disorders (PRIME-MD). It has been translated into more than 80 languages and is widely used throughout the world. Compared with other instruments for screening depression, the PHQ-9 satisfies five practical considerations, which include brevity, self-administered, multipurpose, in the public domain, and easy to score. Four PHQ-9 items related to problems with sleep, fatigability, appetite, and psychomotor agitation/retardation were classified as somatic-affective symptoms, whereas 5 items, related to lack of interest, depressed mood, negative feelings about self, concentration problems and suicidal ideation, were classified as cognitive-affective symptoms of depression. It has demonstrated adequate reliability and validity and has been used in different populations, including Chinese.

Data on anthropometric measurements were collected by trained health technicians. BMI was calculated as body weight in kilograms divided by body height in meters squared (kg/m^2). WC was measured midway between the lowest rib and the superior border of iliac crest at the end of normal expiration with a stretch-resistant measuring tape, and hip circumference (HC) was measured around the widest portion of the buttocks, with the tape parallel to the floor [14]. WHR was calculated as WC in centimeters (cm) divided by HC in cm. Blood pressure was measured three times after the subject had rested for at least 5 minutes prior to measurement, and the mean of the three measurements was used for the analysis.

Blood samples were collected by venipuncture. All participants received an oral glucose tolerance test, and were told to fast for at least 10 h before the test. Plasma glucose, serum triglycerides (TG), total cholesterol (TC), HDL cholesterol (HDL-C), and LDL cholesterol (LDL-C) were measured using an autoanalyser (Cobas 8000 modular analyzer series, Roche Diagnostics, Basel, Switzerland). Hemoglobin A1c (HbA1c) was determined by high-performance liquid chromatography using the VARIANT II Hemoglobin Testing System (Tosoh Corporation, Tokyo, Japan).

Statistical analysis

Statistical analysis was performed using SPSS software, version 19.0 (IBM, Chicago, IL). All continuous variables were presented as mean values and standard deviation (SD). The two-sample t-test was used to compare the differences in baseline characteristics for all continuous variables between the groups with depressive symptoms and the group without, including age, BMI, WC,

WHR, TG, TC, LDL-C, HDL-C, FPG, PPG, HbA1c, systolic blood pressure (SBP), and diastolic blood pressure (DBP). Chi-square test was used for discrete data (alcohol intake, smoking habits, vocation, educational status, and exercise habits). The prevalence of depressive symptoms in each subgroup was standardized for age distribution of the sixth census of population in China by the direct method using 10-year age groupings. The odds ratios (ORs) with 95% confidence intervals (CIs) for depressive symptoms were estimated by conducting logistic regression analyses to test associations between depressive symptoms and BMI, WC, WHR, TG, TC, LDL-C, HDL-C, FPG, PPG, SBP, DBP (all used as continuous variables). First, univariate regression analysis was performed. Second, age was adjusted for (age-adjusted means and 95% CIs). Finally, multiple factors were considered, including age, alcohol intake, smoking habits, vocation, educational status, and exercise habits in the non-diabetic group; family histories of diabetes, various therapies, and duration of diabetes were also considered in the diabetic group, using a forced entry method (multivariable-adjusted means and 95% CIs). In all analyses, $P < 0.05$ was considered to be statistically significant.

Ethics statement

The present study was nested in an ongoing longitudinal (REACTION) study, which is sponsored by the Chinese Society of Endocrinology and led by Rui-Jin Hospital affiliated to School of Medicine, Shanghai Jiao Tong University. All procedures used in this study were in accordance with institutional guidelines. The Committee on Human Research at Rui-Jin Hospital affiliated to School of Medicine, Shanghai Jiao Tong University approved the study protocol, and all study participants provided written informed consents [12].

Results

The baseline characteristics of subjects with and without depression are shown in Table 1. Subjects for analysis were 11,908 females (2,511 with type 2 diabetes, 9,397 without) aged 40–93 years. The prevalence of depressive symptoms (PHQ ≥5) was 8.2%. The socio-demographic characteristics of non-diabetic subjects differed significantly by depressive symptom status except for age, vocation and educational status. The percentages of non-diabetic women who were alcohol drinker or smoker were significantly higher whereas the percentages of adults who exercised regularly were significantly lower among participants with depressive symptoms than among those without ($P < 0.05$ for all comparisons). Non-diabetic subjects with depression had significantly higher values for WHC, TC, HDL-C, FPG and HbA1c compared to those without ($P < 0.05$), while the mean BMI, WC, LDL-C, TG, PPG and SBP among non-diabetic participants with depressive symptoms was not significantly different from those without (all $P > 0.05$). On the other hand, no significant difference between depressive symptoms and BMI, WC, WHC, TC, LDL-C, HDL-C, TG, FPG, PPG, or HbA1c was observed in diabetic women (all $P > 0.05$).

In Table 2, the incidence rates of depressive symptoms were 8.0% for non-diabetic subjects, 8.0% for newly-diagnosed diabetes, and 10.1% for previously-diagnosed diabetes. Compared with non-diabetic subjects, the unadjusted ORs of developing depressive symptoms were 1.00 [95% CI 0.81, 1.25] for newly-diagnosed diabetes, and 1.29 [95% CI 1.06, 1.57] for previously-diagnosed diabetes. The age-adjusted prevalence of depressive symptoms was also significantly higher in previously-diagnosed diabetes (8.9%, age-adjusted OR 1.25 [95% CI 1.02, 1.53]). These relationships remained significant even after controlling for age, alcohol intake, smoking habits, vocation, educational status, and exercise habits (multivariable-adjusted OR 1.23 [95% CI 1.01, 1.50]).

Table 3 shows the unadjusted and age-adjusted prevalence and ORs for depressive symptoms according to the classification of WHC, TC and HbA1c among non-diabetic women. The unadjusted prevalence of depressive symptoms was significantly higher in subjects with WHR ≥0.9 (9.9%, unadjusted OR 1.54 [95% CI 1.19, 1.98]), TC>6.22 mmol/L (9.6% unadjusted OR 1.61 [95% CI 1.12, 2.19]), or HbA1c ≥6.00 mmol/L (9.1%, unadjusted OR 1.72 [95% CI 1.36, 2.16]). The age-adjusted prevalence of depressive symptoms was also higher in subjects with WHR ≥0.9 (8.6%, age-adjusted OR 1.51 [95% CI 1.17, 1.95]), TC>6.22 mmol/L (8.8%, age-adjusted OR 1.58 [95% CI 1.16, 2.15]), or HbA1c ≥6.00 mmol/L (7.7%, unadjusted OR 1.69 [95% CI 1.34, 2.14]). These relationships remained significant even after controlling for age, alcohol intake, smoking habits, vocation, educational status, and exercise habits (WHR ≥0.9: multivariable-adjusted OR 1.39 [95% CI 1.07, 1.80], TC> 6.22 mmol/L: 1.56 [95% CI 1.14, 2.12]), HbA1c ≥6.00 mmol/L: 1.64 [95% CI 1.30, 2.08]. However, no significant trend relationship between depressive symptoms and BMI, WC, TG, or SBP was observed, and the relationship was not "U-shaped" from low to high categories either, among non-diabetic women, (all $P > 0.05$, as shown in Table 3). The relationships remained insignificant after controlling for age or multiple confounding variables. The unadjusted and age-adjusted prevalence of depressive symptoms was significantly lower in subjects with DBP between 80 to 89 mmHg.

Table 4 shows the unadjusted and age-adjusted prevalence and ORs for depressive symptoms according to the classification of WHC, TC, HbA1c, DBP, BMI, WC, TG and SBP among diabetic women. However, none of them was observed to be significantly associated with depressive symptoms in diabetic women (all $P > 0.05$, as shown in Table 4).

Discussion

The prevalence of depressive symptoms (PHQ ≥5) was 8.2% in this study, which is higher than the survey in China (approximately 6%) during 2001–2005 [2]. The first reason for the higher prevalence is the age difference, the mean age of this study is 57.2 which is higher than 44.8 in the 2001–2005 survey. The second reason is this study only includes women, who are more prone to depression. Moreover, the difference may be also attributed to sample size variation and the measurement of depression.

The present cross-sectional study demonstrated a higher prevalence of depressive symptoms in non-diabetic women with higher WHR, TC and HbA1c, while no significant relationships between depressive symptoms and WHR, TC or HbA1c were observed among diabetic women, and no significant trend relationship between depressive symptoms and BMI, WC, TG, or SBP was observed in both non-diabetic and diabetic women, even after controlling for multiple confounding factors. Moreover, the prevalence of depressive symptoms was significantly higher in previously-diagnosed diabetes, compared with non-diabetic subjects, while no significant differences were observed between newly-diagnosed diabetes and non-diabetic subjects. The result suggests that mental health status should be monitored and evaluated in non-diabetic women with high WHR, TC and HbA1c, and the depressive symptoms in diabetic women are more complicated.

Table 1. General characteristics of study participants with and without depressive symptoms.

	Non-diabetic				Diabetic			
	Total	**With depression**	**Without depression**	**P**	**Total**	**With depression**	**Without depression**	**P**
Number	9397	752	8645		2511	228	2283	
Age, year	56.4±7.6	56.8±7.3	56.4±7.6	0.092	60.2±8.5	60.7±8.7	60.2±8.5	0.380
BMI, kg/m^2	25.4±3.6	25.4±3.6	25.4±3.6	0.953	26.7±3.8	26.7±3.6	26.6±3.8	0.704
WC, cm	81.1±8.6	80.9±8.5	81.2±8.6	0.412	85.3±9.0	84.6±8.7	85.3±9.0	0.239
WHC	0.86±0.06	0.87±0.06	0.86±0.06	<0.001	0.90±0.06	0.90±0.06	0.90±0.06	0.906
Vocation, %				0.225				0.462
farmer or worker	7.2	5.7	7.4		3.7	2.2	3.8	
official or soldier or technician	3.9	2.9	3.9		1.2	0.9	1.2	
businessman	0.5	0.3	0.5		0.2	0.0	0.2	
unemployed	4.9	5.5	4.8		4.5	2.6	4.7	
retired	82.7	84.4	82.5		89.8	93.4	89.4	
others	0.9	1.2	0.9		0.7	0.9	0.7	
Educational status, %				0.319				0.970
<high school diploma	38.1	40.7	37.9		52.6	53.1	52.5	
high school diploma	46.7	44.7	46.9		37.8	37.7	37.8	
> high school diploma	15.2	14.6	15.2		9.6	9.2	9.7	
Current alcohol consumption, %	1.3	2.8	1.2	<0.001	1.0	1.8	1.0	0.261
Current smoker, %	2.1	3.6	2	0.004	2.0	2.2	2.0	0.821
Regular exercise, %	6.8	1.6	7.2	<0.001	4.9	1.8	5.3	0.020
History of diabetes, years	–	–	–	–	4.1±6.5	5.2±7.4	4.0±6.4	0.009
Family history of diabetes, %	–	–	–	–	38.5	44.1	37.9	0.071
Hypoglycemic agent use, %	–	–	–	–	38.7	43.4	38.3	0.133
Insulin use, %	–	–	–	–	11.5	15.6	11.1	0.045
FPG, mmol/L	5.35±0.51	5.40±0.52	5.34±0.50	0.004	7.80±2.49	7.78±2.52	7.80±2.50	0.894
PPG, mmol/L	6.94±1.58	6.93±1.59	6.94±1.58	0.937	13.70±4.32	13.60±4.41	13.70±4.31	0.742
HbA$_{1c}$, %	5.78±0.47	5.84±0.43	5.77±0.47	<0.001	7.15±1.48	7.17±1.40	7.15±1.49	0.894
TC, mmol/L	5.33±0.98	5.41±1.02	5.32±0.98	0.013	5.37±1.07	5.44±1.16	5.36±1.07	0.310
LDL-C, mmol/L	3.26±0.83	3.29±0.87	3.26±0.82	0.290	3.30±0.88	3.33±0.94	3.30±0.87	0.618
HDL-C, mmol/L	1.51±0.42	1.54±0.38	1.50±0.42	0.046	1.40±0.34	1.43±0.40	1.40±0.34	0.205
TG, mmol/L	1.52±1.02	1.48±0.95	1.52±1.03	0.311	1.74±1.20	1.77±0.96	1.74±1.22	0.703
SBP, mmHg	128.5±16.2	128.0±16.5	128.5±16.2	0.410	136.7±17.3	137.7±16.8	136.6±17.4	0.351
DBP, mmHg	74.1±9.3	73.0±9.5	74.2±9.2	<0.001	74.6±10.0	74.2±10.2	74.6±10.0	0.563

Table 2. Relationship between diabetes and depressive symptoms in women.

	Unadjusted			Age-adjusted			Multivariable-adjusted*	
	Prevalence (%)	OR (95%CI)	P	Prevalence (%)	OR (95%CI)	P	OR (95%CI)	P
Non-diabetes (n = 9397)	8.0	Reference		7.4	Reference		Reference	
Newly-diagnosed diabetes (n = 1235)	8.0	1.00 (0.81, 1.25)	0.987	7.6	0.98 (0.79, 1.22)	0.848	0.96 (0.77, 1.20)	0.710
Previously-diagnosed diabetes (n = 1276)	10.1	1.29 (1.06, 1.57)	0.010	8.9	1.25 (1.02, 1.53)	0.030	1.23 (1.01, 1.50)	0.044

*Adjusted for age, alcohol intake, smoking habits, vocation, educational status, and exercise habits.

To our best knowledge, the present study is the first report about the relationship between WHR and depressive symptoms, which divided women into diabetic and non-diabetic groups. We found that WHR ≥0.9 was significantly associated with high prevalence and OR of depressive symptoms in non-diabetic women, whereas BMI and WC were not significantly associated with depressive symptoms. The relationship observed between WHR and depressive symptoms is probably explained by abdominal obesity.

Previous studies on the relationship between obesity and depression have generated controversial findings. Some studies have shown that high BMI was associated with lowered risk of depression [15–19]. However, an absent or even an inverse relationship has also been reported. For instance, some studies have shown that BMI is positively related to depression [20–24] and others have shown that increased WC or abdominal obesity is strongly associated with variety of mental disorders, including depression [25],[26]. A drawback of using BMI to investigate the relationship between obesity and depressive symptoms is that it fails to account for the differing ratios of adipose to lean tissue and is easily distorted by muscle mass and bone structure. A limitation of WC alone as a measure is that it takes no account of body composition, whereas WHR is a measure of body shape and to some extent of lower trunk adiposity [27]. Taken together, the present study further suggests that WHR may be a preferred predictor of depression in this population.

Serum lipids and lipoproteins are also argued to be associated with depression, but findings regarding this link have been inconsistent. Some studies have found lower total cholesterol in subjects with depressive symptoms versus controls [28–30], while others have reported higher total cholesterol or found no differences [31],[32]. Levels of LDL-C, HDL-C, and TG were assessed in relation to depression or depressive complaints as well, but less extensively [33],[34].

In the present study, we demonstrated a higher prevalence of depressive symptoms in non-diabetic women with TC> 6.22 mmol/L, while no differences were found for LDL-C, HDL-C or TG levels. The results suggest that the high TC other than LDL-c, HDL-C or TG levels is associated with depressive symptoms in non-diabetic women.

The relationship between glycemic level and depression is still poorly understood. Congruent with prior studies, we found no evidence of a statistically significant relationship between depressive symptoms and glycemic control in type 2 diabetic women [35],[36]. However, we found that high HbA1c level was shown to be associated with depressive symptoms in non-diabetic women, and to our best knowledge, no previous study investigated the relationship between HbA1c level and depressive symptoms in non-diabetic women.

The reported findings on the relationship between blood pressure and the occurrence of depressive symptoms are also conflicting. Low blood pressure has been shown to be associated with depressive symptoms in a number of population studies of both younger and older subjects [37–41], although others also have reported null findings [42],[43].

In the present study, the relationship between DBP and depressive symptoms was also shown to be "U-shaped" from high to low categories, independent of other variables, while SBP was not statistically significant among non-diabetic women. Among diabetic women, neither DBP nor SBP showed significant relationship with depressive symptoms. The result suggests a complex relationship between blood pressure and depression that probably depends on age and race differences.

Table 3. Relationships between metabolic syndrome components and depressive symptoms in non-diabetic women.

	Unadjusted			Age-adjusted			Multivariable-adjusted*	
	Prevalence (%)	OR (95%CI)	P	Prevalence (%)	OR (95%CI)	P	OR (95%CI)	P
BMI								
<18.5 (n = 120)	9.2	1.13 (0.60, 2.12)	0.418	10.0	1.10 (0.59, 2.07)	0.368	1.11 (0.59, 2.10)	0.741
18.5–24.9 (n = 4457)	8.2	Reference		7.3	Reference		Reference	
25.0–29.9 (n = 3892)	7.7	0.94 (0.80, 1.10)	0.993	7.1	0.93 (0.79, 1.09)	0.923	0.91 (0.77, 1.07)	0.246
≥30 (n = 927)	8.2	1.00 (0.77, 1.30)	0.701	7.3	0.99 (0.76, 1.28)	0.765	0.95 (0.73, 1.23)	0.690
WC								
<80 cm (n = 4023)	8.4	Reference		7.5	Reference		Reference	
80–87.9 cm (n = 3368)	7.9	0.94 (0.79, 1.11)	0.459	7.6	0.92 (0.78,1.09)	0.338	0.91 (0.77, 1.08)	0.267
≥88 cm (n = 1999)	7.4	0.87 (0.71, 1.06)	0.160	6.3	0.83 (0.68, 1.02)	0.081	0.81 (0.66, 1.00)	0.041
P value for trend		0.099			0.076		0.608	
WHR								
<0.80 (n = 1314)	6.7	1.00		6.9	1.00		1.00	
0.80–0.85 (n = 2525)	7.2	1.08 (0.83, 1.40)	0.587	6.7	1.07 (0.82, 1.40)	0.607	1.04 (0.80, 1.35)	0.779
0.86–0.89 (n = 3000)	7.7	1.16 (0.90, 1.49)	0.262	7.1	1.15 (0.89, 1.48)	0.293	1.09 (0.84, 1.41)	0.513
≥0.9 (n = 2550)	9.9	1.54 (1.19, 1.98)	0.001	8.6	1.51 (1.17, 1.95)	0.002	1.39 (1.07, 1.80)	0.014
P value for trend		<0.001			<0.001		0.004	
TC								
≤4.14 mmol/L (n = 986)	6.2	1.00		5.7	1.00		1.00	
4.15–5.18 mmol/L (n = 3351)	8.3	1.37 (1.03, 1.83)	0.031	7.8	1.37 (1.03, 1.82)	0.032	1.37 (1.02, 1.82)	0.034
5.19–6.22 mmol/L (n = 3451)	7.5	1.24 (0.93, 1.65)	0.150	6.4	1.22 (0.92, 1.63)	0.173	1.20 (0.90, 1.60)	0.222
>6.22 mmol/L (n = 1598)	9.6	1.61 (1.12, 2.19)	0.003	8.8	1.58 (1.16, 2.15)	0.004	1.56 (1.14, 2.12)	0.005
P value for trend		0.028			0.043		0.064	
LDL-c								
<3.37. mmol/L (n = 5393)	8.0	Reference		7.4	Reference		Reference	
3.37–4.13 mmol/L (n = 2714)	7.6	0.94 (0.79, 1.12)	0.489	6.3	0.93 (0.78, 1.10)	0.393	0.92 (0.77, 1.09)	0.321
≥4.14 mmol/L (n = 1272)	8.8	1.11 (0.89, 1.38)	0.364	7.9	1.09 (0.87, 1.35)	0.466	1.08 (0.87, 1.35)	0.488
P value for trend		0.635			0.787		0.850	
HDL-c								
<1.03 mmol/L (n = 682)	6.5	Reference		6.1	Reference		Reference	
1.03–1.55 mmol/L (n = 4861)	7.8	1.22 (0.88, 1.68)	0.229	6.9	1.22 (0.88, 1.69)	0.228	1.22 (0.88, 1.68)	0.237
≥1.55 mmol/L (n = 3852)	8.6	1.36 (0.98, 1.89)	0.062	7.9	1.37 (0.99, 1.90)	0.059	1.36 (0.98, 1.89)	0.065
P value for trend		0.037			0.033		0.038	
TG								
<1.70 mmol/L (n = 6693)	8.1	Reference		7.3	Reference		Reference	

Table 3. Cont.

	Unadjusted			Age-adjusted			Multivariable-adjusted*	
	Prevalence (%)	OR (95%CI)	P	Prevalence (%)	OR (95%CI)	P	OR (95%CI)	P
1.70–2.82 mmol/L (n = 2033)	7.6	0.93 (0.77, 1.12)	0.451	6.9	0.93 (0.77, 1.12)	0.411	0.93 (0.77, 1.12)	0.419
≥2.83 mmol/L (n = 665)	7.8	0.96 (0.71, 1.29)	0.771	6.6	0.95 (0.70, 1.27)	0.721	0.95 (0.70, 1.28)	0.722
P value for trend		0.960			0.955		0.471	
HbA1c								
<5.50 mmol/L (n = 1999)	5.5	1.00		5.0	1.00		1.00	
5.50–5.74 mmol/L (n = 2662)	8.0	1.49 (1.17, 1.89)	0.001	7.3	1.48 (1.16, 1.87)	0.001	1.48 (1.16, 1.87)	0.001
5.75–5.99 mmol/L (n = 1865)	9.1	1.71 (1.33, 2.20)	<0.001	8.8	1.69 (1.32, 2.18)	<0.001	1.65 (1.28, 2.12)	<0.001
≥6.00 mmol/L (n = 2871)	9.1	1.72 (1.36, 2.16)	<0.001	7.7	1.69 (1.34, 2.14)	<0.001	1.64 (1.30, 2.08)	<0.001
P value for trend		<0.001			<0.001		<0.001	
FPG								
<6.1 mmol/L (n = 8572)	7.9	Reference		7.1	Reference		Reference	
6.1–6.9 mmol/L (n = 825)	8.8	1.13 (0.88, 1.45)	0.349	9.6	1.11 (0.86, 1.43)	0.418	1.07 (0.83, 1.38)	0.620
PPG								
<7.8 mmol/L (n = 6848)	8.0	Reference		7.4	Reference		Reference	
7.8–11.0 mmol/L (n = 2532)	7.9	0.99 (0.83, 1.17)	0.883	6.8	0.96 (0.81, 1.14)	0.668	0.95 (0.80, 1.13)	0.558
SBP								
<120 mmHg (n = 2982)	8.2	Reference		7.3	Reference		Reference	
120–139 mmHg (n = 4323)	8.2	1.01 (0.85, 1.19)	0.936	7.8	0.98 (0.82, 1.16)	0.791	0.96 (0.81, 1.14)	0.645
≥140 mmHg (n = 2071)	7.3	0.89 (0.72, 1.10)	0.273	6.9	0.83 (0.67, 1.04)	0.105	0.82 (0.65, 1.02)	0.072
P value for trend		0.323			0.127		0.085	
DBP								
<80 mmHg (n = 6974)	8.5	Reference		7.6	Reference		Reference	
80–89 mmHg (n = 1963)	6.7	0.77 (0.64, 0.94)	0.010	6.2	0.78 (0.64, 0.95)	0.012	0.78 (0.64, 0.95)	0.013
≥90 mmHg (n = 462)	7.1	0.83 (0.58, 1.20)	0.322	5.8	0.85 (0.59, 1.22)	0.364	0.85 (0.59, 1.22)	0.371
P value for trend		0.018			0.024		0.025	

*Adjusted for age, alcohol intake, smoking habits, vocation, educational status, and exercise habits.

Table 4. Relationships between metabolic syndrome components and depressive symptoms in diabetic women.

	Unadjusted			Age-adjusted			Multivariable-adjusted*	
	Prevalence (%)	OR (95%CI)	P	Prevalence (%)	OR (95%CI)	P	OR (95%CI)	P
BMI								
<18.5 (n = 17)	5.9	0.67 (0.09, 5.16)	0.704	5.8	0.67 (0.09, 5.11)	0.696	0.82 (0.11, 6.42)	0.848
18.5–24.9 (n = 837)	8.5	Reference		6.7	Reference		Reference	
25.0–29.9 (n = 1217)	9.7	1.16 (0.85, 1.58)	0.350	8.9	1.16 (0.85, 1.58)	0.345	1.19 (0.87, 1.63)	0.280
≥30 (n = 439)	8.7	1.02 (0.68, 1.54)	0.916	8.0	1.03 (0.68, 1.56)	0.880	1.10 (0.72, 1.68)	0.651
WC								
<80 cm (n = 621)	9.3	Reference		7.6	Reference		Reference	
80–87.9 cm (n = 942)	10.2	1.10 (0.78, 1.55)	0.581	10.0	1.09 (0.78, 1.54)	0.610 (0.771,1.522)	1.10 (0.78, 1.57)	0.584
≥88 cm (n = 946)	7.8	0.82 (0.58, 1.18)	0.291	7.3	0.81 (0.57, 1.17)	0.259 (0.534,1.173)	0.82 (0.57, 1.19)	0.300
P value for trend		0.228			0.201		0.733	
WHR								
<0.80 (n = 127)	11.0	Reference		8.8	Reference		Reference	
0.80–0.85 (n = 386)	7.3	0.63 (0.32, 1.24)	0.182	6.4	0.63 (0.32, 1.24)	0.178	0.68 (0.34, 1.36)	0.274
0.86–0.89 (n = 791)	9.1	0.81 (0.44, 1.48)	0.491	7.8	0.80 (0.44, 1.47)	0.468	0.89 (0.47, 1.67)	0.719
≥0.9 (n = 1205)	9.5	0.84 (0.47, 1.52)	0.570	9.4	0.82 (0.46, 1.49)	0.519	0.86 (0.46, 1.60)	0.633
P value for trend		0.602			0.690		0.740	
TC								
≤4.14 mmol/L (n = 293)	10.2	Reference		10.3	Reference		Reference	
4.15–5.18 mmol/L (n = 837)	7.6	0.73 (0.46, 1.15)	0.168	7.0	0.73 (0.46, 1.15)	0.177	0.73 (0.46, 1.17)	0.188
5.19–6.22 mmol/L (n = 887)	8.6	0.82 (0.53, 1.28)	0.386	7.0	0.82 (0.53, 1.29)	0.392	0.87 (0.55, 1.37)	0.549
>6.22 mmol/L (n = 491)	11.8	1.17 (0.74, 1.87)	0.500	12.3	1.18 (0.74, 1.88)	0.491	1.28 (0.79, 2.07)	0.318
P value for trend		0.161			0.161		0.069	
LDL-c								
<3.37. mmol/L (n = 1356)	8.8	Reference		7.9	Reference		Reference	
3.37–4.13 mmol/L (n = 733)	9.1	1.05 (0.76, 1.43)	0.780	7.7	1.05 (0.76, 1.43)	0.778	1.13 (0.82, 1.56)	0.452
≥4.14 mmol/L (n = 419)	10.0	1.16 (0.80, 1.68)	0.437	11.7	1.16 (0.80, 1.68)	0.434	1.26 (0.86, 1.83)	0.239
P value for trend		0.451			0.448		0.214	
HDL-c								
<1.03 mmol/L (n = 284)	8.5	Reference		7.0	Reference		Reference	
1.03–1.54 mmol/L (n = 1521)	8.6	1.02 (0.65, 1.61)	0.929	7.8	1.02 (0.65, 1.60)	0.939	1.01 (0.64, 1.60)	0.956
≥1.55 mmol/L (n = 706)	10.3	1.25 (0.77, 2.03)	0.367	9.8	1.24 (0.76, 2.01)	0.384	1.23 (0.76, 2.01)	0.399
P value for trend		0.220			0.235		0.249	
TG								
<1.70 mmol/L (n = 1524)	8.7	Reference		7.5	Reference		Reference	

Table 4. Cont.

	Unadjusted			Age-adjusted			Multivariable-adjusted*	
	Prevalence (%)	OR (95%CI)	P	Prevalence (%)	OR (95%CI)	P	OR (95%CI)	P
1.70–2.82 mmol/L (n = 730)	9.0	1.04 (0.76, 1.42)	0.806	9.2	1.04 (0.77, 1.42)	0.791	1.10 (0.80, 1.50)	0.566
≥2.83 mmol/L (n = 257)	11.3	1.33 (0.87, 2.04)	0.189	8.8	1.34 (0.88, 2.05)	0.179	1.44 (0.94, 2.22)	0.098
P value for trend		0.256			0.243		0.121	
HbA1c								
<6.50 mmol/L (n = 983)	7.9	Reference		6.7	Reference		Reference	
6.50–7.49 mmol/L (n = 852)	10.4	1.36 (0.99, 1.88)	0.061	9.9	1.36 (0.98, 1.88)	0.064	1.24 (0.89, 1.72)	0.208
≥7.50 mmol/L (n = 721)	9.0	1.16 (0.82, 1.64)	0.412	8.3	1.16 (0.82, 1.64)	0.406	0.95 (0.65, 1.39)	0.782
P value for trend		0.358			0.352		0.885	
FPG								
<6.1 mmol/L (n = 547)	9.0	Reference		7.3	Reference		Reference	
6.1–6.9 mmol/L (n = 596)	9.4	1.05 (0.71, 1.58)	0.798	9.6	1.06 (0.71, 1.58)	0.782	1.06 (0.70, 1.60)	0.786
7.0–7.9 mmol/L (n = 575)	8.7	0.97 (0.64, 1.46)	0.877	8.0	0.98 (0.65, 1.48)	0.907	0.98 (0.65, 1.50)	0.938
≥8.0 mmol/L (n = 793)	9.2	1.03 (0.71, 1.51)	0.877	8.7	1.04 (0.71, 1.52)	0.849	0.88 (0.59, 1.31)	0.525
P value for trend		0.978			0.948		0.441	
PPG								
<11.1 mmol/L (n = 532)	10.2	Reference		11.2	Reference		Reference	
11.1–12.9 mmol/L (n = 736)	8.4	0.81 (0.56, 1.19)	0.293	7.3	0.81 (0.56, 1.19)	0.291	0.84 (0.56, 1.25)	0.382
13.0–14.9 mmol/L (n = 523)	7.8	0.75 (0.49, 1.15)	0.191	7.2	0.75 (0.49, 1.15)	0.193	0.78 (0.51, 1.20)	0.259
≥15.0 mmol/L (n = 720)	9.9	0.97 (0.67, 1.41)	0.866	8.1	0.97 (0.67, 1.41)	0.865	0.89 (0.60, 1.31)	0.545
P value for trend		0.954			0.955		0.573	
SBP								
<120 mmHg (n = 384)	7.8	Reference		7.3	Reference		Reference	
120–139 mmHg (n = 1146)	8.8	1.14 (0.75, 1.74)	0.544	7.7	1.13 (0.73, 1.73)	0.590	1.16 (0.75, 1.78)	0.515
≥140 mmHg (n = 973)	10.0	1.31 (0.85, 2.00)	0.220	10.2	1.27 (0.82, 1.97)	0.251	1.31 (0.84, 2.04)	0.232
P value for trend		0.184			0.243		0.207	
DBP								
<80 mmHg (n = 1787)	9.5	Reference		9.0	Reference		Reference	
80–89 mmHg (n = 556)	8.3	0.86 (0.61, 1.21)	0.378	7.3	0.87 (0.62, 1.23)	0.444	0.90 (0.63, 1.28)	0.550
≥90 mmHg (n = 160)	7.5	0.77 (0.42, 1.42)	0.403	7.0	0.79 (0.43, 1.46)	0.454	0.86 (0.46, 1.60)	0.637
P value for trend		0.254			0.318		0.487	

*Adjusted for age, alcohol intake, smoking habits, vocation, educational status, exercise habits, family histories of diabetes, various therapies, and duration of diabetes.

The mechanism of the relationship between depression and abdominal obesity, dyslipidemia and higher glycemic levels is not yet established, and the relationship between them appears to be bi-directional [44]. First, depression has been positively associated with abdominal obesity, dyslipidemia and higher glycemic levels. It can be assumed that visceral adipose tissue plays a key role in the relationship between them via a higher production of inflammatory cytokines (e.g., C-reactive protein and interleukin 6) [45],[46]. Second, depression can activate the hypothalamic-pituitary-adrenocortical (HPA) axis, producing hypersecretion of corticotrophin-releasing hormone, adrenocorticotropic hormone, and cortisol, which could affect abdominal fat accumulation, lipid and glucose metabolism [47–49]. The mechanism of the relationship between lower blood pressure and depressive symptoms is unclear either. It is possible that low blood pressure may lead to depressive symptoms via reduced cerebral perfusion [37]. Taken together, the potential mechanisms are complex, and more studies are needed to explore the mechanisms underlying this reciprocal relation, which will be crucial for the prevention and treatment of depression.

There are several limitations in the present study. First, the causal relationship between WHR, TC, HbA1c or DBP and depressive symptoms cannot be established based on the nature of our cross-sectional study. Second, we used PHQ-9 as a measurement rather than a clinical diagnosis to assess depressive symptoms, which was self-reported and may lead to inevitable recall bias, although the PHQ-9 depression assessment has been validated in the general population including those who are overweight and obese as well as in patients with diabetes. Third, no association between depressive symptoms and metabolic syndrome components in diabetic women was observed, which may be related to small sample size. Further large-scale studies are needed to confirm the result and to fully ascertain the mechanisms underlying the difference between non-diabetic and diabetic women. Forth, the study was performed in middle-aged and elderly Chinese, which limits its generalizability to other ages and ethnics. Finally, there was no information on history of depression and current medication for depression, and antidepressant treatments, which are associated with weight gain, were not taken into account in the present study. Moreover, the differences from other studies could also be attributed to sample size variation, population difference, and the measurement of depression.

In conclusion, the present study indicates that high WHR, TC, HbA1c are significantly associated with increased prevalence and ORs of depressive symptoms in non-diabetic women, while middle DBP is significantly associated with decreased prevalence and ORs of depressive symptoms, even after adjustment of multiple-covariates. The results of the present study have important clinical implications. Considering that high WHR and TC are common in Chinese women, the control of abdominal obesity and hypercholesterolemia may be important for alleviating mood symptoms among non-diabetic women. On the other hand, the cause of depression is more complicated in diabetic women. The prevalence of depressive symptoms was significantly higher in previously-diagnosed diabetes, compared with non-diabetic subjects, while no significant differences were observed between newly-diagnosed diabetes and non-diabetic subjects. Moreover, WHR, TC, HbA1c, DBP may be less important in diabetic women.

Author Contributions

Conceived and designed the experiments: YM. Performed the experiments: YZ QS KC WY CP JL JD ZL JB BW. Analyzed the data: YZ QS KC WY. Wrote the paper: YZ QS KC WY YM.

References

1. Prince M, Patel V, Saxena S, Maj M, Maselko J, et al. (2007) No health without mental health. Lancet 370: 859–877.
2. Phillips MR, Zhang J, Shi Q, Song Z, Ding Z, et al. (2009) Prevalence, treatment, and associated disability of mental disorders in four provinces in China during 2001–05: an epidemiological survey. Lancet 373: 2041–2053.
3. Nolen-Hoeksema S, Larson J, Grayson C (1999) Explaining the gender difference in depressive symptoms. J Pers Soc Psychol 77:1061–1072.
4. Takeuchi T, Nakao M, Nomura K, Yano E (2009) Association of metabolic syndrome with depression and anxiety in Japanese men. Diabetes Metab 35: 32–36.
5. Foley DL, Morley KI, Madden PA, Heath AC, Whitfield JB, et al. (2010) Major depression and the metabolic syndrome. Twin Res. Hum. Genet 13: 347–358.
6. Morikawa M, Okamoto N, Kiuchi K, Tomioka K, Iwamoto J, et al. (2013) Association between depressive symptoms and metabolic syndrome in Japanese community-dwelling older people: a cross-sectional analysis from the baseline results of the Fujiwara-kyo prospective cohort study. Int J Geriatr Psychiatry 28: 1251–1259.
7. Hildrum B, Mykletun A, Midthjell K, Ismail K, Dahl AA (2009) No association of depression and anxiety with the metabolic syndrome: the Norwegian HUNT Study. Acta Psychiatr Scand 120: 14–22.
8. Vogelzangs N, Beekman AT, Dik MG, Bremmer MA, Comijs HC, et al. (2009) Late-life depression, cortisol, and the metabolic syndrome. Am J Geriatr Psychiatry 17: 716–721.
9. Zeman M, Jáchymová M, Jirák R, Vecka M, Tvrzická E, et al. (2010) Polymorphisms of genes for brainderived neurotrophic factor, methylenetetrahydrofolate reductase, tyrosine hydroxylase, and endothelial nitric oxide synthase in depression and metabolic syndrome. Folia Biol (Praha) 56: 19–26.
10. Anderson RJ, Freedland KE, Clouse RE, Lustman PJ (2001) The prevalence of comorbid depression in adults with diabetes: a meta-analysis. Diabetes Care 24: 1069–1078.
11. Golden SH, Lazo M, Carnethon M, Bertoni AG, Schreiner PJ, et al. (2008) Examining a bidirectional association between depressive symptoms and diabetes. JAMA 299: 2751–2759.
12. Ning G; Reaction Study Group (2012) Risk evaluation of cancers in Chinese diabetic Individuals: a IONGitudinal (REACTION) study. J Diabetes 4: 172–173.
13. Kroenke K, Spitzer RL (2002) The PHQ-9: a new depression diagnostic and severity measure. Psychiatric Annals 32: 1–7.
14. Mushtaq MU, Gull S, Abdullah HM, Shahid U, Shad MA, et al. (2011) Waist circumference, waist-hip ratio and waist-height ratio percentiles and central obesity among Pakistani children aged five to twelve years. BMC Pediatr 11:105.
15. Crisp AH, McGuiness B (1976) Jolly fat: relation between obesity and psychoneurosis in general population. BMJ 1: 7–9.
16. Palinkas LA, Wingard DL, Barrett-Connor E (1996) Depression in overweight and obese older adults: a test of the 'jolly fat' hypothesis. J Psychosom Res 40: 59–66.
17. Li ZB, Ho SY, Chan WM, Ho KS, Li MP, et al. (2004) Obesity and depression in Chinese elderly. Int J Geriatr Psychiatry 19: 68–74.
18. Kuriyama S, Koizumi T, Matsuda-Ohmori K, Seki T, Shimazu T, et al. (2006) Obesity and depression in elderly Japanese: the Tsurugaya Project. J Psychosom Res 60: 229–235.
19. Ho R, Niti M, Kua EH, Ng TP (2008) Body mass index, waist circumference, waist-hip ratio and depressive symptoms in Chinese elderly: a population-based study. Int J Geriatr Psychiatry 23: 401–408.
20. Roberts RE, Strawbridge WJ, Kaplan GA (2002) Are the fat more jolly? Ann Behav Med 24: 169–180.
21. Simon GE, Von Korff M, Saunders K, Miglioretti DL, Crane PK, et al. (2006) Association between obesity and psychiatric disorders in the US adult population. Arch Gen Psychiatry 63: 824–830.
22. Olszanecka-Glinianowicz M, Zahorskamarkiewicz B, Kocełak P, Semik-Grabarczyk E, Dabrowski P, et al. (2009) Depression in obese persons before starting complex group weight-reduction programme. Int J Soc Psychiatry 55: 407–413.
23. Pan A, Sun Q, Czernichow S, Kivimaki M, Okereke OI, et al. (2012) Bidirectional association between depression and obesity in middle-aged and older women. Int J Obes 36: 595–602.
24. Jagielski AC, Brown A, Hosseini-Araghi M, Thomas GN, Taheri S (2014) The association between adiposity, mental well-Being, and quality of life in extreme obesity. PLoS One 9: e92859.
25. Zhao G, Ford ES, Li C, Tsai J, Dhingra S, et al. (2011) Waist circumference, abdominal obesity and depression among overweight and obese US. Adults: National Health and Nutrition Examination Survey 2005–2006. BMC 11:130.
26. Grossniklaus DA, Dunbar SB, Gary R, Tohill BC, Frediani JK, et al. (2012) Dietary energy density: A mediator of depressive symptoms and abdominal obesity or independent predictor of abdominal obesity? Eur J Cardiovasc Nurs 11: 423–431.

27. Price G M, Uauy R, Breeze E, Bulpitt CJ, Fletcher AE (2006) Weight, shape, and mortality risk in older persons: elevated waist-hip ratio, not high body mass index, is associated with a greater risk of death. Am J Clin Nutr 84: 449–460.
28. Steegmans PH, Hoes AW, Bak AA, van der Does E, Grobbee DE (2000) Higher prevalence of depressive symptoms in middle-aged men with low serum cholesterol levels. Psychosom Med 62: 205–211.
29. Aijanseppa S, Kivinen P, Helkala EL, Kivelä SL, Tuomilehto J, et al. (2002) Serum cholesterol and depressive symptoms in elderly Finnish men. Int J Geriatr Psychiatry 17: 629–634.
30. Giltay EJ, Reedt Dortland AK, Nissinen A, Giampaoli S, van Veen T, et al. (2009) Serum cholesterol, apolipoprotein E genotype and depressive symptoms in elderly European men: The FINE study. J Affect Disord 115: 471–477.
31. Nakao M, Yano E (2004) Relationship between major depression and high serum cholesterol in Japanese men. Tohoku J Exp Med 204: 273–287.
32. van Reedt Dortland AK, Giltay EJ, Van Veen T, van Pelt J, Zitman FG, et al. (2010) Associations between serum lipids and major depressive disorder: results from the Netherlands Study of Depression and Anxiety (NESDA). J Clin Psychiatry 71: 729–736.
33. Ergün UG, Uguz S, Bozdemir N, Güzel R, Burgut R, et al. (2004) The relationship between cholesterol levels and depression in the elderly. Int J Geriatr Psychiatry 19: 291–296.
34. Huang TL, Chen JF (2004) Lipid and lipoprotein levels in depressive disorders with melancholic feature or atypical feature and dysthymia. Psychiatry Clin Neurosci 58: 295–299.
35. Fisher L, Mullan JT, Arean P, Glasgow RE, Hessler D, et al. (2010) Diabetes distress but not clinical depression or depressive symptoms is associated with glycemic control in both cross-sectional and longitudinal analyses. Diabetes Care 33: 23–28.
36. Tsujii S, Hayashino Y, Ishii H; Diabetes Distress and Care Registry at Tenri Study Group (2012) Diabetes distress, but not depressive symptoms, is associated with glycaemic control among Japanese patients with Type 2 diabetes: Diabetes Distress and Care Registry at Tenri (DDCRT 1). Diabet Med 29: 1451–1455.
37. Ng TP, Feng L, Niti M, Yap KB (2010) Low blood pressure and depressive symptoms among Chinese older subjects: a population-based study. Am J Med 123: 342–349.
38. Licht CMM, Geus EJC, Seldenrijk A, van Hout HP, Zitman FG, et al. (2009) Depression is associated with decreased blood pressure, but antidepressant use increases the risk for hypertension. Hypertension 53: 631–638.
39. Niu K, Hozawa A, Awata S, Guo H, Kuriyama S, et al. (2008) Low blood pressure is associated with depressive symptoms in an elderly population aged 70 years and over: a population-based, cross-sectional analysis. Hypertens Res 31: 409–416.
40. Lenoir H, Lacombe JM, Dufouil C, Ducimetière P, Hanon O, et al. (2008) Relationship between blood pressure and depression in the elderly. The three-city study. J Hypertens 26: 1765–1772.
41. Hildrum B, Mykletun A, Holmen J, Dahl AA (2008) Effect of anxiety and depression on blood pressure: 11-year longitudinal population study. Br J Psychiatry 193: 108–113.
42. Donner-Banzhoff N, Chan Y, Szalai JP, Hilditch JR (1997) Low blood pressure associated with low mood: a red herring? J Clin Epidemiol 50: 1175–1181.
43. Gilmore C, Green BH, Copeland JR, Dewey ME, Davidson IA, et al. (1995) Blood pressure as a risk factor for depression in elderly people: a prospective study. Acta Psychiatr Scand 91: 126–129.
44. Pan A, Keum N, Okereke OI, Sun Q, Kivimaki M, et al. (2012) Bidirectional association between depression and metabolic syndrome: a systematic review and meta-analysis of epidemiological studies. Diabetes Care 35: 1171–1180.
45. Eckel RH, Grundy SM, Zimmet PZ (2005) The metabolic syndrome. Lancet 365: 1415–1428.
46. Capuron L, Su S, Millesr AH, Bremner JD, Goldberg J, et al. (2008) Depressive symptoms and metabolic syndrome: is inflammation the underlying link? Biol Psychiatry 64: 896–900.
47. Musselman DL, Evans DL, Nemeroff CB (1998) The relationship of depression to cardiovascular disease: epidemiology, biology, and treatment. Arch Gen Psychiatry 55: 580–592.
48. Bjorntorp P, Rosmond R (2000) The metabolic syndrome: a neuroendocrine disorder? Br J Nutr 83 (Suppl. 1): S49–S57.
49. Anagnostis P, Athyros VG, Tziomalos K, Karagiannis A, Mikhailidis DP (2009) Clinical review: The pathogenetic role of cortisol in themetabolic syndrome: a hypothesis. J Clin Endocrinol Metab 94: 2692–2701.

Therapeutic Effect of Vagus Nerve Stimulation on Depressive-Like Behavior, Hyperglycemia and Insulin Receptor Expression in Zucker Fatty Rats

Shaoyuan Li[1,2], Xu Zhai[1]**, Peijing Rong[1*], Michael F. McCabe[3], Xing Wang[2], Jingjun Zhao[1], Hui Ben[1], Shuxing Wang[1,2,3,4,5*]**

1 Department of Physiology, Institute of Acupuncture and Moxibustion, China Academy of Chinese Medical Sciences, Beijing, China, 2 Department of Anatomy, Xinxiang Medical University, Xinxiang, Henan, China, 3 Department of Anesthesia, Critical Care, and Pain Medicine, Massachusetts General Hospital, Harvard Medical School, Boston, MA, United States of America, 4 Primate Research Center, Guangdong Entomological Institute, Guangzhou, Guangdong, China, 5 Guangdong Landau Biotechnology Co. Ltd, Guangzhou, Guangdong, China

Abstract

Depression and type 2 diabetes (T2D) are common comorbid diseases and highly prevalent in the clinical setting with an unclarified mechanism. Zucker diabetic fatty (ZDF, fa/fa) rats natively develop T2D with hyperglycemia and hyperinsulinemia. Here we studied whether ZDF rats also innately develop depression, what a correlation is between depression and T2D, whether insulin receptor (IR) expression is involved in, and whether transcutaneous auricular vagus nerve stimulation (taVNS) would be beneficial in amelioration of the comorbidity. Six week old male ZDF and Zucker lean (ZL, fa/+) littermates were randomly divided into naïve (ZDF, n = 6; ZL, n = 7) and taVNS (ZDF-taVNS, n = 8; ZL-taVNS, n = 6) groups. Once daily 30 min-taVNS sessions were administrated under anesthesia for 34 consecutive days in taVNS groups. Blood glucose levels were tested weekly, and plasma glycosylated hemoglobin (HbAlc) level and immobility time in forced swimming test were determined on day 35 in all groups. The expression of insulin receptor (IR) in various tissues was also detected by immunostaining and Western blot. We found that naïve ZDF rats developed hyperglycemia steadily. These ZDF rats showed a strong positive correlation between longer immobility time and higher plasma HbAlC level. Long term taVNS treatment simultaneously prevented the development of depression-like behavior and progression of hyperglycemia in ZDF rats. The expression of IR in various tissues of naïve ZDF rats is lower than in naïve ZL and long-term taVNS treated ZDF rats. Collectively, our results indicate that in ZDF rats, i) depression and T2D develop simultaneously, ii) immobility time and HbAlc concentrations are highly and positively correlated, iii) a low expression of IR may be involved in the comorbidity of depression and T2D, and iv) taVNS is antidiabetic and antidepressive possibly through IR expression upregulation.

Editor: David A. Slattery, University of Regensburg, Germany

Funding: This work was supported by National Natural Science Foundation of China, 81271243; National Basic Research Program of China (973 Program), 2012CB518503; and Project Supported National Science and Technology Ministry, 2012BAF14B10. The funders had no role in study design, data collection and analysis, decision to publish, or preparation of the manuscript.

Competing Interests: The authors have declared that no competing interests exist.

* Email: rongpj@hotmail.com (PR); 13718103762@139.com (SW)

These authors contributed equally to this work.

Introduction

Type 2 diabetes (T2D) is a metabolic disorder characterized by high blood sugar level in the context of insulin resistance, in which body cells have lost the ability to respond adequately to relatively normal levels of insulin [1]. Rates of T2D have been increasing markedly since 1960 in parallel with obesity. To make things worse, ongoing epidemiological studies estimate that greater than 60% of adult US population may be categorized as either overweight or obese, which is a major risk factor of T2D [2,3]. Furthermore, there is a growing appreciation that the complications of obesity extend to the central nervous system (CNS) and may result in increased risk for neurological comorbidities such as depressive illness. Depression is a state of low mood that affects thoughts, behavior, feelings and sense of well-being. Patients with depression may lose interest of life and contemplate, attempt, or commit suicide [4].

During the past two decades, studies found an increased prevalence of depression in the diabetic population, and vice versa [4,5]. Despite the high prevalence of and common comorbidity between depression and T2D [6,7], the mechanism behind the phenomena is unclear. The increasing burden of T2D and major depressive disorder makes the search for an extended understanding of etiology and for the development of additional treatments highly significant.

As a kind of complementary and alternative medicine, acupuncture is generally accepted as a beneficial, well-tolerated, and safe monotherapy for depression in animal models, clinical patients, and eldercare facility residents [8–11]. Specifically, the taVNS, which stimulates the afferent auricular branches of vagus

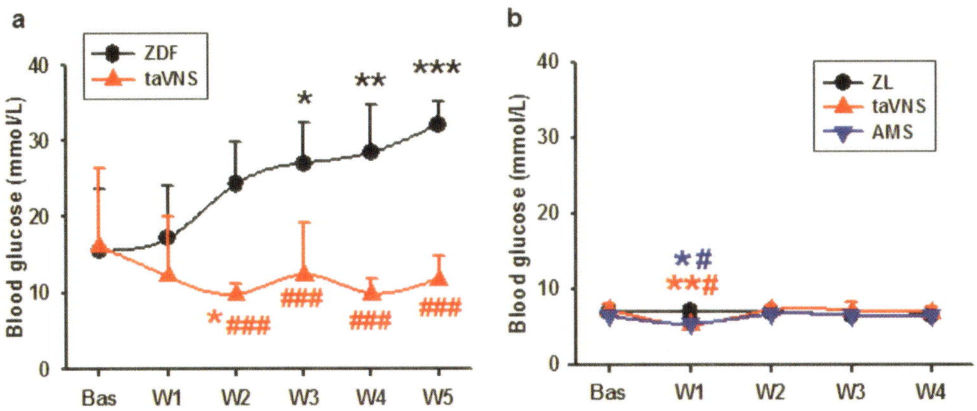

Figure 1. Blood glucose change in naïve and taVNS treated rats. Showing the development of hyperglycemia in ZDF rats with or without the taVNS treatment (a) and the effect of taVNS in ZL rats. ZDF, naïve ZDF rats; ZL, naïve ZL rats; taVNS, transcutaneous auricular vagus nerve stimulation; AMS, auricular margin stimulation; Bas, baseline; W1-5, week 1 to week 5 of the experiment. *, **, ***, $P<0.05$, 0.01, 0.001 *vs.* Bas; #, ###, $P<0.05$, 0.001 *vs.* naïve rats, respectively.

nerve that project to solitary nucleus [12]. Neurons in solitary nucleus further project, mono- or multi-synaptically, to the limbic and the autonomic nervous system structures, including the pineal gland, ventral tegmental area, the hypothalamus, amygdala, anterior cingulate cortex, nucleus accumbens, and the lateral prefrontal cortex [12]. Fibers from the solitary nucleus also project to the locus ceruleus and dorsal raphe nucleus, respectively major nuclei related to noradrenergic and serotonergic innervations of the entire brain cortex. It is clear that the serotonergic, dopaminergic, and noradrenergic systems are commonly involved in the pathophysiology of depression and in the neuromechanisms of action of antidepressants [12]. Acupuncture has also been shown to decrease blood glucose level in T2D [13] and is beneficial in the treatment of obesity [14,15], which is a primary cause of T2D in genetically predisposed people [3].

Based on the existence of overt depression in Zucker diabetic fatty (ZDF, fa/fa) rats [12] as well as the increasingly prevalent and high comorbidity of obesity and depression [16], in this study we used ZDF rats as a diabetes and depression rodent model to explore the correlation of the illnesses, the antidiabetic and antidepressive effectiveness of taVNS, and focused on a possible involvement of IR expression in the mechanism of the comorbidity between T2D and depression.

Materials and Methods

Animal model

Male ZDF rats (n = 14) and ZL littermates (n = 13) were purchased from Vital River Laboratories International Inc. (Beijing, China). Littermates from the same or foster mother were housed in one large cage with water and normal food pellets available ad libitum except during taVNS session. Animal room was maintained at 22±1°C and artificially illuminated from 7:00 A.M. to 7:00 P.M. There was no previous handling of the rats. Rats entered the experimental procedure at 6 weeks of age and were separated into ZDF and ZL groups according to the genotype, the appearance, and the first tested glucose concentration. The initial body weight was 175±15 grams for ZDF and 130±10 for ZL rats. The rats were raised in groups of three to four. The cages and beddings were changed every other day. The person in charge of the animal's welfare was also the same person who carried out the experiments. The experimental protocol was approved by Institutional Animal Care and Use Committee in China Academy of Chinese Medical Sciences.

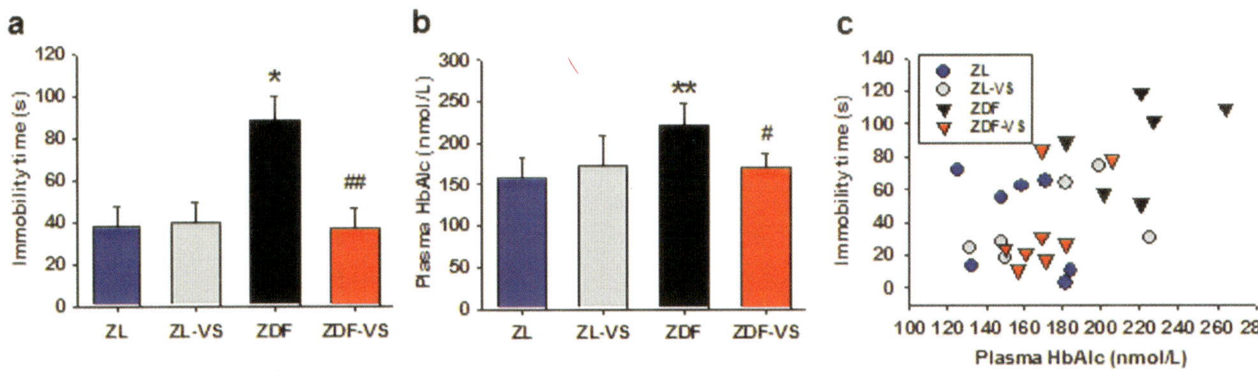

Figure 2. Correlation of depressive behavior and glucose metabolism dysfunction. Showing the immobility time of rats in FST (a) and the HbAlc concentration (b) on day 35 and their correlation in linear regression. ZL, naïve ZL rats; ZL-VS, taVNS in ZL rats; ZDF, naïve ZDF rats; ZDF-VS, taVNS in naïve ZDF rats. *, **, $P<0.05$, 0.01 *vs. ZL*; #, ##, $P<0.05$, 0.01 *vs.* ZDF, respectively.

Table 1. Immobility time in FST on day 35.

Rat group	Naïve ZDF	ZDF-taVNS	Naïve ZL	ZL-taVNS
Mean	87.833	36.625	40	39.667
Standard deviation (SD)	28.032	28.096	29.878	23.304
Sample size (N)	6	8	7	6
Std. error of mean(SEM)	11.444	9.934	11.292	9.514
Lower 95% conf. limit	58.411	13.312	12.367	15.207
Upper 95% conf. limit	117.26	60.118	67.633	64.126
Tukey-Kramer multiple comparisons test P value *vs.* Naïve ZDF		<0.01	<0.05	<0.05

Blood glucose concentration test

By using Ascensia Breeze Blood Glucose Monitoring System (Newbury, Berks, UK), the progression of T2D was determined by weekly tested non-fasted blood glucose concentration from week 0 (baseline) to week 5. In an electronic stimulation experiment room, a rat was tenderly put into the plexiglass box linked to the inhalation anesthesia system. Under 2% isoflurane anesthesia, glucose concentration was tested from tail tip blood immediately before taVNS session. The test range was 0.6–33.3 mmol/L. Any concentration over the testing limit was recorded as 33.3 mmol/L for statistical purposes.

Administration of taVNS

All the time points recorded in this study are in accordance with the taVNS occurrences, i.e. the beginning of taVNS is day 1. For taVNS, under 2% isoflurane inhalation anesthesia, two opposite magnetic electrodes (+/−) were placed over the right side auricular concha region, inside and outside respectively so that electronic current can conduct through the tissue, including the vagus nerve fibers. Saline was applied between an electrode and the skin to improve electronic conduction. A 30 min taVNS procedure at a frequency of 2/15 Hz (2 and 15 Hz, switched every second) and an intensity of 2 mA was administered once daily via an electrical stimulator (HANS-100, Nanjing, China). The parameters had been proven effective previously [17]. The procedures were performed in the afternoon after blood glucose test and blood sample collection at designed time points, for 34 consecutive days for ZDF rats and 27 days for ZL rats. Because the glucose concentration of ZL rats showed no detectable fluctuations for over two weeks, the experimental period in them was one week shorter for the benefit of rats. Auricular margin was used as sham acupoint.

ELISA

Concentration of plasma HbAlc was evaluated upon sacrifice at day 28 for ZL rats and day 35 for ZDF rats. ELISA kits were purchased from R&D System (Beijing, China) and analyzed by Huanya Biomedicine Technology Co. LTD (Beijing, China). The results were read using a microplate reader (Multiskan MK3, Thermo Scientific, Beijing, China) at wavelengths of 450 nm.

Forced swimming test (FST)

The FST was modified based on the methods previously used in our study [18,19] but omitted the pre-test session, which we found to be a confounding factor to the final results such that the pre-tested rats tended to stay still in the formal test and the immobility time was extremely prolonged to obscure the difference between animal groups. Briefly, a rat was placed in a clear plastic tank (45×35×60 cm) containing 30 cm of water (24±0.5°C) for 5 min. The total duration of non-swimming time within the 5-min session was recorded with a stopwatch as immobility score (in seconds) and compared among groups. A rat was judged to be non-swimming when no attempt was made to escape the tank and the rat was hunched forward (a floating position). Both ZL and ZDF rats underwent the same test procedure. Following FST session, the rat was removed from the water tank, dried with a towel, and returned to the home cage. All tests took place between 2 PM and 5 PM in a behavior testing room and were observed by the experimenter who blinded to the group assignment in order to minimize between-experimenter and between-session variations.

Immunohistochemical staining

Rats were anesthetized with sodium pentobarbital and transcardially perfused with 200 ml of saline followed by 200–300 ml of cold 4% paraformaldehyde in 0.1 M phosphate buffer (PB). Brain

Table 2. HbAlc concentration on day 35.

Rat groups	Naïve ZDF	ZDF-taVNS	Naïve ZL	ZL-taVNS
Mean	219.57	170.94	157.68	172.91
Standard deviation (SD)	27.465	17.187	23.461	35.620
Sample size (N)	6	8	7	6
Std. error of mean(SEM)	11.213	6.076	8.867	14.542
Lower 95% conf. limit	190.74	156.57	135.98	135.53
Upper 95% conf. limit	248.40	185.31	179.38	210.30
Tukey-Kramer multiple comparisons test P value *vs.* Naïve ZDF		<0.05	<0.01	<0.05

Table 3. Correlations between HbAlc level and immobility time in FST on day 35.

Rat groups	ZDF	ZL
Estimated HbAlc level from immobility time	$y=153.244+0.685x$	$y=173.732-0.231x$
Estimated immobility time from HbAlc level	$y=-108.276+0.87x$	$y=69.655-0.186x$
Correlation	$R=0.757$	$R=-0.207$
P value	$P=0.002$	$P=0.497$

sections from bregma −1.4 to −4 [20] were dissected, postfixed for 2 hr, and kept in 30% sucrose in 0.1 M PB until sank to the bottom. Tissues were then mounted in OCT compound and frozen on dry ice.

Brain (30 μm) sections were cut on a cryostat, mounted serially onto microscope slides, and stored at −80°C. Immunohistochemical staining was used to detect IR (mouse monoclonal, 1:1000; Abcam, Cambridge, MA), NeuN (neuronal marker, rabbit monoclonal, 1:1000; Abcam, Cambridge, MA), and GFAP (astrocyte marker, chicken polyclonal, 1:1000; Abcam, Cambridge, MA). Sections were blocked with 1% goat serum in 0.3% Triton for 1 hr at room temperature and incubated overnight at 4°C with a primary antibody. For controls, a primary antibody was omitted. The sections were then incubated for 1 hr at room temperature with corresponding FITC- or CY3-conjugated secondary antibody (1:200; Jackson ImmunoResearch, West Grove, PA). Four to six nonadjacent brain or spinal sections were randomly selected, analyzed using a LEXT OLS4000 3D Laser Measuring Microscope (Olympus), recorded using a digital camera, and processed using Adobe Photoshop.

Western blot

The expression of IR in hypothalamus, liver, and skeletal muscle was tested by Western blot. Rats (n = 3 each group) were decapitated under anesthesia and samples were collected. The segments were homogenized in SDS sample buffer containing a mixture of proteinase inhibitors (Sigma). Protein samples were separated on SDS-PAGE gel (4–15% gradient gel; Bio-Rad, Hercules, CA) and transferred to polyvinylidene difluoride filters (Millipore, Bedford, MA). The filters were blocked with 3% milk and incubated overnight at 4°C with a primary antibody of IR (mouse monoclonal, 1:4000; Abcam, Cambridge, MA) for 1 hr at room temperature with HRP-conjugated secondary antibody (1:7000; Abcam, Cambridge, MA). The blots were visualized in ECL solution (NEN, Boston, MA) for 1 min and exposed onto hyperfilms (Amersham Biosciences) for 1–10 min. The blots were then incubated in a stripping buffer (67.5 mM Tris, pH 6.8, 2% SDS, and 0.7% β-mercaptoethanol) for 30 min at 50°C and reprobed with a polyclonal rabbit anti-GADPH antibody (1:20,000; Abcam, Cambridge, MA) as loading control. Western analysis was made in triplicates. The density of specific bands was measured with a computer-assisted imaging analysis system and normalized against loading controls. Differences were compared using One-way ANOVA.

Statistical analysis

By running GraphPad InStat version 3 for Windows, raw data of glucose concentration, immobility, and ELISA results were compared using repeated measure One-way ANOVA to detect differences among treatment groups, followed by Tukey-Kramer Multiple Comparisons Test to determine sources of differences. Data were presented as mean ± standard deviation. Differences were considered to be statistically significant at the level of $\alpha = 0.05$. The correlation between HbAlc concentration and immobility time was acquired by linear regression.

Results

The development of hyperglycemia in naïve ZDF rats and the preventive effect of taVNS on the progression

As determined by the weekly blood glucose concentration, the naïve ZDF rats (n = 6) developed hyperglycemia steadily with age, in contrast with a euglycemia in taVNS treated ZDF rats (Fig. 1a, n = 6). The results were also compared with that of ZL rats, naïve, and taVNS or AMS (auricular margin stimulation) treated rats (n = 4, each), in which no hyperglycemia developed (Fig. 1b).

Effects of long term taVNS on depression-like behavior and plasma HbAlc concentration in rats

As determined by the FST on day 35, the naïve ZDF rats performed poorly in the tank with an immobility time of 87.83±28.03 (mean ± SD, n = 6). This immobility time is much longer than that of ZL rats and of taVNS treated ZDF rats (One-way ANOVA $P = 0.006$, Fig. 2a, Table 1). Simultaneously, the HbAlc concentration in taVNS treated rats is significantly lower than that in naïve ZDF rats (One-way ANOVA $P = 0.0019$, Fig. 2b, Table 2).

The antidepressive and antidiabetic effects of taVNS were also evaluated in ZL rats. While it is antidepressive and antidiabetic in ZDF rats, the taVNS shows no effects in ZL rats, possibly due to normal swimming time and glucose metabolism condition in the latter ($P>0.05$, Fig. 2a, Table 1).

The correlation between the immobility time and the HbAlc concentration on day 35 is shown in Fig. 2c. As analyzed in linear regression, a strong positive correlation exists between the immobility time and the HbAlc concentration in ZDF rats ($y = 153.244+0.685x$), in contrast to ZL rats in which a weak negative correlation ($y = 173.732-0.231x$) is shown (Fig. 2C, Table 3). Alternatively, a higher HbAlc concentration can predicate a longer immobility time in ZDF rats ($y = -108.276+0.87x$), in contrast to that in ZL rats ($y = 69.655-0.186x$).

IR expression in naïve ZDF and the effect of taVNS on the expression of IR

As detected by immunostaining and by Western blots, the expression of IR in the hypothalamus, liver, and skeletal muscle is lower in naïve ZDF rats than that in ZL. However, in the same tissues of the taVNS treated ZDF rats, the IR expression was upregulated (Fig. 3).

In double labelling immunofluorescence brain sections, the IR was colocalized with NeuN (Fig. 4a–d) but not GFAP (Fig. 4e–h), indicating that the IR-immunopositive cells in the brain is

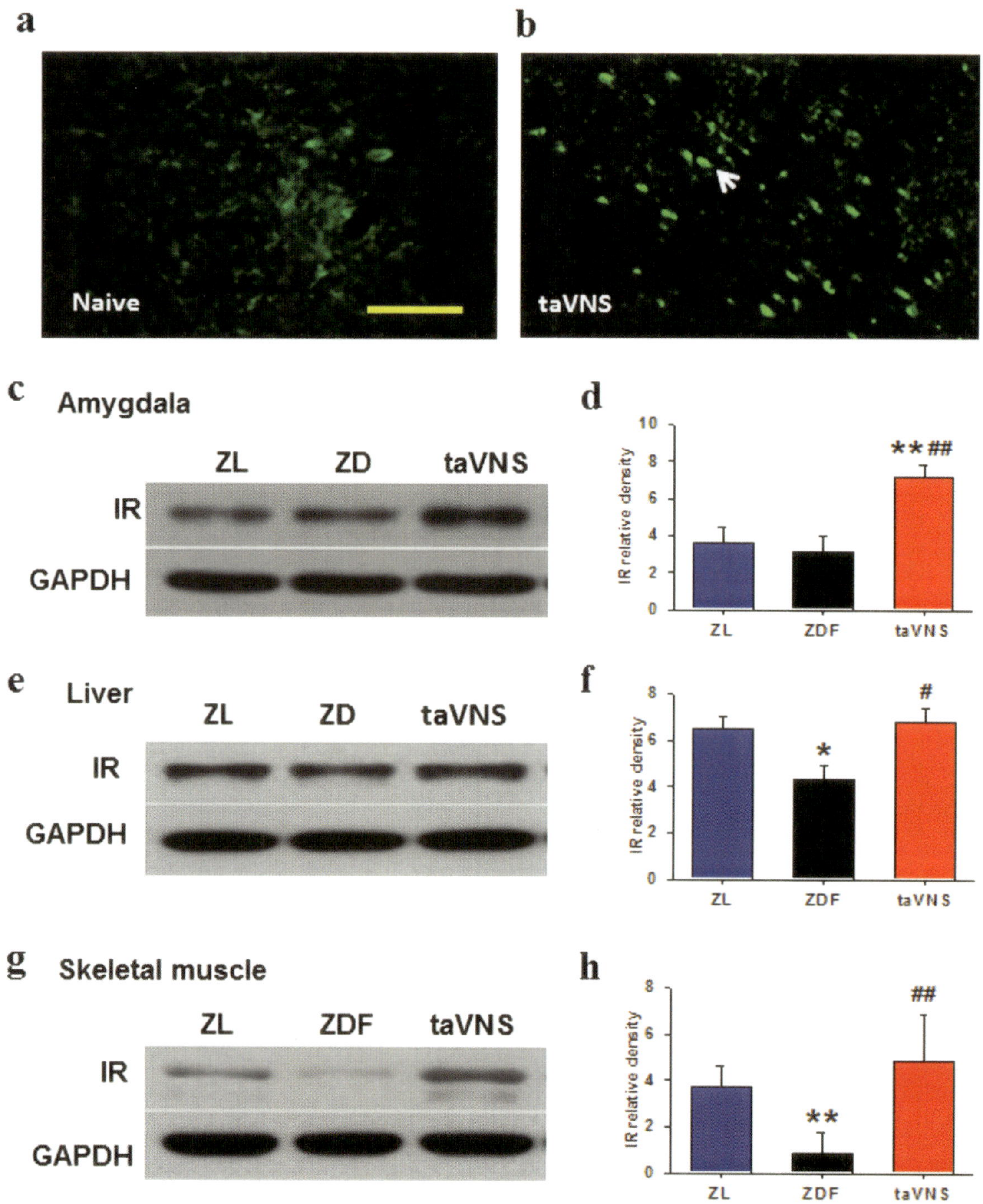

Figure 3. Expression of insulin receptor in various tissues of rats. (a, b) Immunofluorescent results showing the expression of insulin receptor **(IR)** in amygdala of naïve ZDF rats (a) and of ZDF rats treated for 5 consecutive weeks with daily half hour taVNS treatment (b). Arrow head, IR-immunopositive neurons. Bar, 100 μm. (c–h) Western blot results showing the expression of insulin receptor in hypothalamus (c, d), liver (e, f), and skeletal muscle (g, h) of naïve rats, or rats treated with taVNS for 34 consecutive days. ZL, naïve ZL rats; ZDF, naïve ZDF rats; taVNS, auricular vagus electronic stimulation. n = 3 each group, Western blot triplicated for each sample. *,** $P<0.05$, 0.01 *vs.* ZL; #,## $P<0.05$, 0.01 *vs.* ZDF.

neuronal in characteristics. The IR expressed in the membrane of neurons.

Discussion

In this study we report that the ZDF rats not only develop diabetes innately, they also develop depressive-like behaviors and that taVNS simultaneously prevent the progression of depressive behavior and hyperglycemia in ZDF rats.

A number of epidemiological studies have established a link between insulin resistance and the prevalence of depression. However, at this time it is not conclusive as to whether insulin resistance induces depression or the opposite. Although a study found that downregulation of hypothalamic insulin receptor

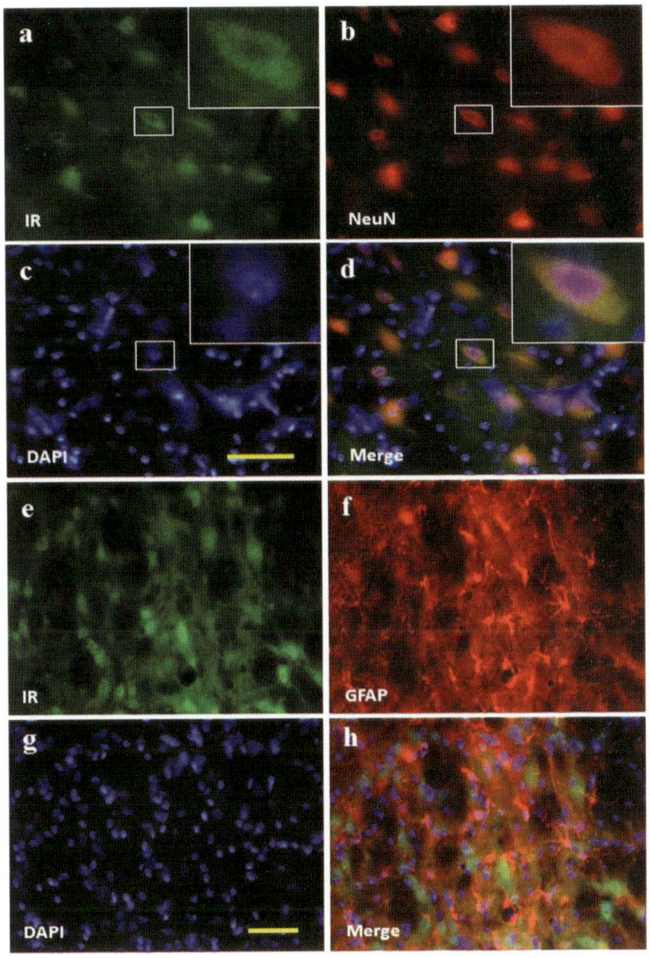

Figure 4. Neurochemical characteristics of insulin receptor positive cells in the brain. Double labelling immunofluorescence results showing that the IR is colocalized with NeuN (a–d) but not GFAP (e–h). Bar, 100 μm.

expression elicits depressive-like behaviors in rats [21], others found that the occurrence of depression precede the onset of diabetes [22], and that insulin resistance can be reversed by antidepressant treatment [23]. Meanwhile, not only are depressive symptoms a risk factor for the development of T2D, they have also been shown to contribute to hyperglycemia, diabetic complications, functional disability and all-cause mortality among diabetic patients [4,5]. Taken together, these reports indicate that the depression and insulin resistance may be bidirectional in cause.

Leptin is an adipocytokine or hormone secreted by white adipose tissue. Mediated through leptin receptor, leptin works together with insulin to decrease blood glucose level. Genetically, ZDF rats are leptin receptor deficient in and resistant to leptin, and therefor develop T2D with hyperglycemia and hyperinsulinemia. It is reported that hyperinsulinemia increases sympathetic nerve activity in obesity and diabetes [24] and that an increased sympathetic tone is closely related to depression [4]. From this point of view, we propose that depression in ZDF rats might be a result of hyperinsulinemia and glucose metabolism dysfunction in the CNS and that antidepressive effect of taVNS may be elicited by decreasing sympathetic tone or increasing parasympathetic activity; in turn, this antidepressive effect would also be helpful in reducing the insulin resistance. Indeed, the activity of the vagus nerve is negatively associated with risk factors such as stress and smoking, morbidity and mortality, and accordingly, taVNS which directly stimulates the afferent vagus branches at the auricular concha region, has been used in the therapeutic intervention in depression and epilepsy [23,25,26].

IR is necessary for the insulin to activate the intracellular signaling system both in the CNS and the peripheral cells. It is known that insulin performs unique functions within the CNS [27]. Produced nearly exclusively by the pancreas, insulin crosses the blood-brain barrier using a saturable transporter, affecting feeding and cognition through CNS mechanisms largely independent of glucose utilization. While peripheral insulin acts primarily as a metabolic regulatory hormone, CNS insulin has an array of effects on the brain that may more closely resemble the actions of the ancestral insulin molecule [28,29]. Resistance to insulin action within the CNS may be in parallel or associated with peripheral insulin resistance, but it is also possible that variable insulin resistance syndromes exist so that resistance at one tissue may be independent from that of others. In this study, the expression of IR was low in various tissues including the hypothalamus, the liver, and the skeletal muscle of naïve ZDF rats and it was upregulated in taVNS treated rats. These results, while indicating that IR is involved in the pathogenesis mechanism of depression and T2D, also support the theory that taVNS is helpful in ameliorating both the depressive and the diabetic syndromes in these rats. It is very likely that, the upregulated expression of IR in the peripheral tissue such as liver and skeletal muscle is related to the amelioration of T2D, and in the CNS it is beneficial in the antidepressive effect of taVNS.

Although we demonstrate that taVNS is antidiabetic and antidepressive in ZDF rats, it has limited efficiency in ZL rats, a similar phenomenon as in melatonin treated experimental animals [30]. This may be due to a reduced parasympathetic activity in ZDF but not ZL rats. Further investigation would be focused on detection of the secretion change of hormones that are easily affected by the autonomic nervous system. One such hormone candidate is melatonin, which is related to both depression [19,20,31,32] and T2D [33–35] with nonsufficient concentration in the circulating blood.

Conclusions

Our results show that downregulated expression of IR and the compensatory hyperinsulinemia may be involved in the comorbidity between depression and T2D and that taVNS has a potential antidiabetic and antidepressive in ZDF rats.

Acknowledgments

Many thanks to Dr. J. Mao (Massachusetts General Hospital, Harvard Medical School), Dr. B. Zhu (Institute of Acupuncture and Moxibustion, China Academy of Chinese Medical Sciences), Drs. Z.K. Guo, W.C. Yang, and X.H. Cai (Xinxiang Medical Univ.) and members of their laboratories for generous assistance.

Author Contributions

Conceived and designed the experiments: SW PR. Performed the experiments: SL XZ PR JZ HB XW. Analyzed the data: SW. Contributed reagents/materials/analysis tools: SW. Wrote the paper: SW PR MFM.

References

1. Fu Z, Gilbert ER, Li D (2013) Regulation of insulin synthesis and secretion and pancreatic Beta-cell dysfunction in diabetes. Curr Diabetes Rev 9: 25–53.
2. Wilding JP (2014) The importance of weight management in type 2 diabetes mellitus. Int J Clin Pract 68:682–691.
3. Smyth S, Heron A (2006) Diabetes and obesity: the twin epidemics. Nat Med 12:75–80.
4. Lang UE, Borgwardt S (2013) Molecular mechanisms of depression: perspectives on new treatment strategies. Cell Physiol Biochem 31:761–777.
5. Rustad JK, Musselman DL, Nemeroff CB (2011) The relationship of depression and diabetes: Pathophysiological and treatment implications. Psychoneuroendocrinology 36: 1276–1286.
6. Foran E, Hannigan A, Glynn L (2014) Prevalence of depression in patients with type 2 diabetes mellitus in Irish primary care and the impact of depression on the control of diabetes. Ir J Med Sci. [Epub ahead of print] PubMed PMID: 24723006.;
7. Mendenhall E, Norris SA, Shidhaye R, Prabhakaran D (2014) Depression and type 2 diabetes in low- and middle-income countries: a systematic review. Diabetes Res Clin Pract 103:276–285.
8. Lyons Z, van der Watt G, Shen Z, Janca A (2012) Acupuncture and Chinese herbs as treatments for depression: an Australian pilot study. Complement Ther Clin Pract 18:216–220
9. Mischoulon D, Brill CD, Ameral VE, Fava M, Yeung AS (2012) A pilot study of acupuncture monotherapy in patients with major depressive disorder. J Affect Disord 141:469–473.
10. Yeung AS, Ameral VE, Chuzi SE, Fava M, Mischoulon D (2011) A pilot study of acupuncture augmentation therapy in antidepressant partial and non-responders with major depressive disorder. J Affect Disord 130:285–289.
11. Zhang ZJ, Chen HY, Yip KC, Ng R, Wong VT (2010) The effectiveness and safety of acupuncture therapy in depressive disorders: systematic review and meta-analysis. J Affect Disord 124:9–21.
12. Liu RP, Fang JL, Rong PJ, Zhao Y, Meng H, et al. (2013) Effects of electroacupuncture at auricular concha region on the depressive status of unpredictable chronic mild stress rat models. Evid Based Complement Alternat Med 2013:789674
13. Peplow PV, Baxter GD (2012) Electroacupuncture for control of blood glucose in diabetes: literature review. J Acupunct Meridian Stud 5:1–10.
14. Belivani M, Dimitroula C, Katsiki N, Apostolopoulou M, Cummings M, et al. (2013) Acupuncture in the treatment of obesity: a narrative review of the literature. Acupunct Med 31: 88–97.
15. Wang Q, Li WH, Zhou QH, Tang XD, Zhang XX, et al. (2012) Weight reduction effects of acupuncture for obese women with or without perimenopausal syndrome: a pilot observational study. Am J Chin Med 40:1157–1166.
16. Preiss K, Brennan L, Clarke D (2013) A systematic review of variables associated with the relationship between obesity and depression. Obes Rev 14:906–918.
17. Huang F, Dong J, Kong J, Wang H, Meng H (2014) Effect of transcutaneous auricular vagus nerve stimulation on impaired glucose tolerance: a pilot randomized study. BMC Complement Altern Med 14:203.
18. Wang S, Tian Y, Song L, Lim G, Tan Y, et al. (2012) Exacerbated mechanical hyperalgesia in rats with genetically predisposed depressive behavior: role of melatonin and NMDA receptors. Pain 153: 2448–2457.
19. Zeng Q, Wang S, Lim G, Yang L, Mao J, et al. (2008) Exacerbated mechanical allodynia in rats with depression-like behavior. Brain Res 1200:27–38.
20. Paxinos G, Watson C (1997) The rat brain in stereotaxic coordinates, 3rd ed. New York: Academic Press.
21. Grillo CA, Piroli GG, Kaigler KF, Wilson SP, Wilson MA, et al. (2011) Downregulation of hypothalamic insulin receptor expression elicits depressive-like behaviors in rats. Behav Brain Res 222:230–235.
22. Cline BH, Steinbusch HW, Malin D, Revishchin AV, Pavlova GV, et al. (2012) The neuronal insulin sensitizer dicholine succinate reduces stress-induced depressive traits and memory deficit: possible role of insulin-like growth factor 2. BMC Neurosci 13:110.
23. Buhl ES, Jensen TK, Jessen N, Elfving B, Buhl CS, et al. (2010) Treatment with an SSRI antidepressant restores hippocampo-hypothalamic corticosteroid feedback and reverses insulin resistance in low-birth-weight rats. Am J Physiol Endocrinol Metab 298:E920–929.
24. Ward KR, Bardgett JF, Wolfgang L, Stocker SD (2011) Sympathetic response to insulin is mediated by melanocortin 3/4 receptors in the hypothalamic paraventricular nucleus. Hypertension 57:435–441.
25. Rong P, Fang J, Kong J, Wang L, Meng H, et al. (2012) Trancutanous vagus nerve stimulation for the treatment of depression: a study protocol for a double blinded randomized clinical trails. BMC Complement Altern Med 12:255.
26. He W, Rong PJ, Li L, Ben H, Zhu B, et al. (2012) Auricular acupuncture may suppress epileptic seizures via activating the parasympathetic nervous system: a hypothesis based on innovative methods. Evid Based Complement Alternat Med 2012:615476.
27. La Marca R, Nedeljkovic M, Yuan L, Maercker A, Elhert U (2010) Effects of auricular electrical stimulation on vagal activity in healthy men: evidence from a three-armed randomized trial. Clin Sci (Lond) 118:537–546.
28. Zhao WQ, Chen H, Quon MJ, Alkon DL (2004) Insulin and the insulin receptor in experimental models of learning and memory. Eur J Pharmacol 490:71–81.
29. Banks WA, Owen JB, Erickson MA (2012) Insulin in the brain: there and back again. Pharmacol Ther 136:82–93.
30. Langenberg C, Pascoe L, Mari A, Tura A, Laakso M, et al. (2009) Common genetic variation in the melatonin receptor 1B gene (MTNR1B) is associated with decreased early-phase insulin response. Diabetologia 52:1537–1542.
31. Maurizi CP (1984) Disorder of the pineal gland associated with depression, peptic ulcers, and sexual dysfunction. South Med J 77:1516–1518.
32. Cardinali DP, Srinivasan V, Brzezinski A, Brown GM (2012) Melatonin and its analogs in insomnia and depression. J Pineal Res 52:365–375.
33. Frese T, Bach AG, Mühlbauer E, Pönicke K, Brömme HJ, et al. (2009) Pineal melatonin synthesis is decreased in type 2 diabetic Goto-Kakizaki rats. Life Sci 85:526–533.
34. McMullan CJ, Schernhammer ES, Rimm EB, Hu FB, Forman JP (2013) Melatonin secretion and the incidence of type 2 diabetes. JAMA 309:1388–1396.
35. Agil A, Rosado I, Ruiz R, Figueroa A, Zen N, et al. (2012) Melatonin improves glucose homeostasis in young Zucker diabetic fatty rats. J Pineal Res 52:203–210.

7

Assessing Regional Cerebral Blood Flow in Depression Using 320-Slice Computed Tomography

Yiming Wang[1*], Hongming Zhang[2], Songlin Tang[1,3], Xingde Liu[4*], Adrienne O'Neil[5,6], Alyna Turner[5,7,8], Fangxian Chai[1], Fanying Chen[9], Michael Berk[5,6,7,10,11]

1 Department of Psychiatry, Hospital Affiliated to Guiyang Medical University, Guiyang, Guizhou, China, **2** Department of Cardiology, The General Hospital of Jinan Military Region, Jinan, China, **3** Department of Neurology, First People's Hospital of Shaoyang, Shaoyang, Hunan, China, **4** Department of Cardiology, Hospital Affiliated to Guiyang Medical University, Guiyang City, Guizhou, China, **5** IMPACT Strategic Research Centre, School of Medicine, Deakin University, Geelong, Australia, **6** School of Public Health and Preventive Medicine, Monash University, Melbourne, Australia, **7** Department of Psychiatry, The University of Melbourne, Parkville, Victoria, Australia, **8** School of Medicine and Public Health, The University of Newcastle, Callaghan, New South Wales, Australia, **9** Mental Health Education And Counseling Center, Guiyang Medical University, Guiyang City, Guizhou, China, **10** Department of Psychiatry, Orygen Youth Health Research Centre, The University of Melbourne, Parkville, Victoria, Australia, **11** Florey Institute of Neuroscience and Mental Health, University of Melbourne, Parkville, Victoria, Australia

Abstract

While there is evidence that the development and course of major depressive disorder (MDD) symptomatology is associated with vascular disease, and that there are changes in energy utilization in the disorder, the extent to which cerebral blood flow is changed in this condition is not clear. This study utilized a novel imaging technique previously used in coronary and stroke patients, 320-slice Computed-Tomography (CT), to assess regional cerebral blood flow (rCBF) in those with MDD and examine the pattern of regional cerebral perfusion. Thirty nine participants with depressive symptoms (Hamilton Depression Rating Scale 24 (HAMD24) score >20, and Self-Rating Depression Scale (SDS) score >53) and 41 healthy volunteers were studied. For all subjects, 3 ml of venous blood was collected to assess hematological parameters. Trancranial Doppler (TCD) ultrasound was utilized to measure parameters of cerebral artery rCBFV and analyse the Pulsatility Index (PI). 16 subjects (8 = MDD; 8 = healthy) also had rCBF measured in different cerebral artery regions using 320-slice CT. Differences among groups were analyzed using ANOVA and Pearson's tests were employed in our statistical analyses. Compared with the control group, whole blood viscosity (including high\middle\low shear rate)and hematocrit (HCT) were significantly increased in the MDD group. PI values in different cerebral artery regions and parameters of rCBFV in the cerebral arteries were decreased in depressive participants, and there was a positive relationship between rCBFV and the corresponding vascular rCBF in both gray and white matter. rCBF of the left gray matter was lower than that of the right in MDD. Major depression is characterized by a wide range of CBF impairments and prominent changes in gray matter blood flow. 320-slice CT appears to be a valid and promising tool for measuring rCBF, and could thus be employed in psychiatric settings for biomarker and treatment response purposes.

Editor: Huafu Chen, University of Electronic Science and Technology of China, China

Funding: This study was supported by a Grant for YW from National Natural Science Foundation of China, (Project Grant 2012 31260237), YW has received Grant/Research Support from the Science and Technology Fund of Guizhou Province, China, Qiankehe Diquhe (2012) 7001, Qiankehe (LG, 2011, 005, J, 2006, 2065, SY, 2008, 3063), which was supported by High-Level Personnel Research Conditions, Special Assistant Funding (TZJF-2008 55), Guizhou Province Special Fund for Outstanding Scientific and Technology Education Talents 2012, 35, Guizhou Province Overseas Students studying science and technology activities funded projects 0011 006 and Scientific and Technology Projects in Guiyang City, China, 2009, Zhu subjects agriculture in Contract 3-008 for study design, the collection, analysis, and interpretation of data and the writing of the manuscript. MB is supported by a NHMRC Senior Principal Research Fellowship 1059660.

Competing Interests: The authors have declared that no competing interests exist.

* Email: yimingw66@yahoo.com (YW); lxd@gmc.edu.cn (XL)

These authors contributed equally to this work.

Introduction

In major depressive disorder (MDD), symptom development and course are influenced by brain circuits associated with vascular disease [1]. Studies conducted in depressed populations suggest that patients may exhibit impairments in regional cerebral blood flow (rCBF) and dysfunction in cortical and subcortical brain structures [2]; a close relationship has been observed between mild cognitive impairment and brain hypoperfusion [3]. rCBF is improved by treatment including cognitive-behavioral and electroconvulsive therapy (ECT) in MDD [4–5], suggesting a state related change. This may be linked to reduced mitochondrial energy generation and dysfunction in the disorder [6–7]. In parallel, there is a large literature showing alterations in brain glucose utilization in depression [8]. Therefore, monitoring rCBF in psychiatric populations and settings may be useful in the context of monitoring treatment response.

Imaging studies have previously utilized techniques such as functional magnetic resonance imaging (fMRI) and have demonstrated changes in hemodynamics of the limbic system and subcortical regions in those with depression [9]. Single-photon

Table 1. The comparison of demographic data between control and depression groups (Mean ± SEM).

Items	control (n = 41)	depression (n = 39)
Ages(years)	46.22±11.68	46.74±11.42
(Ranges)	18–60	18–60
Sex(M/F)(n)	9/32	8/31
Resting SBP (mm Hg)	120±25	125±27
Resting DBP (mm Hg)	80±10	76±8
Smokers/non-smokers (n)	20/21(49%/51%)	21/18 (54%/46%)

Note: no significant differences in the demographic variables (age, sex, blood pressure, smoking) between two groups, SBP: systolic blood pressure, DBP: diastolic blood pressure.

emission computed tomography (SPECT) has also been employed to document hypoperfusion of the frontal and prefrontal regions in late-life depressed patients [10–13], as well as improvements in rCBF following treatment with antidepressants [14] and ECT [15]. Similarly, MRI with arterial spin labeling has demonstrated significant CBF elevation in white matter in those for whom depression remits following antidepressant use [16].

The use of heterogeneous imaging techniques has, in some instances, yielded inconsistent results. For example, studies of depressed patients using positron emission tomography (PET) have indicated decreased glucose utilization in temporal lobe cortex [17], while others have found increased cerebral glucose metabolism in older patient populations [18]. While these studies suggest that there is a potential relationship between cognitive impairment and altered rCBF, most studies are subject to limitations including their use of semi-quantitative measurement that do not objectively reflect rCBF changes.

In contrast, the Toshiba Aquilion ONE 320 slice dynamic volume CT [19] is a refined diagnostic imaging test which utilizes dynamic volume Computed Tomography (CT) technology. It has the capacity to display soft tissue, bones and blood vessels in a singular, high resolution image and can also capture dynamic processes including blood flow and organ function, in three-dimensional real-time. This technology has advanced patient care in a range of medical settings by reducing time to diagnosis in heart disease and stroke populations. If applied in psychiatry, this technique allows for the acquisition of data pertaining to brain blood circulation and perfusion maps, including unenhanced, enhanced, delayed patterns, and assessment of arterial and venous diagrams in the same phase. It uses relatively low radiation doses and could quickly and accurately determine changes in cerebral hemodynamics as well as quantitative examination of cerebral perfusion. To date, several studies have been conducted using One 320 slice CT in coronary artery and pulmonary vascular populations [20–21]. While the advantages of employing whole brain CT perfusion in acute stroke, ahronic ischemia and arteriovenous malformation have been acknowledged [22], no publications investigating its utility in psychiatric populations were found at the time of writing. To our knowledge, this study will be the first to utilize 320-slice CT imaging previously used in coronary and stroke patients to assess rCBF in those with MDD and analyze the extent which it corresponds with regional cerebral blood flow velocity (rCBFV) as measured by Trancranial Doppler (TCD) ultrasound. We also aimed to compare rCBF in depressed patients to healthy control subjects to clarify regional cerebral perfusion patterns in the cerebral hemispheres, in order to explore its potential utility in psychiatric settings for possible diagnostic and treatment response purposes.

Materials and Methods

Subjects

The sample comprised patients (n = 39, 8 men and 31 women, aged 18–60 years, mean ages 46.74±11.42). They were hospitalized patients or outpatients with major depression seen in the Psychiatry Department of the affiliated hospital of Guiyang Medical University between April and December, 2009. Patients who met diagnostic criteria for a depressive disorder as defined by the Diagnostic and Statistical Manual of Mental Disorders-IV (DSM-IV) (diagnosed by two clinicians), had a Hamilton Depression Rating Scale 24 (HAMD24) score of >20 points, and a Self-Rating Depression Scale (SDS) score >53 were included in this study. Exclusion criteria included taking psychotropic substances or drugs influencing vessel compliance function

Table 2. The comparison of demographic data between control and depression groups using the 320 slice CT (Mean ±SEM).

Items	control (n = 8)	depression (n = 8)
Ages(years)	44.13±10.37	43.12±12.09
(Ranges)	18–60	18–60
Sex(M/F)(n)	1/8	1/8
Resting SBP (mm Hg)	118±22	120±27
Resting DBP (mm Hg)	75±10	78±8
Smokers/non-smokers (n)	1/7(13%/87%)	1/7 (13%/87%)

Note: no significant differences in the demographic variables (age, sex, blood pressure, smoking) between two groups, SBP: systolic blood pressure, DBP: diastolic blood pressure.

Table 3. The comparison of hemorheological parameters between depression and control groups (Mean ±SEM).

Items	Control (n = 41)	Depression(n = 39)
High shear rate (mPa.s/150S^{-1})	3.92±0.31	4.63±0.39*
Middle shear rate (mPa.s/60S^{-1})	4.38±0.36	5.72±0.47**
Low shear rate (mPa.s/10S^{-})	6.43±0.70	7.75±1.10**
Hematocrit	41.32±2.91	43.34±4.68*
Red blood cell sedimentation (mm/h)	39.34±6.62	38.07±8.90

Note: Compared with control group *P<0.05, **P<0.01.

upon enrollment (such as stimulants, hypnotics or sedatives), diseases of the nervous system (Aneurysms involving the supra-aortic vessels, chronic cerebral venous insufficiency), somatic diseases (e.g. diabetes, hypertension, coronary heart disease, atherosclerosis), or other mental disorders.

Forty one healthy volunteers, who were healthy and underwent physical examination in the physical examination center of the affiliated hospital of Guiyang Medical University between April and December 2009 were recruited concurrently as a control group. They were matched for age and gender (9 men and 32 women, aged 18–60 years, Mean age 46.22±11.68), with a

Table 4. The comparison of parameters of rCBFV between control and depression groups (Mean ± SEM, cm/s).

Items	Control (n = 41)	Depression(n = 39)
ACA-R-Vs	96.31±11.76	79.85±20.41**
ACA-R-Vm	63.95±8.15	54.44±14.80**
ACA-R-Vd	40.67±6.93	37.00±11.40
ACA-L-Vs	96.64±12.21	77.31±14.26**
ACA-L-Vm	64.10±7.82	52.90±11.17**
ACA-L-Vd	41.64±5.98	36.54±8.70**
TICA-R-Vs	114.03±13.44	95.87±17.40**
TICA-R-Vm	76.85±9.69	69.11±21.98*
TICA-R-Vd	51.28±7.18	46.46±10.30*
TICA-L-Vs	112.54±12.32	97.69±20.41**
TICA-L-Vm	75.28±9.16	67.90±15.47*
TICA-L-Vd	50.46±7.22	47.85±12.17
MCA-R-Vs	117.05±13.87	98.15±17.60**
MCA-R-Vm	78.97±10.24	68.62±12.39**
MCA-R-Vd	52.95±7.46	47.87±10.15*
MCA-L-Vs	114.59±12.94	98.10±20.17**
MCA-L-Vm	77.31±9.51	68.72±14.69**
MCA-L-Vd	51.72±7.70	48.46±11.41
VA-R-Vs	71.85±10.06	61.87±11.68**
VA-R-Vm	48.49±6.55	43.87±8.42**
VA-R-Vd	32.62±4.42	30.64±6.82
VA-L-Vs	72.59±8.93	62.79±10.77**
VA-L-Vm	49.67±6.04	45.08±7.56**
VA-L-Vd	33.49±4.18	32.08±5.56
BA-Vs	71.85±10.06	67.82±11.68**
BA-Vm	52.59±6.57	48.21±9.06*
BA-Vd	35.38±4.97	34.12±7.23

Note: compared to the control group, *P<0.05, **P<0.01.
rCBFV: regional cerebral blood flow velocity.
MCA: middle cerebral artery, ACA: anterior cerebral artery.
PCA: posterior cerebral artery, TICA: the tip of internal carotid artery.
VA: vertebral artery, BA: basilar artery, L: Left, R: Right,
Vs: systolic peak velocity, Vm: mean flow velocity, Vd: diastolic velocity.

Table 5. The comparison of the values of PI between control and depression groups (Mean±SEM).

Items	Control (n=41)	Depression(n=39)
ACA-R	0.89±0.10	0.80±0.18*
ACA-L	0.86±0.79	0.78±0.15*
TICA-R	0.88±0.08	0.76±0.12**
TICA-L	0.87±0.09	0.75±0.12**
MCA-R	0.82±0.08	0.74±0.11*
MCA-L	0.82±0.09	0.73±0.11*
VA-R	0.83±0.11	0.72±0.10**
VA-L	0.79±0.09	0.68±0.09**
BA	0.77±0.10	0.70±0.11*

Note: Compared with control group *P<0.05, ** P<0.01.
PI: Pulsatility index, ACA: anterior cerebral artery,
TICA: the tip of internal carotid artery, MCA: middle cerebral artery,
VA: vertebral artery, BA: basilar artery, L: Left, R: Right.

HAMD24 score <20 and Hamilton Anxiety score <8, and had no history of depression, anxiety or somatic disorders.

Ethics statement and consent

The study was approved by the Ethics of Human Investigation Committee at Guiyang Medical University (NO: 20090016) and all experiments were performed in accordance with relevant guidelines and regulations. The participants themselves or a legally authorized representative gave written informed consent to participate in the study and obtained safeguards in this study. The procedures followed were in accordance with the revised Declaration of Helsinki [23].

Hemorheologic measures

All subjects had 3 ml of venous blood collected in the early morning (07:00–08:00) to assess blood rheology parameters (blood viscosity and hemoconcentration). Heparin was used as an anticoagulant; whole blood viscosity (including high\middle\low shear rates), hematocrit (HCT) and red blood cell sedimentation were checked [24] by an automatic blood rheometer (LBY-N6B, Beijing Precil Instrument Co. Ltd.).

TCD screening methods

In a quiescent condition, all participants were assessed using the 2 MHz probe transcranial color-coded Doppler (TCD) sonography (Germany, DWL-X type), in accordance with Hua-Yang TCD ultrasound practices and diagnostic criteria guidelines [25]. The middle cerebral artery (MCA) and the anterior cerebral artery (ACA) were insonated through the temporal bone acoustic windows while the participant was in the conventional supine position. The vertebral artery (VA) and basilar artery (BA) were insonated through the occipital acoustic window while the participant was in the sitting position. Data were generated via the trace envelope of the measured arterial spectrum and a series

Table 6. The comparison of rCBF between control and depression groups (Mean ±SEM, ml·min-1·100 g-1, n=8).

Items	Control	Depression
ACA-R-GM	46.11±12.41	36.96±10.20*
ACA-L-GM	44.72±10.95	36.45±11.67*
ACA-R-WM	23.74±6.74	20.20±5.71*
ACA-L-WM	25.21±6.63	21.67±6.68*
MCA-R-GM	49.63±10.78	44.09±12.76*
MCA-L-GM	49.71±15.61	41.19±13.77**
MCA-R-WM	25.05±6.94	21.97±5.71
MCA-L-WM	26.17±6.91	22.52±5.75*
PCA-R-GM	46.63±10.06	39.02±10.92*
PCA-L-GM	45.76±11.91	34.32±12.21**
PCA-R-WM	27.73±11.44	24.73±8.61
PCA-L-WM	28.33±10.85	25.65±8.45

Note: Compared with control group * P<0.05, ** P<0.01.
rCBF: regional cerebral blood flow, ACA: anterior.
cerebral artery, MCA: middle cerebral artery.
PCA: posterior cerebral artery, L: Left, R: Right.
GM: gray matter, WM: white matter.

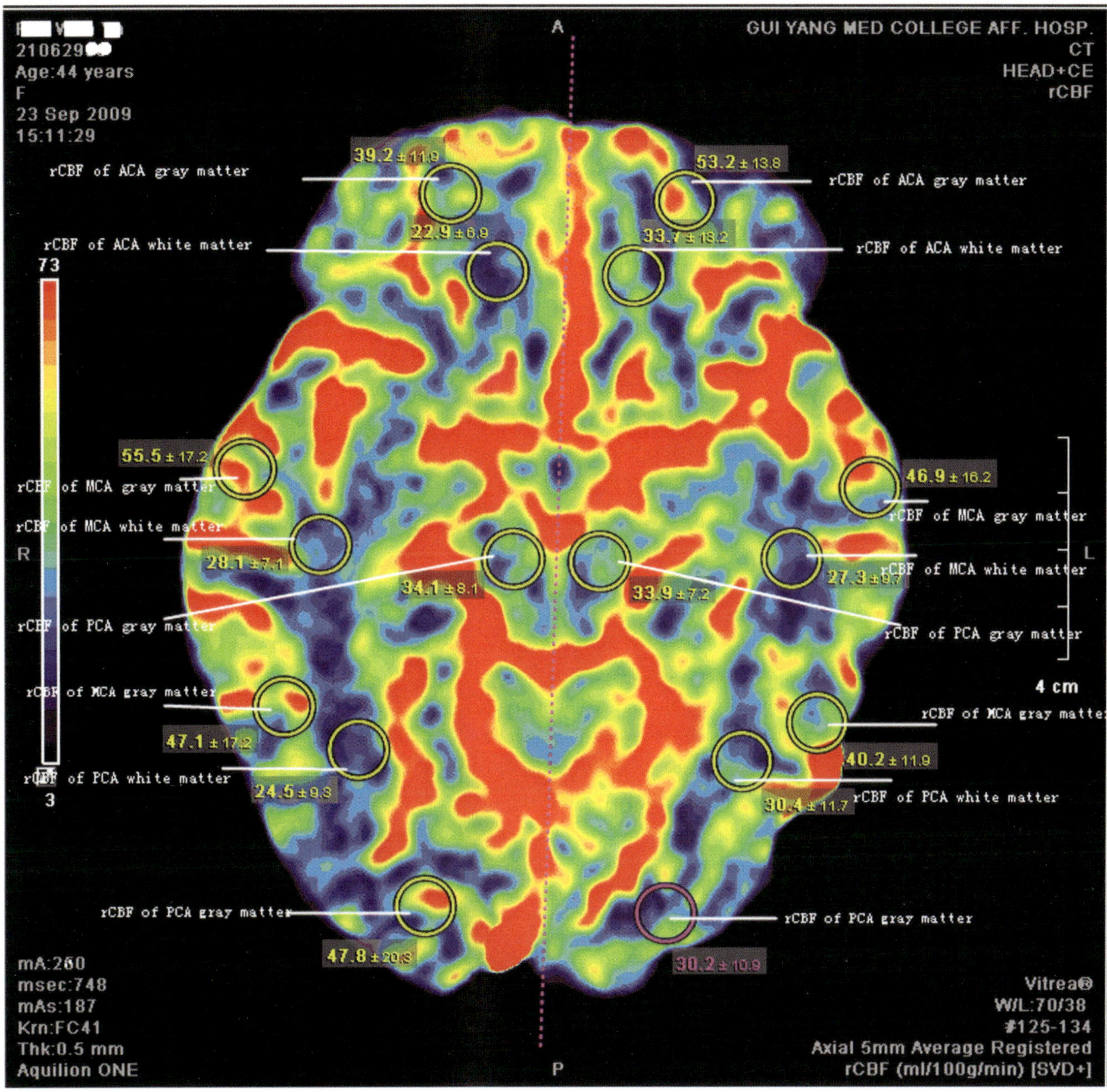

Figure 1. Case example: Coronal slices from dynamic CT angiography taken from a 44-year-old woman with depression. Circles represent regions of interest, with the mean ± SEM from 19 volume data presented. In MCA (middle cerebral artery) regions, the values of rCBF (regional cerebral blood flow) in left gray matter were lower than in the right [Left: 46.9 and 40.2 ml/(min·100 g),Right: 55.5 and 47.1 ml/(min·100 g)]. In PCA (posterior cerebral artery) regions, the values of rCBF in left gray matter were lower than in the right [Left: 30.2 ml/(min·100 g), Right: 47.8 ml/(min·100 g)].

of blood flow parameter values by the machine's software analyzer system. The Pulsatility Index (PI) was calculated as PI = (peak systolic velocity–end diastolic velocity)/mean blood flow velocity.

rCBF measurement methods

Sixteen subjects (8 = depressed, 1 men and 7 women, mean ages 43.12±12.09; 8 = healthy, 1 men and 7 women, mean ages 44.13±10.37) were randomly selected to undergo rCBF assessment using the 320 slice CT [26] (Japan's Toshiba Aquilion ONE; non-helical scan mode, 912-channel, 16 cm coverage, lap rotation time 0.5 s, slice thickness 0.5 mm, vision 240 mm), After iodine allergy testing, participants were asked to lie in the supine position, where a 20 th catheter tube was placed in the cubital vein before the scan. A plastic tube was connected to the Empower 9900P type binocular high-pressure syringe, and participants were injected with a nonionic contrast agent (iodine Pa Alcohol Injection 37 g(I)/100 ml/bottle, Shanghai Bracco Xinyi Pharmaceutical Co. Ltd.). 50 ml and 20 ml saline was administered intravenously in the cubital fossa with an injection rate of 6 ml/s. Scan parameters were as follows: 80 kv, 100 mA. Next, brain volumes were acquired after the injection of contrast medium, scan parameters as follows: 120 kv, 200 mA, dynamic volume scanning

Table 7. The comparison of rCBF between the left and right cerebral hemispheres in depression group (Mean ±SEM, ml·min-1·100 g-1, n=8).

Items	Left	Right
ACA -GM	36.45±11.67	36.96±10.20
ACA -WM	21.67±6.67	20.21±5.71
MCA-GM	41.49±13.77*	44.09±12.77
MCA-WM	22.52±5.75	21.97±5.71
PCA-GM	34.32±12.21*	39.02±10.92
PCA-WM	25.64±8.45	24.73±8.61

Note: Compared with Right * P<0.05.
rCBF: region cerebral blood flow, ACA: anterior cerebral artery.
MCA: middle cerebral artery, PCA: posterior cerebral artery.
L: Left, R: Right, GM: gray matter, WM: white matter.

was delayed 5 s. The time series was as follows: volume scanning was delayed 7 s, during scan across the artery was 11 s, the scan interval was 1 s, 35 s to 60 s venous and delayed scans, during every other scan interval was 5 s. A total of 19 volume data were obtained, each consisting of 320 images. Each inspection obtained a total of 6080 images (each volume data =0.5 min, total time =9.5 min). Concordant with the national standard, the total radiation dose of CT plain scan and perfusion scan was approximately 4.6 mSv.

Perfusion image analysis methods

Nineteen volume data were imported into the perfusion fx special package for processing. The right ACA was selected as the input artery and superior sagittal sinus as an output vein. The time-density curves of the dynamic region of interest were automatically analyzed by the software. Perfusion parameters, including cerebral blood volume (CBV), CBF, mean transit time (MTT) and the time to peak (TTP), were generated using the deconvolution mathematical model. The CBV, CBF, MTT, TTP of CT perfusion images in the cross-section, sagittal and coronal plane in the whole brain were obtained by the computer pseudo-color processing. The specific hemodynamic portion of the brain in depression was obtained by drawing various regions of interests (ROIs) encompassing the regions of gray and white matter which were perfused by blood supply at every level of the ACA, MCA, and PCA, and then comparing them with the ROIs of the normal brain. The ROIs (100±5 Pix) were distributed in gray and white matter of regions of blood supply at every level of the ACA, MCA and PCA.

Statistical analyses

Data were analyzed using SPSS Version 22.0. All measurement indicators were expressed as Means ± SEM with independent samples t-tests used to determine significant differences between the depression and control groups, where $P<0.05$ was considered statistically significant. Differences among groups were analyzed using one-way ANOVA. Stepwise linear regression was conducted to calculate the regression equation. A series of Pearson's correlations were undertaken to observe the strength and direction of the relationship between rCBF and rCBFV parameters. 95% confidence intervals were used in the study.

Results

Demographic features

No significant differences between the control and depression groups were observed for demographic variables (age, sex, blood pressure, smoking), (Table 1, 2).

Comparison of hematological parameters between the depression and control groups

Compared with the control group, whole blood viscosity (including high\middle\low shear rate) and hematocrit were significantly increased in those with depression, however no significant difference was observed between the groups for red blood cell sedimentation (Table 3).

Comparison of parameters of rCBFV between the depression and control groups

Compared with the control group, selected rCBFV parameters in the majority of cerebral arteries were decreased for those with depressive disorder (Table 4). For example, peak systolic flow velocity (Vs) and mean flow velocity (Vm) in bilateral ACA and MCA regions, and in TICA, VA and BA regions were statistically different. Further, statistically significant between group-differences showing decreased end-diastolic flow velocity (Vd) in the left ACA and the right TICA were observed. PI values were significantly lower for the depressed group in all the cerebral artery regions when compared with the control group (Table 5).

Comparison of rCBF between the depression and control group

Compared with the control group, the values of rCBF in bilateral gray and white matter of the cerebral hemispheres were lower for those with a depressive disorder; with the exception of white matter in the left and right PCA region and white matter of the right MCA region (Table 6).

Comparison of rCBF between left and right cerebral hemisphere in depression

Compared with the right cerebral hemisphere, rCBF values in left gray matter in MCA and PCA regions were significantly lower in those with depressive disorder (Table 7, Figure 1).

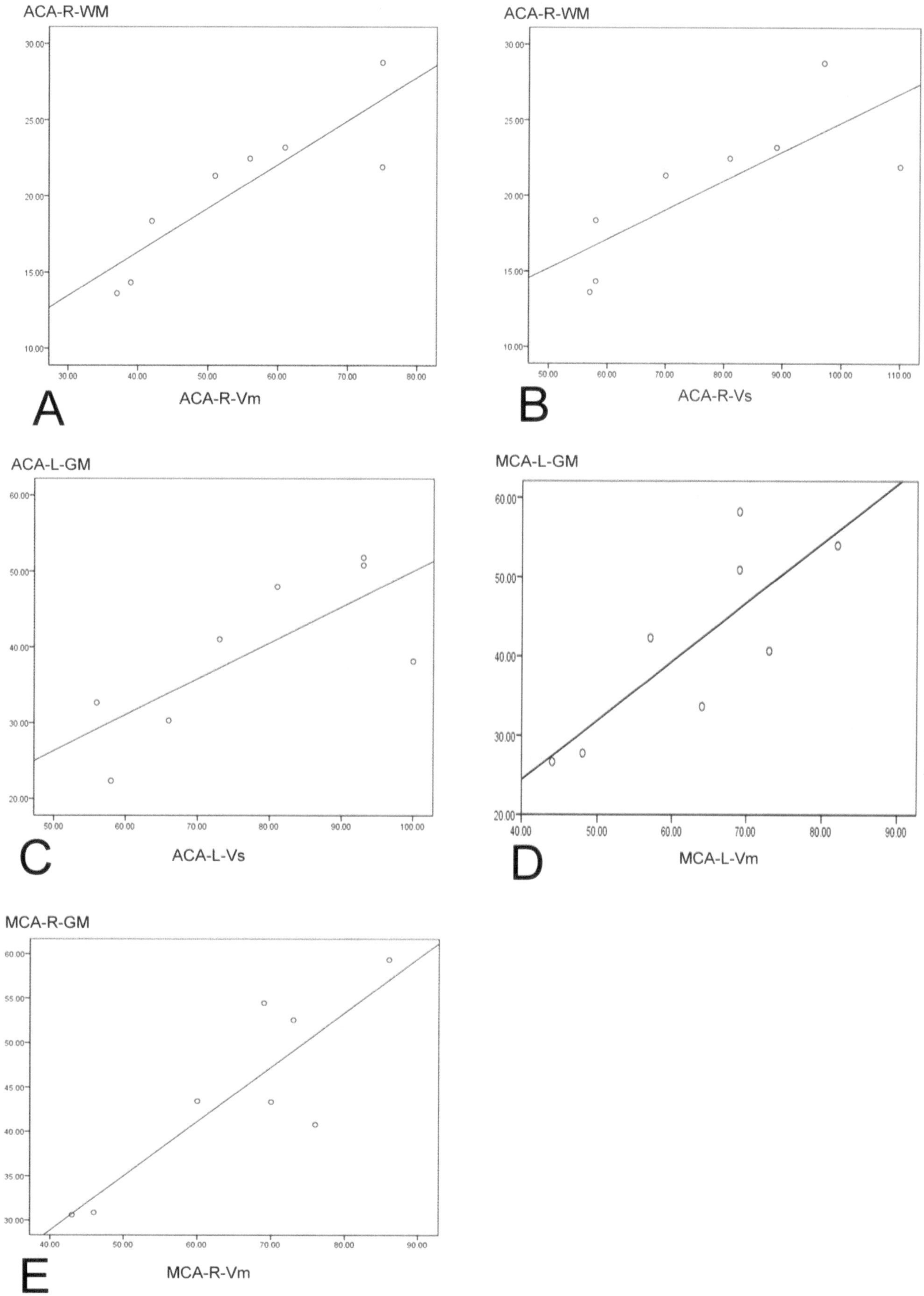
ACA-R-WM
30.00
25.00
20.00
15.00
10.00
30.00
40.00
50.00
60.00
70.00
80.00
A
ACA-R-Vm
ACA-R-WM
30.00
25.00
20.00
15.00
10.00
50.00
60.00
70.00
80.00
90.00
100.00
110.00
B
ACA-R-Vs
ACA-L-GM
60.00
50.00
40.00
30.00
20.00
50.00
60.00
70.00
80.00
90.00
100.00
C
ACA-L-Vs
MCA-L-GM
60.00
50.00
40.00
30.00
20.00
40.00
50.00
60.00
70.00
80.00
90.00
D
MCA-L-Vm
MCA-R-GM
60.00
55.00
50.00
45.00
40.00
35.00
30.00
40.00
50.00
60.00
70.00
80.00
90.00
E
MCA-R-Vm

Figure 2. The correlation between rCBFV and rCBF in cerebral artery regions. A: A positive correlation between mean flow velocity (Vm) and rCBF in white matter (WM) of right ACA (anterior cerebral artery) (P<0.01; r = 0.874). B: A positive correlation between systolic peak velocity (Vs) and rCBF in WM of right ACA (P<0.01; r = 0.778). C: A positive correlation between Vs and rCBF in gray matter (GM) of left ACA (P<0.05; r = 0.758). D: A positive correlation between Vm and rCBF in GM of left MCA (middle cerebral artery) (P<0.05; r = 0.802). E: A positive correlation between Vm and rCBF in GM of right MCA (P<0.01; r = 0.859). rCBFV: regional cerebral blood flow velocity, rCBF: region cerebral blood flow.

The relationship between rCBF and rCBFV in MDD group

When exploring the strength and direction of the association between rCBF and rCBFV in the MDD group, we found a positive correlation for gray matter of the bilateral ACA and MCA regions, except for the right ACA (Vs, Vm, Vd) and left ACA (Vd); and in white matter of the right ACA (Vs, Vm, Vd) and right MCA (Vm). The strongest correlation coefficients were produced for right ACA (Vm r = 0.874, Vd r = 0.839 for white matter) and right MCA Vm (r = 0.859 for gray matter), left MCA (Vs r = 0.760, Vm r = 0.802, Vd r = 0.748 for gray matter). Overall, the strength of the relationships were most consistent for gray matter. The correlation coefficients are displayed in Table 8, the regression equation between rCBFV and rCBF in Table 9 and illustrated in Figures 2.

Discussion

For the first time to our knowledge, we have provided data on the potential utility and novel application of the 320 slice Dynamic volumes CT in a clinically depressed population, a tool validated in coronary and stroke populations. These data demonstrate that patients with depression are characterized by a wide range of CBF impairments, in particular prominent changes in gray matter, when compared with healthy controls. rCBF data generated using this technology in a sub-sample of MDD patients was shown to correlate well with those generated by other measures (TCD ultrasound), suggesting that it could be employed in psychiatric settings for potential diagnostic and treatment response purposes.

Previous studies have suggested reduced rCBF in MDD, illustrated by hypoperfusion in the frontal lobe, temporal lobe, and in the limbic system [27–28]. Indeed, our results are consistent with other functional imaging studies conducted in this area using SPECT imaging [29,12] and a range of other techniques. As these techniques are often hampered by limitations including accessibility, poor resolution and subjectivity, this study provides some support for the use of CT perfusion imaging for rapid imaging and assessment to determine the CBF dynamics quickly, accurately and in 3 dimensional high resolution in a psychiatric setting [30–31]. The resulting image aligns with real data [32]. Therefore, the use of 320-slice CT for the objective study of cerebral perfusion appears to have clinical value potentially supplanting older techniques.

We found that there was decreased rCBFV in the majority of cerebral arteries in depressive patients, for example, Vs and Vm differed in the bilateral ACA, CA, TICA, VA and BA regions, while Vd differed in the left ACA and right TICA regions. Furthermore, in patients with depression, there was a positive relationship between the rCBFV and the corresponding vascular rCBF in the gray matter of bilateral ACA and MCA regions (with the exception of right ACA (Vs, Vm, Vd) and left ACA (Vd)), and the white matter of the right ACA (Vs, Vm, Vd) and MCA (Vm) regions. We also demonstrated that the rCBF values of left gray matter in MCA and PCA regions were lower than that of right in those with depressive disorder. Hardoy's results [33], in MDD showing hypoperfusion in the left frontal and temporal areas and perfusion asymmetry, was consistent with the findings in our cohort.

A reduction in blood flow could be due to either functional or structural deficiencies. TCD PI reflects cerebrovascular resistance by the flow velocity waveform [34]. Kwater et al. [35] reported a strong association between higher PI and systemic arterial stiffness in patients with atherosclerosis, however atherosclerosis reduces cerebrovascular reactivity, leading to higher PI values. In our study, however, PI was decreased in the depressive group compared with controls, suggesting that the reason for the reduced

Table 8. The correlation coefficients between rCBF and rCBFV in depression group (n = 8).

rCBFV items	rCBF of Gray matter	rCBF of White matter
ACA-R-Vs	0.599	0.778*
ACA-R-Vm	0.674	0.874**
ACA-R-Vd	0.624	0.839**
ACA-L-Vs	0.758*	0.607
ACA-L-Vm	0.720*	0.568
ACA-L-Vd	0.575	0.569
MCA-R-Vs	0.706*	0.520
MCA-R-Vm	0.859**	0.718*
MCA-R-Vd	0.748*	0.683
MCA-L-Vs	0.760**	0.426
MCA-L-Vm	0.802**	0.535
MCA-L-Vd	0.748**	0.538

Note: The correlation coefficient t test * P<0.05. ** P<0.01.
rCBFV: regional cerebral blood flow velocity, rCBF: region cerebral blood flow.
ACA: anterior cerebral artery, MCA: middle cerebral artery, L: Left, R: Right.
Vs: systolic peak velocity, Vm: mean flow velocity, Vd: diastolic velocity.

Table 9. Regression equation between rCBFV and rCBF in depression group (n = 8).

Regression equation	*P* value
ACA-L-GM-rCBF = 2.636+0.474(ACA-L-Vs)	0.029
ACA-R-WM-rCBF = 4.852+0.287(ACA-R-Vm)	0.005
ACA-R-WM-rCBF = 7.831+0.86(ACA-R-Vm)-0.441(ACA-R-Vs)	0.003
MCA-L-GM-rCBF = 0.745(MCA-L-Vm)-5.333	0.017
MCA-R-GM-rCBF = 4.420+0.612(MCA-R-Vm)	0.006

rCBFV: regional cerebral blood flow velocity, rCBF: region cerebral blood flow.
ACA: anterior cerebral artery, MCA: middle cerebral artery, L: Left, R: Right.
GM: gray matter, WM: white matter, Vs: systolic peak velocity, Vm: mean flow velocity.

blood flow in the depressive group may be functional rather than structural.

We also observed that the whole blood viscosity and hematocrit were significantly increased in the depressed patients. Blood viscosity is a measure of the thickness and stickiness of blood, and increased levels of blood viscosity has been associated with arterial disease including myocardial infarction and stroke [36–37]. It has been suggested that stress is associated with hemoconcentration of the cerebral hemispheres in patients with MDD [38]. Lechin [39] argued that blood viscosity is positively involved with the levels of neural sympathetic and cholinergic activity in MDD, while Wong et at. found that decreased blood viscosity is correlated with the improvement of depressive symptoms after antidepressant treatment in MDD.

There is evidence of significant hypoperfusion in the gray matter of the cerebral hemispheres in people with depression [40]. The reason for this may be concordant with the proximal relationship between the dominant hemisphere cortex and human cognition, emotion and related functions, while its relationship to deep white matter appears more peripheral. Botteron [41] reported that elderly depressed people with memory impairment showed changes in the medial temporal lobe and its adjacent structures.

Su liang et al [42] proposed that elderly depressive patients with cognitive impairment exhibited decreased local glucose metabolism in the caudate nucleus bilaterally, the inferior frontal gyrus, left cingulate and anterior central gyrus regions, and the decline in both executive function and memory function was related to low local glucose metabolism in the caudate nucleus bilaterally, the frontal lobe, temporal lobe, the left central gyrus and limbic brain regions of deep white matter. Indeed, our results were concordant with this study.

Limitations of both the technique and of the study

The specific hemodynamic regions of the brain in depression was obtained by drawing various regions of interests encompassing the regions of gray and white matter which were perfused by ACA, MCA, and PCA blood supply, and then comparing them with the ROIs of the normal brain. This captured representative regional cerebral blood flow, but not the actual value of the lobes of the brain. Secondly, because relatively few subjects had rCBF assessment, this could result in possible bias. While changes in rCBF were seen, potential clinical applications require further study. Lastly a multivariate ANOVA analysis testing multiple correlations was not performed, and differences between groups were analyzed using one-way ANOVA.

Conclusions

These data suggest that people with depression are characterized by a wide range of cerebral blood flow impairments and there appear to be more prominent changes in left gray matter. The 320 slice Dynamic volumes CT appears to be a potentially useful tool for measuring rCBF, with advantages over existing instruments. This technique could be employed in psychiatric settings for biomarker, diagnostic and treatment response purposes. Future studies should replicate this study in a larger sample, acquiring additional data to determine the factors influencing blood supply to the region of the brain of patients affected in those with depression. The relationship to treatment response in particular needs to be explored.

Acknowledgments

The manuscript is original, Data has not previously published, including in an abstract or poster, the figures, tables, and/or data that haven't been published elsewhere, and are also not under concurrent consideration elsewhere. The authors YW, HZ, ST, FC, AO, AT, XL, MB have personally reviewed and given final approval of the version submitted, and all authors have declared that there are no biomedical financial interest or potential conflicts of interest.

Author Contributions

Conceived and designed the experiments: YW XL ST. Performed the experiments: ST FC FC. Analyzed the data: YW ST FC FC. Contributed reagents/materials/analysis tools: YW ST MB. Wrote the paper: YW HZ ST FC AO AT XL FC MB.

References

1. Taylor WD, Aizenstein HJ, Alexopoulos GS (2013) The vascular depression hypothesis: mechanisms linking vascular disease with depression. Mol Psychiatry. 18: 964–974.
2. Oda K, Okubo Y, Ishida R, Murata Y, Ohta K, et al. (2003) Regional cerebral blood flow in depressed patients with white matter magnetic resonance hyperintensity. Biol Psychiatry 53: 150–156.
3. Kume K, Hanyu H, Murakami M, Sato T, Hirao K, et al. (2011) Frontal Assessment Battery and brain perfusion images in amnestic mild cognitive impairment. Geriatr Gerontol Int. 11: 77–82.
4. Aihua N, Yanzhu B, Chunying J, Shumiao G, Xiufen W (2007) Study of Regional Cerebral Blood Flow in the Patients with Depression Treated by Cognitive Behavioral Therapy or Citalopram. Chin Gen Prac (Chin) 10: 1944–1945.
5. Takano H, Kato M, Inagaki A, Watanabe K, Kashima H (2006) Time course of cerebral blood flow changes following electroconvulsive therapy in depressive patients measured at 3 time points using single photon emission computed tomography. Keio J Med 55: 153–160.
6. Hroudová J, Fišar Z, Kitzlerová E, Zvěřová M, Raboch J (2013) Mitochondrial respiration in blood platelets of depressive patients. Mitochondrion 13: 795–800.

7. Manji H, Kato T, Di Prospero NA, Ness S, Beal MF, et al. (2012) Impaired mitochondrial function in psychiatric disorders. Nat Rev Neurosci 13: 293–307.
8. Sacher J, Neumann J, Fünfstück T, Soliman A, Villringer A, et al. (2012) Mapping the depressed brain: a meta-analysis of structural and functional alterations in major depressive disorder. J Affect Disord 140: 142–148.
9. Kessler H, Taubner S, Buchheim A, Münte TF, Stasch M, et al. (2011) Individualized and Clinically Derived Stimuli Activate Limbic Structures in Depression: An fMRI Study. PLoS One 6: e15712.
10. Awata S, Ito H, Konno M, Ono S, Kawashima R, et al. (1998) Regional cerebral blood flow abnormalities in late-life depression: relation to refractoriness and chronification. Psychiatry Clin Neurosci 52: 97–105.
11. Ishizaki J, Yamamoto H, Takahashi T, Takeda M, Yano M, et al. (2008) Changes in regional cerebral blood flow following antidepressant treatment in late-life depression. Int J Geriatr Psychiatry 23: 805–811.
12. Navarro V, Gastó C, Lomeña F, Mateos JJ, Marcos T (2001) Frontal cerebral perfusion dysfunction in elderly late-onset major depression assessed by 99MTC-HMPAO SPECT. Neuroimage 14: 202–205.
13. Nobler MS, Roose SP, Prohovnik I, Moeller JR, Louie J, et al. (2000) Sackeim HA. Regional cerebral blood flow in mood disorders, V: Effects of antidepressant medication in late-life depression. Am J Geriatr Psychiatry 8: 289–296.
14. Davies J, Lloyd KR, Jones IK, Barnes A, Pilowsky LS (2003) Changes in regional cerebral blood flow With Venlafaxine in the Treatment of Major Depression. Am J Psychiatry 160: 374–376.
15. Milo TJ, Kaufman GE, Barnes WE, Konopka LM, Crayton JW, et al. (2001) Changes in RCBF After Electroconvulsive Therapy for Depression. J ECT 17: 15–21.
16. Colloby SJ, Firbank MJ, He J, Thomas AJ, Vasudev A, et al. (2012) Regional cerebral blood flow in late-life depression: arterial spin labelling magnetic resonance study. Br J Psychiatry 200: 150–155.
17. Post RM, DeLisi LE, Holcomb HH, Uhde TW, Cohen R, et al. (1987) Glucose utilization in the temporal cortex of affectively ill patients: positron emission tomography. Biol Psychiatry 22: 545–553.
18. Smith GS, Kramer E, Ma Y, Kingsley P, Dhawan V, et al (2009) The functional neuroanatomy of geriatric depression. Int J Geriatr Psychiatry 24: 798–808.
19. Coolens C, Breen S, Purdie TG, Owrangi A, Publicover J, et al. (2009) Implementation and characterization of a 320-slice volumetric CT scanner for simulation in radiation oncology. Med Phys 36: 5120–5127.
20. Evangelista A, Pelliccia F, Arrivi A, Gaudio C (2011) Images in 320-slice CT and myocardial bridge. BMJ Case Rep doi:10.1136/bcr.05.2011.4200
21. Song ZJ, Chen GF, Lin Jia CY, Cao JX, Ao GK (2013) The ultra-early protective effect of ulinastatin on rabbit acute lung injury induced by paraquat. BMC Emerg Med. (suppl 1): S7.
22. Shankar JJ, Lum C (2011) Whole brain CT perfusion on a 320-slice CT scanner. Indian J Radiol Imaging 21: 209–214.
23. Rickham PP (1964) Human Experimentation: code of ethics of the World Medical Association. Br Med J 18, 2: 177.
24. Baskurt OK, Boynard M, Cokelet GC, Connes P, Cooke BM, et al. (2009) New guidelines for hemorheological laboratory techniques. Clin Hemorheol Microcirc 42: 75–97.
25. Guideline developed in conjunction with the American College of Radiology (ACR), the Society for Pediatric Radiology (SPR), and the Society of Radiologists in Ultrasound (SRU) (2012) AIUM Practice Guideline for the Performance of a Transcranial Doppler Ultrasound Examination for Adults and Children, 2 th ed. American Institute of Ultrasound in Medicine Press.
26. Siebert E, Bohner G, Dewey M, Masuhr F, Hoffmann KT, et al. (2009) 320-slice CT neuroimaging: initial clinical experience and image quality evaluation. Br J Radiol. 82: 561–70.
27. Vangu MDT, Esser JD, Boyd IH, Berk M (2003) Effects of electroconvulsive therapy on regional cerebral blood flow measured by 99mtechnetium HMPAO SPECT. Progr Neuro-Psychoph 27: 15–19.
28. Kawakatsu S, Komatani A (1994) Xe-133 inhalation single photon emission computerized tomography in manic-depressive illness. Nippon Rinsho 52: 1180–1184.
29. Brockmann H, Zobel A, Joe A, Biermann K, Scheef L, et al. (2009) The value of HMPAO SPECT in predicting treatment response to citalopram in patients with major depression. Psychiatry Res 173: 107–112.
30. Cenic A, Nabavi DG, Craen RA, Gelb AW, Lee TY (1999) Dynamic CT measurement of cerebral blood flow: A validation study. AJNR Am J Neuroradiol 20: 63–73.
31. Koenig M, Kraus M, Theek C, Klotz E, Gehlen W, et al. (2001) Quantitative assessment of the ischemic brain by means of perfusion-related parameters derived from perfusion CT. Stroke 32: 431–437.
32. Cody DD, Mahesh M (2007) AAPM/RSNA physics tutorial for residents: technologic advances in multidetector CT with a focus on cardiac imaging. RadioGraphics 27: 1829–1837.
33. Hardoy MC, Cadeddu M, Serra A, Moro MF, Mura G, et al. (2011) A pattern of cerebral perfusion anomalies between major depressive disorder and Hashimoto thyroiditis. BMC Psychiatry 11: 148.
34. Gosling RG, King DH (1974) Arterial assessment by Doppler shift ultrasound. Proc R Soc Med 67: 447–449.
35. Kwater A, Gsowski J, Gryglewska B, Wizner B, Grodzicki T (2009) Is blood flow in the middle cerebral artery determined by systemic arterial stiffness? Blood Pressure 18: 130–134.
36. Lowe GD (1986) Blood rheology in arterial disease. Clin Sci 71: 137–146.
37. Jan KM, Chien S, Bigger JT Jr (1975) Observations on blood viscosity changes after acute myocardial infarction. Circulation 51: 1079–1084.
38. Wong ML, Dong C, Esposito K, Thakur S, Liu W, et al. (2008) Elevated stress-hemoconcentration in major depression is normalized by antidepressant treatment: secondary analysis from a randomized, double-blind clinical trial and relevance to cardiovascular disease risk. PLoS One 3: e2350-2355. http://dx.doi.org/doi:10.1080/08037050902975114.
39. Lechin F, van der Dijs B, Orozco B, Lechin ME, Báez S, et al. (1995) Plasma neurotransmitters, blood pressure, and heart rate during supine-resting, orthostasis, and moderate exercise conditions in major depressed patients. Biol Psychiatry 38: 166–173.
40. Orosz A, Jann K, Federspiel A, Horn H, Höfle O, et al. (2012) Reduced cerebral blood flow within the default-mode network and within total gray matter in major depression. Brain Connect 2: 303–310.
41. Botteron KN, Raichle ME, Drevets WC, Heath AC, Todd RD (2002) Volumetric reduction in left subgenual prefrontal cortex in early onset depression. Biol Psychiatry 51: 342–344.
42. Liang S. Shenxun S, Yihui G, Chuantao Z, Mingyuan Z (2006) Depression in the elderly patients with brain positron emission tomography. Chin J Psychia 39: 81–84. http://dx.doi.org/doi:10.1080/08037050902975114.

8

Psychological Factors as Predictors of Suicidal Ideation among Adolescents

Norhayati Ibrahim, Noh Amit*, Melia Wong Yuin Suen

Faculty of Health Sciences, National University of Malaysia (UKM), Kuala Lumpur, Malaysia

Abstract

Background: There has been a drastic increase in the rate of suicides over the past 45 years in Malaysia. The statistics show that adolescents aged between 16 and 19 years old are at high risk of committing suicide. This could be attributed to issues relating to the developmental stage of adolescents. During this stage, adolescents face challenges and are exposed to various stressful experiences and risk factors relating to suicide.

Method: The present study examined psychological factors (i.e., depression, anxiety and stress) as predictors for suicidal ideation among adolescents. A cross-sectional study was conducted on 190 students (103 males and 87 females), aged 15 to 19 years old from two different schools in Kuala Lumpur. The Depression Anxiety Stress Scale 21-item version (DASS-21) was used to measure depression, anxiety and stress among the students, and the Beck Scale for Suicide Ideation (BSS) to measure suicidal ideation. The data were analysed using Pearson's correlation and multiple regression analysis.

Results: The results show that 11.10%, 10.00%, and 9.50% of the students reported that they were experiencing severe depression, anxiety and stress, respectively. There were significant correlations between depression, anxiety, and stress with suicidal ideation. However, only depression was identified as a predictor for suicidal ideation.

Conclusion: Hence, this study extends the role of depression in predicting suicidal ideation among adolescents in the Malaysian context. The findings imply that teenagers should be assisted in strengthening their positive coping strategies in managing distress to reduce depression and suicidal ideation.

Editor: Marianna Mazza, Catholic University of Sacred Heart of Rome, Italy

Funding: The authors have no support or funding to report.

Competing Interests: The authors have declared that no competing interests exist.

* Email: nohamit@ukm.edu.my

Introduction

Suicide can be considered as a 'silent enemy'. Although it is common to find that people do not admit to having suicidal thoughts, some of them have the potential to die by committing suicide. In fact, there is a common public misperception that only those who are diagnosed with depression are at risk of committing suicide. However, almost 40% of the people who commit complete suicide are not clinically depressed, which indicates that various psychological conditions could potentially increase the risk of suicide. These include post-traumatic stress disorder, eating disorders and bipolar disorder [1]. In 2010, suicide was found to be the tenth leading cause of death (38,364 people a year) in the United States of America [2]. In fact, 90% of the suicides are committed by people suffering from psychological disorders, 60% are associated with mood disorders, 25%–50%% are associated with alcohol use and abuse, and 10% are associated with borderline personality disorder [3].

In developing countries, there is a dearth of research on suicide and suicidal ideation. This could be attributed to the taboo related to suicide. For instance, in Malaysia, committing suicide is a taboo and the topic is not openly discussed. In recent years, the suicide rate has increased and appears to be an emerging social problem in Malaysia. Indeed, statistics show that the suicidal rate has increased by 60% over the past 45 years and it is estimated that 140 people attempt suicide daily [4]. The Malaysian Psychiatric Association estimated that seven people, who mostly comprise youth and young adults, are killing themselves daily [5]. This is indeed a shocking statistic. It implies that within 24 hours, seven lives are lost due to suicide.

According to the National Health and Morbidity Survey conducted by the Ministry of Health Malaysia [6], 6.3% of the participants reported having suicide ideation. In this survey, it was found that the youngest aged group – 16 to 19 years old – was most disposed to suicidal thoughts followed by the 20 to 24 years age group. The findings also showed that females reported higher suicidal ideation. However, there was no difference between the urban and rural population concerning suicidal ideation [5], [6]. In addition, the National Suicide Registry Malaysia (NSRM) estimated that between January and August 2010, a total of 425 people had committed suicide [7]. In addition, a local study by Tam et al. [8] reported that there were 445 suicide cases in Malaysia for the first eight months of 2010 compared to 290 cases in 2008. These figures were only based on legal cases or cases reported to the police, indicating that there are still many unreported cases. Therefore, it is important to examine the nature and extent of suicidal ideation in the Malaysian context.

There are various risk and protective factors associated with suicide and suicidal ideation among young people [9]. For instance, Gutierrez and Osman [9] classified the risk factors into individual risk factors and family risk factors, and protective factors into personal protective factors and environmental protective factors. However, notwithstanding the above factors, the psychological related factors play an important role in understanding the psychological wellbeing of those who have the potential to be involved in suicide and suicidal ideation; and, understanding these factors, helps to determine the tendency of young people to engage in suicidal ideation and suicide-related behaviour [10].

Some of the major psychological factors associated with suicidal ideation are depression, anxiety, and stress. Most of the findings on the relationship between psychological factors and suicide as well as suicidal ideation are based on the evidence of the psychological autopsy conducted among those who have committed suicide [11]. Depression is one of the important psychological factors related to suicide and suicidal ideation. Evidence from the psychological autopsy showed that, at the time of suicide or attempted suicide, some people were suffering from depression [11]. Furthermore, research conducted in a clinical setting, which was based on clinical screening of approximately 1000 patients in a cardiology clinic for depression and suicidality, showed that 109 patients (12%) expressed suicidal ideation [12]. Research also indicated that depression is positively associated with suicidal ideation [13], [14], [15]. The depression could be attributed to individuals' feelings of hopelessness, helplessness, and a lack of social support and coping skills when they face difficulties and stressful life experiences.

Another common risk factor for suicidal ideation is anxiety. Anxiety is one of the most common psychiatric illnesses seen in general practice [16]. Although anxiety is found to be positively associated with suicidal ideation, the relationship between anxiety and suicidal ideation is inconclusive [17]. This is because anxiety may elicit symptoms of depression and may also lead to suicidal thoughts [18]. In a meta-analysis, Kanwar et al. [17] examined the relationship between anxiety and suicidal ideation. They found that patients with anxiety were more likely to have suicidal ideation, attempted suicide, and completed suicide compared to those without anxiety [17].

Stress is another risk factor for suicidal ideation, and research has indicated that stress is positively associated with suicidal ideation [19], [20]. In the literature concerning suicide, stress is commonly linked to negative life events and/or negative life experience. There are various work-and-life related stressors, such as stressful life events, loss, unemployment, and other environmental stressors, which could be associated with suicidal ideation [13], [20]. The interactions of various aspects of stressors have the potential to make stress management difficult and have the potential to lead to suicidal ideation [21]. Therefore, stress management requires the integration of a good quality of life, coping skills, and problem solving skills. The way a person copes with stress may indicate how much stress may affect their psychological well-being, how much stress may lead them to feeling a sense of hopelessness or of not being supported, and how they may define stress as a potential contributor to suicidal ideation.

Understanding the psychological factors is important for prevention and treatment in relation to suicide among young people in a specific cultural context. This is because by having a proper understanding about the risk of suicide among adolescents, an appropriate assessment process will facilitate the appropriate treatment being given to those who are at risk. This research has the potential to identify the proper support and psychological needs for those who are having suicidal ideation and at risk of suicide. Therefore, the aims of this study are, firstly, to examine the association between depression, anxiety, stress and suicidal ideation. Secondly, to examine the role of depression, anxiety, and stress in predicting suicidal ideation. In this research, we hypothesize that, firstly, there will be positive correlation between depression, anxiety, stress and suicidal ideation, and, secondly, depression will predict suicidal ideation.

Method

Ethical Approval

This study was approved by the Research Ethics Committee, National University of Malaysia (UKM) [Ethics Approval no: NN-064-2013].

Research Design

The research design was cross-sectional using the survey method. Each participant underwent two psychological tests and a demographic profile.

A total of 190 adolescents, consisting of 103 males and 87 females with an overall mean age of 16.04 (SD = 1.16), participated in this study. The participants were Form 3 to Form 6 students from two schools in Kuala Lumpur. The respondents had obtained parental (including caregivers, and guardians) consent prior to participating in this study. The random sampling method was adopted in this study.

The informed consent of the participants was obtained from parents, caregivers, and guardians on behalf of the minors/ children enrolled in this study. As the written informed consent forms were gathered, no verbal consent method was used in this study. The consent of the participants was recorded using informed consent forms distributed to parents, caregivers, and guardians of the participants. The consent procedure and informed consent form were approved by the Research Ethics Committee, National University of Malaysia (UKM).

Instruments

Two psychological instruments were used in this study – Depression Anxiety Stress Scale 21-item version (DASS-21), and the Beck Scale for Suicide Ideation (BSS).

Depression Anxiety Stress Scale 21-item version (DASS-21)

DASS-21 is a self-administered psychometric test that gauges the levels of depression, anxiety and stress in the previous week. It is applicable in a clinical or non-clinical setting. There are 21 items in DASS-21 with seven items for each variable measure. The scoring is from 0 to 3 whereby 0 – did not apply to me at all, 1 – applied to me to some degree or some of the time, 2 – applied to me to a considerable degree or a good part of the time, and 3 – applied to me very much or most of the time.

This test takes approximately 10 to 15 minutes to complete. DASS-21 is the most widely validated version of the DASS. Translation to the Malay language was conducted and its psychometric properties were proven [22]. The DASS-21 indicated an alpha coefficient of.74 to.84. The DASS-21 was further validated through factor analysis, which ranged from.39 to.73. The correlation among the scales was between.54 and.68.

Table 1. Demographic characteristics of the sample (N = 190).

Demographic Variable	Frequency	Percentage
Age		
Means	16.04	
SD	1.16	
Level of secondary education/form		
Form 3	71	37.40
Form 4	60	31.60
Form 5	43	22.60
Form 6	16	8.40
Religion		
Islam	14	7.40
Buddhism	113	59.50
Hinduism	18	9.50
Christianity	37	19.50
Others	6	3.20
Number of siblings		
1	18	9.50
2	61	32.10
3	72	37.90
4	26	13.70
5	5	2.60
6	4	2.10
10	1	0.50

Beck Scale for Suicide Ideation (BSS)

BSS is a 21-item self-administered test to detect and measure the severity of suicidal ideation in adults and adolescents. Both clinical and non-clinical settings are applicable for the usage of BSS. There are three statements under each item in which the intensity ranges from 0 to 2. Participants are asked to circle the statement that best describes their feelings in the past week including the day of administration. The minimum score is 0, while the maximum score is 42. [11].

BSS only takes 10 minutes to complete. It is considered to have good internal consistency at.90 and.87 using Cronbach's Alpha. According to Beck and Steer [23], it is proven that BSS has good content validity with the Suicide Scale of Ideation (SSI) and concurrent validity between SSI and BSS (r = .90).

Data Analysis

All the raw data were keyed into the SPSS 16.0 program (*Statistical Package for the Social Sciences version 16*) and analysed. Descriptive analysis was mainly used to describe the findings of the data, such as mean, standard deviation and percentage of the demographic data. In addition, inferential analysis was used to test the hypotheses developed. Pearson's correlation was used to test the relationship between the variables. The multiple regression procedure using the 'Enter step' was conducted to predict the influence of depression, anxiety and stress on the suicidal ideation of the students.

Results

Table 1 shows that all the students were aged between 15 and 19 years old (Form 3 to Form 6), with a mean age of 16.04, *SD* = 1.16. There were 71 students (37.40%) in Form 3, 60 students

Table 2. Frequency for the levels of depression, anxiety and stress.

Severity	Depression (%)	Anxiety (%)	Stress (%)
Normal	89 (46.80)	76 (40.00)	109 (57.40)
Mild	24 (12.60)	22 (11.60)	27 (14.20)
Moderate	41 (21.60)	40 (21.10)	20 (10.50)
Severe	21 (11.10)	19 (10.00)	18 (9.50)
Extremely Severe	8 (4.20)	23 (12.10)	2 (1.10)

Table 3. Correlation between depression, anxiety, stress and suicidal ideation.

	Suicidal Ideation
Depression	.56*
Anxiety	.42*
Stress	.47*

* $p<0.05$.

(31.60%) in Form 4, 43 students in Form 5 (22.60%) and 16 students (8.40%) in Form 6. In terms of the distribution of the students according to religion, there were 14 Muslims (7.40%), 18 Hindus (9.50%), 37 Christians (19.50%) and 113 Buddhists (59.50%) who formed the majority. Most of the participants reported having 2 to 3 siblings, which comprised 32.10% and 37.90%, respectively. Only one student reported having 10 siblings while the others had a number of siblings ranging from 1 to 6. In addition, the findings showed that only 16 students (8.4%) reported having a history of seeking psychological services while 17 students (8.9%) reported that their family members were previously or currently receiving ongoing psychological treatment.

Table 2 illustrates that the majority of the students scored within the normal range for depression, anxiety and stress, with 46.80%, 40.00% and 57.40%, respectively. There were 24 students (12.60%) who scored mild for depression, while 21 students (11.10%) were in severe depression. The second largest group of students, with 41 students (21.60%), fell in the moderate range of depression, whereas only 8 students (4.20%) fell in the extremely severe depression range. In brief, there was a high percentage of students who experienced moderate to extremely severe depression, although the majority of them (59.40%) were under the normal to mild range. The mean score for the depression scale was 10.98, *SD* = 9.11.

As for the anxiety scale, 22 students (11.60%) reported mild anxiety, while 23 students (12.10%) were found to be in the extremely severe anxiety region. Similar to the depression scale, 40 (21.10%) of the students fell in the moderate range, whereas only 19 students (10.00%) reported experiencing severe anxiety. The findings demonstrated that there was an almost equal distribution of students who were anxious as well as students who were less anxious. The mean score for the anxiety scale was 10.03, *SD* = 7.73.

The majority of the students reported no or mild stress with 109 students (57.40%) and 27 students (14.20%) for each level. There were 20 students (10.50%) who fell in the moderate range, whereas 18 students (9.50%) reported severe stress. Only two students (1.10%) reported extremely severe stress. Generally, most of the students were under the normal to mild stress level, which signified better stress management. The mean score for the stress scale was 13.88, *SD* = 7.94.

The results show that 128 students (67.40%) reported no suicidal ideation at all with a score of zero. Approximately 50 students (26.30%) scored 1 to 5 points indicating that, in total, more than two-thirds of the students (93.7%) had no significant suicidal ideation, while 12.6% scored more than 5 points, thereby indicating that they were at risk of suicide.

Table 3 shows that there were positive significant relationships between depression and suicidal ideation; anxiety with suicidal ideation; and stress with suicidal ideation. The results indicated that Pearson's coefficient of depression, anxiety and stress with suicidal ideation were r = .56, r = .42 and r = .47, respectively ($p<.05$). This means that high rates of depression, anxiety and stress result in higher suicidal ideation. These results support the first hypothesis concerning the positive relationship between depression, anxiety, stress and suicidal ideation in the present study.

The results in table 4 indicate that only one predictor, which was depression, explained a 32.60% of the variance [$R^2 = .33$, $F(3, 159) = 25.61$, $p<.05$]. It was found that only depression significantly predicted suicidal ideation ($\beta = .45$, $p<.05$). However, anxiety ($\beta = .08$, n.s.) and stress ($\beta = .08$, n.s.) were not significant predictors of suicidal ideation. These results support the second hypothesis in that depression is a significant predictor for suicidal ideation in the present study.

Discussion

The aims of this study are to examine the correlation between depression, anxiety, stress, and suicidal ideation, and to identify role of depression, anxiety, and stress in predicting suicidal ideation.

The findings show that there are moderate positive correlations between depression, anxiety, stress, and suicidal ideation. The results suggest that the respondents who reported high levels of depression tended to report high levels of suicidal ideation. This finding is consistent with other studies concerning the positive association between depression and suicidal ideation, as reported by Yen et al. [15]. In addition, the results also suggest that anxiety is positively associated with suicidal ideation. This suggests that those who reported high levels of stress tended to report high levels of suicidal ideation. This finding is consistent with Kanwar et al. [17]. The correlation analysis also indicates that stress is positively associated with suicidal ideation. This suggests that those who reported high levels of stress tended to report high levels of suicidal ideation. This finding supports other studies concerning the positive association between stress and suicidal ideation [13], [19], [20]. Based on these findings, depression, anxiety, and stress can be considered as the risk factors for suicidal ideation among adolescents in this research.

Table 4. Multiple regression analysis of psychological factors influencing suicidal ideation.

Predictors	B	B	t	p
Constant	−.65		−2.26*	.03*
Depression	.11	.45*	4.36*	.00*
Anxiety	.02	.08	.77	.45
Stress	.02	.08	.73	.47

$R^2 = 0.33$.
* $p<0.05$.

Although previous studies showed that depression, anxiety and stress were predictors of suicidal ideation [24], [25], in this study, the results indicate that only depression predicts suicidal ideation. This suggests that depression could be regarded as one of the potential predictors for suicidal ideation among adolescents. This means that those who feel depressed may perceive themselves as lacking control over the situation and persistently feeling defeated. In fact, their perception towards their current situation is negative and overwhelming, and they tend to be preoccupied with a sense of guilt and worthlessness. Therefore, depression could be a potential risk for suicidal ideation and suicidal related behaviour among adolescents [26].

However, the findings indicate that anxiety and stress did not predict suicidal ideation. The insignificant predicting role of anxiety could be attributed to the sensitivity of the measure to tap the worry construct. In another study, Carter et al. [24] assessed anxiety, which primarily reflected on worry. For instance, I worry what my parents will say; I worry about what other people think. Worry refers to overwhelming and excessive thoughts about the future, past behaviour and competencies, and peer relationships. Worry is the essential indicator in anxiety disorders and it is present in clinically referred anxious youth that possess suicidal ideation [24]. However, although in the present study DASS-21 was used to measure the anxiety scale, most of the items only reflected anxiety symptoms, such as dryness of mouth, and trembling in the hands. There was only one item that measured the reason for their anxiety. This could partially explain why anxiety could not predict suicidal ideation in the present study. This is because the measurement lacked the indication of worry, which is the key to suicidal ideation in anxious youth. Anxiety symptoms might not be strong indicators of suicidal tendency as they only explain the outcome of worry.

In addition, stress was not a significant predictor of suicidal tendency. This finding contradicted the findings reported by Zhang et al. [27], and Bender et al. [28]. The insignificant predicting role of stress could be partially attributed to the sensitivity of the measure to tap the stress-related construct. Nonetheless, the stress scale in the present study only measures general stress as opposed to adverse life stress as reported by Zhang and colleagues [27]. Hence, the type and intensity of stress, as measured in this study, might not be significant for predicting suicidal ideation. Furthermore, only a handful of studies found that stress directly predicts suicidal ideation. Numerous studies reported that stress and stressful life events were strongly associated with depressive symptoms, which then increased the suicidal risk [25], [29], [30].

Furthermore, it is important to acknowledge the complexity in predicting the role and relationship between depression, anxiety, stress and suicidal ideation. As reported by O'Connor et al. [15], the relationship between depression and suicide ideation is moderated by acute life stress. This means that stress has a vague direct effect on depression, even towards suicidal ideation. This is because stress may precede depression. Therefore, high stress levels could not significantly predict suicidal ideation [15]. In fact, stress is often mediated by other different factors (such as negative appraisal and poor social support) in relation to suicidal ideation. Hence, stress might lead to depression and anxiety but not towards suicidal ideation. Under a stressful environment, suicidal ideation has the potential to increase and individuals will only consider suicidal related behaviour in the presence of the depressive element.

Limitations and future research

There are a few limitations to the present study. Firstly, as the design of this study is a cross-sectional study, no cause and effect relationship could be established. Secondly, this study did not measure changes in suicide ideation at different time points; therefore, no patterns of change in depression, anxiety, stress, and suicide ideation could be established. Third, the majority of the participants are from urban schools in Malaysia; therefore, the findings could not be generalized to other adolescent populations in Malaysia. Lastly, the current research was limited in terms of its exploration of suicide and suicide related behaviours, as it only focused on suicidal ideation among adolescents.

Given these preliminary findings, future research may focus on longitudinal design and interventional studies in order to explain suicidal ideation more precisely. Other risk and protective factors related to suicidal ideation, such as social support, religiosity, coping and problem solving skills, should be taken into consideration in studying suicidal ideation among adolescents.

Conclusions

Since prevention is better than cure, identifying risk factors for suicidal ideation is a way to prevent suicide among adolescents. As there are moderate positive correlations between depression, anxiety, stress, and suicidal ideation in the prevention of adolescents' suicide, these risks factors should be assessed and addressed accordingly. As depression predicts suicidal ideation, it is important to screen depression and suicidal ideation among students who are at high risk of suicide. This screening facilitates the prevention of suicide by referring those high-risk students to mental health services. In addition, school counsellors and other mental health professionals play an important role in screening for depression and suicidal ideation among adolescents and offering and/or referring them for the appropriate psychological preventions and interventions.

Acknowledgments

We would like to thank all the students who participated in this research. We are also very thankful to the Kuala Lumpur Federal Territory Education Department, Ministry of Education, and teachers from both schools for their permission to collect the data.

Author Contributions

Conceived and designed the experiments: NI NA. Performed the experiments: NI MWYS. Analyzed the data: NI MWYS. Contributed reagents/materials/analysis tools: NI MWYS. Wrote the paper: NI NA.

References

1. Smith BL (2014) Psychologists need more training in suicide risk assessment. Monitor on Psychology 45: 42–42.
2. McIntosh JL, Drapeau CW (for the American Association of Suicidology) (2012) U.S.A. suicide 2010: Official final data. Washington, DC: American Association of Suicidology. Available: http://www.suicidology.org. Accessed 2014 Aug 17.
3. Barlow DH, Durand VM (2009) Abnormal psychology: An integrative approach (5th ed.). Belmont, CA: Wadsworth Cengage Learning.
4. Ramachandra S (2010) Suicide rates in Malaysia are on the rise. New Straits Times, 29 August.
5. Aishvarya S, Maniam T, Hatta Sidi, Oei TPS (2013) Suicide ideation and intent in Malaysia: A review of the literature. Compr Psychiatry 55: 1–6.
6. Institute for Public Health. (2011) National Health and Morbidity Survey 2011. Kuala Lumpur: Ministry of Health Malaysia.
7. Lum M (2011) I'm gonna jump. *The Star Online*, 20 November. Available: http://thestar.com.my/health/story.asp?file=/2011/11/20/health/9917622&sechealth. Accessed 17 August 2014.
8. Tam CL, Lee TH, Har WM, Chan LC (2011) Perception of suicidal attempts among college students in Malaysia. Asian Soc Sci 7: 30–41.

9. Gutierrez PM, Osman A (2008) Adolescent suicide: an integrated approach to the assessment of risk and protective factors. DeKalb, IL: Northern Illinois University Press.
10. Gutierrez PM, Osman A, Kopper BA, Barrios FX (2000) Why young people do not kill themselves: the Reasons for Living Inventory for Adolescents. J Clin Child Psychol 29: 177–187.
11. Phillips MR, Li XY, Zhang YP (2002) Suicide rates in China 1995–99. Lancet 359: 835–40.
12. Shemesh E, Annunziato RA, Rubinstein D, Sultan S, Malhotra J, et al. (2009) Screening for depression and suicidality in patients with cardiovascular illnesses. Am J Cardiol 104: 1194–1197.
13. Rohtash S, Hardeep LJ (2008) Suicidal Ideation in Relation to Depression, Life Stress and Personality among College Students. J Indian Acad Appl Psychol 34: 259–265.
14. Takeuchi T, Nakao M (2013) The relationship between suicidal ideation and symptoms of depression in Japanese workers: a cross-sectional study. BMJ Open 3: e003643 doi:10.1136/bmjopen-2013-003643.
15. Yen S, Shea MT, Pagno M, Sanislow CA, Grilo CM (2003) Axis I and axis II disorders as predictors of prospective suicide attempts: findings from the collaborative longitudinal personality disorders study. J Abnorm Psychol 112: 375–381.
16. McDowell AK, Lineberry TW, Bostwick JM (2011) Practical Suicide-Risk Management for the Busy Primary Care Physician. Mayo Clin Proc 86: 792–800 doi: 10.4065/mcp.2011.0076.
17. Malik S, Kanwar A, Sim LA, Prokop LJ, Wang Z, et al. (2014) The association between sleep disturbances and suicidal behaviors in patients with psychiatric diagnoses: a systematic review and meta-analysis. Syst Rev 3: 18 doi: 10.1186/2046-4053-3-18.
18. Davidson CL, Wingate LR, Grant DM, Judah MR, Mills AC (2011) Interpersonal Suicide Risk and Ideation: The Influence of Depression and Social Anxiety. J Soc Clin Psychol 30: 842–855.
19. Gould MS, Greenberg T, Velting D, Shaffer D (2003) Youth suicide risk and preventive interventions: a review of the past 10 years. J Am Acad Child Adolesc Psychiatry 42: 386–405.
20. Overholser JC (2003) Predisposing factors in suicide attempts: life stressors. In A. Spirito & J. Overholser (Eds), Evaluating and Treating Adolescent Suicide Attempters: From Research to Practice (pp. 42–49). New York: Academic Press.
21. Lee SI, Jung H (2006) Psychosocial Risk Factors for Suicide. Psychiatr Invest 3: 15–22.
22. Ramli M, Mohd AF, Zaini Z (2007) Translation, validation andpsychometric properties of Bahasa Malaysia version of the DepressionAnxiety and Stress Scale (DASS). ASEAN J Psychiatr 8: 82–89.
23. Beck AT, Steer RA (1993) Beck Scale for Suicide Ideation: Manual. San Antonio, TX: The Psychological Corporation.
24. Carter R, Silverman WK, Allen A, Ham L (2008) Measures matter: The relative contribution of anxiety and depression to suicidal ideation in clinically referred anxious youth using brief versus full length questionnaires. Depress Anxiety 25: E27–E35.
25. O'Connor RC, Rasmussen S, Hawton K (2010) Predicting depression, anxiety and self-harm in adolescents: The role of perfectionism and acute life stress. Behav Res Ther 48: 52–59.
26. Lai YC, Shek TL (2010) Personal and family correlates of suicidal ideation in Chinese adolescents in Hong Kong. Soc Indic Res 95: 407–419.
27. Zhang XY, Wang HP, Xia Y, Liu XH, Jung EJ (2011) Stress, coping and suicide ideation in Chinese college students. J Adolesc 35: 1–8.
28. Bender WN, Rosenkrans CB, Crane MK (1999) Stress, depression and suicideamong students with learning disabilities: Assessing the risk. Learn Disabil Q 22: 143–156.
29. Hernandez BN (2006) Psychosocial predictors of depressive symptoms in Mexican American middle school girls. Thesis Ph.D. University of Houston.
30. You Z, Chen M, Yang S, Zhou Z, Qin P (2014) Childhood Adversity, Recent Life Stressors and Suicidal Behavior in Chinese College Students. PLoS ONE 9(3): e86672 doi:10.1371/journal.pone.0086672.

9

Prevalence and Risk Factors for Depressive Reaction among Resident Survivors after the Tsunami following the Great East Japan Earthquake, March 11, 2011

Chieko Matsubara[1]*, Hitoshi Murakami[1], Koubun Imai[2], Tetsuya Mizoue[3], Hidechika Akashi[1], Chiaki Miyoshi[1], Tamotsu Nakasa[1]

1 Bureau of International Medical Cooperation, National Center for Global Health and Medicine, Shinjuku-ku, Tokyo, Japan, **2** Department of Psychiatry, National Center for Global Health and Medicine, Shinjuku-ku, Tokyo, Japan, **3** Department of Epidemiology and Prevention, National Center for Global Health and Medicine, Shinjuku-ku, Tokyo, Japan

Abstract

Objectives: The Great East Japan Earthquake caused a gigantic tsunami which devastated coastal areas of northern Japan on 11 March 2011. Despite the large number of 'resident survivors' who continued to reside in their damaged houses on the second or upper floors, research on the mental health of these individuals has been limited. This study explored the prevalence of depressive reaction and risk factors for depressive reaction among these resident survivors.

Methods: A cross-sectional household health support needs screening was conducted for resident survivors in Higashi-Matsushima city, Miyagi prefecture, two to four months after the tsunami. The health interview that was conducted including mental status, assessed by the Patient Health Questionnaire-2 (PHQ-2).

Results: Of 5,454 respondents, 8.1% had depressive reaction. After adjustment by the number of weeks from the tsunami and the mortality rate at each respondent's place of residence, depressive reaction was significantly associated with house flooding below or above the ground floor (odds ratios of 1.92, 2.36, respectively), the unavailability of gas supply (odds ratio, 1.67), being female (odds ratio, 1.47), middle aged or elderly (odds ratios of 2.41, 2.42, respectively), regular intake of psychotropic medicine(s) since before the tsunami (odds ratio, 2.53) and the presence of one to five or more than six cohabiters (odds ratios of 0.61, 0.52, respectively).

Conclusions: The results suggest a considerable psychological burden (depressive reaction) following the tsunami among resident survivors. Special supports for families with psychiatric problems need to be considered among resident survivors. Restoration of lifeline utilities and the strengthening of social ties of persons living alone may help prevent depressive reaction among resident survivors after a tsunami.

Editor: Kenji Hashimoto, Chiba University Center for Forensic Mental Health, Japan

Funding: This study was funded by Research Grant for International Health, H23-6, by the Ministry of Health, Labor and Welfare, Japan (http://www.ncgm.go.jp/kaihatsu/). This work was also supported in part by Grants-in-Aid for Research from the National Center for Global Health and Medicine (26A-201). The funders had no role in study design, data collection and analysis, decision to publish, or preparation of the manuscript.

Competing Interests: The authors have declared that no competing interests exist.

* Email: c-matsubara@it.ncgm.go.jp

Introduction

On the afternoon of 11 March 2011, a massive magnitude 9.0 undersea earthquake (the Great East Japan Earthquake), with an epicenter approximately 70 km off the Pacific coast, caused a gigantic tsunami that devastated the coastal areas of northern Japan. Tsunami waves reached a height of 40 m. By the end of 11 March 2013, 15,882 people had been confirmed dead, and 2,668 were missing [1]. The predominant cause of death was drowning (90.6%) [2].

The coastal city of Higashi-Matsushima in Miyagi prefecture had 65% of its urban areas engulfed by the tsunami, which travelled inland as far as 3 km from the coast. Inundation rates were highest in municipalities hit by the tsunami [3]. The city office reported that 1,061 of its 43,000 residents had died and 76% of its houses were completely or partially destroyed [3].

In the wake of the tsunami, evacuation centers were overcrowded with a large number of displaced people who accounted for up to one-third of the inhabitants [4]. However, some survivors continued to reside in their damaged houses, while some returned from the evacuation centers to their damaged homes when the floodwaters had subsided. These survivors, who often lived on the second or upper floors of their homes even though the first floor had been destroyed by the tsunami, were known as 'resident survivors'. With distribution channels and medical institutions in the city clearly damaged and lifeline utilities cut off, the resident survivors struggled to survive on insufficient medical care and/or emergency support in their homes, many of which were almost entirely covered in mud at the ground floor, according to anecdotal reports [4].

To assess this situation, a household health support needs screening survey was conducted by the local health office in areas inundated by the tsunami, except those in which all homes had been disappeared [4]. The health interview that was conducted with resident survivors also looked at their mental status. The highest priority of this screening was to both determine depressive reaction among the resident survivors and meet their underlying needs for various types of health services. The screened survivors were then referred to regional medical services and offered health services, e.g. examination by medical doctors including psychiatric specialists, prescribed medication and/or home-care assistance.

Mental health issues are a significant concern after tsunamis, such as the one that occurred following a massive undersea earthquake along Sumatra's northwest coast in Indonesia in 2004. Researches have shown a greater prevalence of depression among displaced persons after a tsunami than non-displaced persons [5–7], as well as decreases in prevalence along with the time that had elapsed [5,8]. The predictors of depression were the loss of livelihood [5], witnessing of others' suffering [9], and direct exposure to the disaster [9,10]. Among those who were displaced, geriatrics showed unexpectedly less depression compared to non-geriatrics [11].

Previous studies have reported that social ties are linked to a lower risk of mental health problems [12–16]. Moreover, recent research demonstrated that social ties reduced depression symptoms following the disasters of the 1999 Chi-Chi earthquake in Taiwan [17] and the 2001 terrorist attacks in New York City [18]. In contrast, Akiyama et al. showed that perceived social ties did not significantly affect the prevalence of depression or anxiety among Burmese refugee students living in boarding houses in Thailand [19]. To date, information on the social contexts of resident survivors after a tsunami has been scant, and how social ties affect the mental health of these individuals when vital community links have been severely devastated remains largely unknown.

A better understanding of the impact of tsunamis on the mental health of resident survivors is required for designing and implementing effective public health responses that meet underlying needs for care and support. Therefore, this study aimed to explore the prevalence and correlates of depressive reaction among resident survivors after the tsunami following the Great East Japan Earthquake in 2011.

Methods

We conducted a cross-sectional household health support needs screening.

Study Sites

The sites targeted for the household screening included 31 local administrative areas that had been completely or partially flooded by the tsunami. In total, 7,084 registered households were targeted, and 4,672 (59.9%) households were finally confirmed to reside by the screening [4].

Data Collection

The local health office started the household screening on April 26 and finished on July 29, 2011. Public health nurses in Higashi-Matsushima city conducted the screening, together with public health nurses from across the country who had come to assist local health officers. There was a tendency for areas with more severe destruction to be screened earlier in order to meet potentially greater demands there as rapidly as possible.

The Target Population

The target population of the screening was composed of individuals who continued to reside in their damaged houses in tsunami-flooded areas. Because of the way in which the census was administered in the areas which were completely or partially flooded, participants whose houses were not flooded were included in the screening. People were included in the study if they resided in the targeted areas, were aged 15 years or above, and were contactable in person at home. The exclusion criteria included people who had evacuated to temporary shelters or moved outside the tsunami flooded areas, were below 15 years of age, or could not be contacted at home. Older adults who had difficulty forming answers to these questions on their own, e.g., dementia, were also excluded from this mental health screening.

Although a total of 15,503 registered residents of all ages were screened, ultimately 5,455 residents 15 years old or above were contacted in person at home. More than half of the household members were absent at the time of the survey because of work or school. Therefore, the individuals included in the screening were also likely to have been persons who were home at the time of the tsunami (Friday afternoon).

Questionnaire

A questionnaire comprise of 11 categories that obtained demographic data such as age and gender; physical status (e.g., any chronic medical conditions, blood pressure, cough, need of nursing care); mental status, including depressive reaction and/or posttraumatic stress reactivity; and the impact of the tsunami, including flooding in the house, destruction of the house, disruption of lifeline utilities (water, electricity and/or gas), food intake frequency and direct exposure to sea water at the time of the tsunami was administered to participants. However, variables related to deceased or missing family members and lost jobs were not included in the questionnaire, as the public health nurses had determined that the survivors were reluctant to talk about such matters during the pre-visits they had conducted.

Dependent Variable

The dependent variable in this study was "depressive reaction," which we assessed with the Patient Health Questionnaire-2 (PHQ-2). The PHQ-2 has been validated with with general population [20], outpatients [21], college students [22], adults living with HIV/AIDS [23] and primary care [24]. The Japanese PHQ-2 was validated its sensitivity and specificity and applied into primary care [24]. It consists of the following two symptom items for major depressive episodes in the Diagnostic and Statistical Manual of Mental Disorders, Fourth Edition (the DSM-IV) [25]: "Do you feel depressed or melancholic?" and "Is there anything you used to enjoy, but are not able to now?"

We made adjustments to the response categories. The adjustments were put back to the PHQ-2's original questionnaire (PRIME-MD) [26]. Dichotomous (yes/no) rather than four-point Likert-type response sets were used in the assessment (0 = "not at all," 1 = "several days," 2 = "more than half the number of days," and 3 = "nearly every day" over the last two weeks). Then, instead of using the PHQ-2 cutoff point of ≥3, we asked respondents who had ticked off both items whether these problems made it difficult for them to perform common activities of daily living, e.g. being afraid to go out after the tsunami. These adjustments were made because the public health nurses and psychiatric specialists had found that most respondents who ticked off both problems experienced these more than half the number of days over the last two weeks. This modification allowed the interviewers (the public health nurses) to identify the individuals who needed to be diagnosed and treated immediately, further ensuring the instrument's strategic practicality.

Respondents were deemed to have depressive reaction if they agreed with both items and reported difficulty performing common activities of daily living.

Independent Variables

In the questionnaire, social tie indicators were addressed by numbers of cohabiters. Social ties are often provided by cohabiting families, communities, schools, and places of work, but the tsunami had destroyed many previously existing community links and resident survivors were now sporadically distributed across devastated areas. Therefore, the public health nurses decided not to ask questions regarding community, school, or workplace ties, which they had determined would distress the respondents. The number of cohabiters was categorised into tertile groups to explore if a bigger number of cohabiters was differently associated with the risk of depressive reaction.

The impact of the tsunami was assessed by number of weeks from the tsunami to the screening and degree of flooding in the house. Data on flooding in the house was categorised into three groups, in descending order of severity: above the ground floor, below the ground floor, and no flooding.

The availability of lifeline utilities (water, electricity and gas) was also examined to determine whether each of these was available. Behaviour and attitudes were expected to be influenced by any limited availability of lifeline utilities under post-disaster conditions. We considered the availability of water, electricity, and gas in adjusting for the impact of the tsunami on mental health.

The demographic information collected in this study included age and gender. Age was also categorized into three groups (15 to 39 years, 40 to 64 years, and 65 years or older) according to the criteria outlined by the World Health Organization (WHO) for people of middle age and the elderly [27]. We categorised age into three groups to consider the possibility of differences in risks for the middle aged and elderly compared to those who were younger.

There may have been individuals that had developed depression before the tsunami and thought it would be desirable to exclude these people from the target population. However, as the majority of medical records were lost in the tsunami, we could not identify these people through the normal means. While many of those in the target population could not remember the exact names of the medicines they had been regularly taking, most were able to recall the broad categories of their medicines (e.g., psychotropic or diabetic medicine). Therefore, in order to understand the respondents' mental health status prior to the tsunami, we asked whether respondents regularly took or were regularly taking any kinds of psychotropic medicines, such as for epilepsy or schizophrenia, or a tranquilizer or sleep inducer, since before the tsunami.

Analysis

IBM SPSS Statistics version 21 for Windows was used to analyse the data. We conducted chi-square tests for univariate analyses. We also performed two logistic regression analyses to explore the association of the tsunami with depressive reaction using the forced-entry method, after examining multicollinearity.

Logistic regression models were conducted for depressive reaction after adjusting for number of weeks since the tsunami and the mortality rate at each respondent's place of residence [28]. The morality rate was applied into the regression model to consider the prevalence of depression in a residential community with numbers of casualties, as we avoid harming the respondents emotionally by asking any items regarding deceased or missing family members at that point in time.

P-values of ≤ 0.05 were considered to be statistically significant.

Ethics Statement

All participants were informed about the objectives, the screening procedures, the possibility that the results would be utilized for a study, and the confidentiality of the study, with the aid of a prepared information sheet. The participants were explained an opportunity to refuse inclusion at any time during the screening. Verbal consent was obtained prior to enrolment, although the Ethical Guidelines for noninterventional epidemiological studies without human specimen collection does not require informed consent stipulated by the Ministry of Education, Culture, Sports, Science and Technology and the Ministry of Health, Welfare, Labour and Welfare, Japan. Written consent was not obtained, as it was not the requirement for noninterventional epidemiological studies without human specimen collection. For subjects aged below 18 years, we conducted the screening after obtaining parental agreement and that of their children. We prepared and retained a name list of the participants who agreed to participate in the screening. All household screening protocols and procedures, including the informed consent procedure, were reviewed and approved by the Research Ethics Committee of the National Center for Global Health and Medicine, Japan (Ethics approval code: NCGM-G-001103-00). The National Center for Global Health and Medicine acted in collaboration with the city of Higashi-Matsushima with regard to the restoration of public health. A total of 87 household members declined to participate in the screening. Numerical codes were used in place of names at the time of analysis to ensure confidentiality.

Results

Table 1 lists the univariate analyses for depressive reaction. Among the 5454 respondents, 10.0% respondents ticked off both items of the PHQ-2 and 8.1% of them had difficulties in daily common activities, regarded as depressive reaction. There were more respondents who were female (67.2%) and aged 65 years or older (39.6%) than in the city's population. The houses of more than 80% of the respondents had been inundated by the tsunami at the screening areas. The mean number of weeks from the tsunami was 12.7 weeks (Standard Deviation, 2.9). Covariates associate with depressive reaction were gender ($p = 0.009$), age ($p < 0.001$), regular taking of psychotropic medicine(s) since before the tsunami ($p < 0.001$), the height of house flooding ($p < 0.001$), the number of cohabiters ($p = 0.012$) and the unavailability of gas supply ($p = 0.002$).

Table 2 shows the results of the multivariate regression analysis for depressive reaction. After adjusting for number of weeks from the tsunami and the mortality rate at each respondent's place of residence, we found that depressive reaction was significantly associated with being female (odds ratio, 1.47), middle aged or elderly (odds ratios of 2.41 and 2.42, respectively), regular taking psychotropic medicine(s) since before the tsunami (odds ratio, 2.53), house flooding below or above the ground floor (odds ratios of 1.92 and 2.36, respectively), the presence of 1 to 6 or more than

Table 1. Univariate analysis of depressive reactivity in various variables among the resident survivors after the tsunami.

		Number of respondents[†]	Depressive reactivity	
			%	*p*-value[‡]
Total		5454	8.1	
The mortality rate at the place of residence	0 to 0.50%	1724	7.9	0.631
	0.51 to 1.0%	1671	7.7	
	1.1 to 5.0%	1212	8.7	
	5.1 to 10.0%	0	0	
	10.1% and over	129	10.1	
Gender	Male	1790	6.6	**0.009**
	Female	3664	8.8	
Age	15 to 39 years old	947	3.3	**<0.001**
	40 to 64 years old	2347	9.2	
	65 years old and over	2160	9.1	
Direct exposure to sea water	Yes	597	9.6	0.196
	No	4742	7.9	
Regular intake of psychotropic medicine(s) since before the tsunami	Yes	176	3.2	**<0.001**
	No	5278	96.8	
House flooding	Above the ground floor	3418	9.6	**<0.001**
	Below the ground floor	673	8.0	
	No flooding	927	4.0	
The number of cohabiters	More than 6 persons	296	8.1	**0.012**
	1 to 6 person(s)	4632	7.7	
	None	526	11.7	
Water supply	Yes	4224	8.3	0.488
	No	152	9.9	
Electricity supply	Yes	4252	8.3	0.130
	No	95	12.6	
Gas supply	Yes	4035	8.0	**0.002**
	No	231	13.9	

†: Number may not be add up to 5454 because not all the respondents answered all the questions.
‡: Chi-square test.

6 cohabiters (odds ratios, 0.61, 0.50, respectively), and the unavailability of gas supply (odds ratio, 1.67).

Discussion

The results of this study demonstrated that 8.1% of the resident survivors had depressive reaction from two to four months after the 11 March tsunami. To our knowledge, this is the first study to report on depressive reaction among resident survivors after a tsunami.

The results showed a much higher prevalence of depressive reaction among respondents than in the general population (as shown in the benchmark World Mental Health Japan Survey 2002–2003 with the DSM-IV). That study showed that, within the previous year, the prevalence rates of depression were 2.9% (95% CI = 2.1, 3.7) [29].

The prevalence of depressive reaction decreased along with the increase in the number of weeks from the tsunami. These results were consistent with previous studies [5,8,30], and suggested that depressive reaction would diminish over time.

The height of house flooding was a significant predictor of depressive reaction. The result suggested that the level of house damage would reflect the level of distress among resident survivors, who continued to live in their damaged houses. Since it is common for Japanese to put off their shoes in the house, the resident survivors whose houses were flooded above the ground floor would be inconvenient in their houses. Even if the distance from the coast was the same, the level of flooding in the house could be different depending on the landscape. Therefore, the data obtained through the household screening could provide substantial information on levels of flooding in houses, which would reflect the eventual impact of the tsunami more accurately.

However, direct exposure to sea water at the time of the tsunami was not associated with depressive reaction in this study. Future studies to be conducted if an approach can be found to assess the height of exposure to sea water with less burdensome to respondents.

Table 2. Logistic regression analysis for depressive reactivity using forced-entry method.

		Depressive reactivity (n = 4634)				
		B	S.E.	*p*-value	OR	95%CI
Week		−0.05	0.02	**0.014**	0.95	(0.91–0.99)
The mortality rate at the the place of residence	0 to 0.5%	Ref.				
	More than 0.5 to 1.0%	0.08	0.14	0.578	1.08	(0.82–1.43)
	More than 1.0 to 5.0%	−0.02	0.15	0.894	0.98	(0.73–1.32)
	10.0% and over	0.57	0.43	0.178	1.78	(0.77–4.09)
Gender	Male	Ref.				
	Female	0.39	0.13	**0.003**	1.47	(1.14–1.90)
Age	15 to 39	Ref.				
	40 to 64	0.88	0.22	**<0.001**	2.41	(1.56–3.72)
	65+	0.88	0.22	**<0.001**	2.42	(1.56–3.76)
Regular intake of psychotropic medicine since before the tsunami	No	Ref.				
	Yes	0.93	0.23	**<0.001**	2.53	(1.62–3.97)
House flooding	No	Ref.				
	Below the ground floor	0.64	0.25	**0.010**	1.92	(1.17–3.10)
	Above the ground floor	0.86	0.21	**<0.001**	2.36	(1.57–3.54)
The number of cohabiter(s)	None	Ref.				
	1 to 6 person(s)	−0.50	0.17	**0.003**	0.61	(0.44–0.85)
	More than 6 persons	−0.65	0.33	**0.050**	0.52	(0.28–1.00)
Direct exposure to sea water	No	Ref.				
	Yes	0.06	0.17	0.750	1.06	(0.75–1.49)
Water supply	Yes	Ref.				
	No	0.15	0.37	0.676	1.17	(0.56–2.42)
Electricity supply	Yes	Ref.				
	No	0.16	0.37	0.676	1.17	(0.56–2.41)
Gas supply	Yes	Ref.				
	No	0.51	0.25	**0.038**	1.67	(1.03–2.71)
Cox-Snell R^2		0.02				
Nagelkerke R^2		0.06				

We found a significant association between the female gender and depressive reaction among the resident survivors. These results were consistent with the results of most previous reports [18,31–33].

A higher risk was found for depressive reaction among persons aged 40 to 64 years and 65 years or older than those aged 15 to 39 years. Approximately 140,000 to 200,000 persons were estimated to have lost their jobs as a result of the Great East Japan Earthquake [34], and many of them were residents in the devastated coastal areas [35]. This lost job might be related to a burden for those who lost their jobs because of the tsunami, as shown in a previous study conducted after a terrorist attack [18].

A significant association was found between depressive reaction and regular intake of psychotropic medicine(s) since before the tsunami. We used "regular intake of psychotropic medicine since before the tsunami" instead of "developed depression since before the tsunami", as we could not identify persons who had developed depression before the tsunami by medical records. Given that persons engaged in "regular intake of psychotropic medicine since before the tsunami" included those with depression, a significant association between "depressive reaction" and "regular intake of psychotropic medicine since before the tsunami" would be expected.

According to anecdotal reports, some resident survivors had hoped to continue staying at the evacuation centers but could not due to conditions their family members had, such as autism and schizophrenia. Therefore, it would be necessary to consider special support for such families coping with psychiatric problems to further ensure the efficacy of public health programs geared toward survivors of the tsunami.

The results of this study offer insight into the protective effects of social ties provided by cohabiters in terms of the incidence of depressive reaction among resident survivors. Associations between weaker social ties and the development of depression have been also reported after a terrorist attack [18] and an aircraft accident [36].

The effect exerted by the presence of cohabiters might be due to the following two reasons. First, the cohabiters might play an important role in allowing the survivors to share their traumatic experiences, and thus provide critically needed emotional support in the form of person-to-person contact. It is reasonable to speculate that cohabiters helped mitigate the sense of loneliness and isolation felt by resident survivors through their reactions in the aftermath of the crisis. As mentioned earlier, the resident survivors exhibited noticeable difficulties in retelling their experiences at the time of screening. Anecdotal reports by international counsellors, who had immediately been dispatched to the scene after the tsunami, also described how profound their sense of helplessness was, and the survivors' inability to talk about what had happened or how they felt.

Second, cohabiters could have shared crucial information on the social context with each other in the post-disaster situation. Given the circumstances, this information is potentially more critical for resident survivors than for refugees at the evacuation centers. This is because the tsunami destroyed their community links and communication networks which had existed previously; therefore, support depended to a large extent on the resources available via social ties. For example, food supply and/or medical services were mainly available at the evacuation centers, and resident survivors needed to know the schedules for these services as well as their locations. Cohabiters, even children, can help obtain more information and establish more dense social networks [37]. Thus, cohabiters would be expected to play important roles in the formation of rudimentary social ties and networks after a catastrophe such as a tsunami.

Further, the characteristics of social ties of residents of Miyagi prefecture may have worked supportively after the tsunami. In general, the people living in Miyagi tend to participate more frequently in civic activities such as volunteer work and be associated with people at school or the office, but perform fewer activities with others in the neighbourhood or society [38]. As a result, the information brought by cohabiters from across the residential community would take on an even greater importance for the resident survivors.

Finally, the prevalence of depressive reaction was also associated with the disruption of lifeline utilities, particularly gas supply. As of 31 March 2011, the rate of restoration was more than 90% for electricity and 70% for water, but only 30% for gas in Miyagi prefecture [39]. Even though most households in Higashi-Matsushima city were provided with liquefied petroleum gas, the gas supply was only restarted two weeks after the tsunami. This was because an electrical power outage after the tsunami disturbed the gas filling instruments [40]. This disruption of the gas supply exerted a major impact on the lives of the victims in terms of their cooking, bathing, and heating, all of which are closely related to the quality of life in a wintry region. Anecdotes confirmed that efforts to restore lifeline utilities post-disaster encouraged the resident survivors who experienced prolonged difficulties in their lives after the tsunami.

In conducting this study, we noted several limitations which may have had an effect on the scope and generalizability of the results. First, a greater percentage of elderly women were included in this study than that in the city's population. These elderly female residents were also more likely to have been affected by the tsunami while at home, as the earthquake happened at 14:46. Second, the screening was conducted earlier in areas where destruction was greater, so the regression analysis was adjusted for the number of weeks since the tsunami. Third, the questionnaire did not include any variables about deceased or missing family members, lost jobs because of the tsunami, or other variables related to the survivors' social networks other than the number of cohabiters, or variables related to peritraumatic distress [41], because it was apparent in the pre-interviews that the respondents were reluctant to answer such questions. It would be a probable reason why the regression model in this study did not explain depressive reaction well, even though we applied the mortality rate at the each respondent's place of residence and did not found significant association between the depressive reactivity and the mortality rate. In previous papers, Adams et al. has explained depression with an R square of 0.24 using a regression model that included perievent panic after the terrorist attacks in New York City [42], and Akiyama et al. depression with an R square of 0.23 using a regression model that included traumatic events distribution among Burmese refugee students [19]. Future studies that include these variables are needed if an approach can be found to make such inquiries less burdensome. Fourth, this screening could not exclude respondents who have depressive problem before the tsunami and who have mild cognitive impairment as with previous studies.

Conclusions

The results suggest that there is a considerable psychological burden (depressive reaction) among resident survivors after a tsunami. The predictors of depressive reaction were being female, middle-aged or elderly, regular intake of psychotropic medicine(s) since before the tsunami, house flooding (especially above the ground floor), an unavailability of gas supply, and living alone. Special supports for families with psychiatric problems need to be considered among resident survivors. Strengthening of social ties for persons living alone and restoration of lifeline utilities to their normal state would ameliorate the development of depression among resident survivors who continue to reside in their homes in the aftermath of a tsunami.

Acknowledgments

We would like to express our sincere gratitude to Higashi-Matsushima city, Miyagi prefecture, for their invaluable cooperation with the National Center for Global Health and Medicine.

Author Contributions

Conceived and designed the experiments: C. Matsubara KI HM TM HA C. Miyoshi TN. Performed the experiments: KI TM HA. Analyzed the data: C. Matsubara. Contributed reagents/materials/analysis tools: KI TM HA. Wrote the paper: C. Matsubara. Contributed substantially to manuscript revisions: C. Matsubara KI HM TM HA. Monitored and supervised study progress: C. Miyoshi TN.

References

1. The National Police Agency (2013) Police measures and damage situation of the tohoku-pacific ocean earthquake, 2011 (as of March 11, 2013). 2013. Available at: http://www.npa.go.jp/archive/keibi/biki/higaijokyo.pdf. Accessed 2014 March 28.
2. Cabinet Office, Government of Japan (2011) White paper on disaster management 2011. 2013. Available at: http://www.bousai.go.jp/kaigirep/hakusho/h23/bousai2011/html/honbun/index.htm. Accessed 2014 March 28.
3. Higashi-Matsushima city (2013) The situation of the earthquake damage. 2013.
4. Department of Health and Welfare, Higashi-matsushima city, Miyagi Prefecture (2013) Overcome togetherthe great east japan earthquake: Report of public health nurse, dietitian activity at Higashi-matsushima city.
5. van Griensven F, Chakkraband ML, Thienkrua W, Pengjuntr W, Lopes Cardozo B, et al. (2006) Mental health problems among adults in tsunami-affected areas in southern thailand. JAMA 296: 537–548.

6. Udomratn P (2009) Prevalence of tsunami-related PTSD and MDD in Thailand. Asian J Psychiatr 2: 124–127.
7. Tayama J, Ichikawa T, Eguchi K, Yamamoto T, Shirabe S (2012) Tsunami damage and its impact on mental health. Psychosomatics 53: 196–197.
8. Thavichachart N, Tangwongchai S, Worakul P, Kanchanatawan B, Suppapitiporn S, et al. (2009) Posttraumatic mental health establishment of the tsunami survivors in thailand. Clin Pract Epidemiol Ment Health 5: 11-0179-5-11.
9. Rosendal S, Salcioglu E, Andersen HS, Mortensen EL (2011) Exposure characteristics and peri-trauma emotional reactions during the 2004 tsunami in southeast asia what predicts posttraumatic stress and depressive symptoms? Compr Psychiatry 52: 630–637.
10. Kristensen P, Weisaeth L, Heir T (2009) Psychiatric disorders among disaster bereaved: An interview study of individuals directly or not directly exposed to the 2004 tsunami. Depress Anxiety 26: 1127–1133.
11. Viswanath B, Maroky AS, Math SB, John JP, Benegal V, et al. (2012) Psychological impact of the tsunami on elderly survivors. Am J Geriatr Psychiatry 20: 402–407.
12. Kawachi I, Berkman LF (2001) Social ties and mental health. J Urban Health 78: 458–467.
13. Schweitzer R, Melville F, Steel Z, Lacherez P (2006) Trauma, post-migration living difficulties, and social support as predictors of psychological adjustment in resettled sudanese refugees. Aust N Z J Psychiatry 40: 179–187.
14. Sicotte M, Alvarado BE, Leon EM, Zunzunegui MV (2008) Social networks and depressive symptoms among elderly women and men in havana, cuba. Aging Ment Health 12: 193–201.
15. Cluver L, Fincham DS, Seedat S (2009) Posttraumatic stress in AIDS-orphaned children exposed to high levels of trauma: The protective role of perceived social support. J Trauma Stress 22: 106–112.
16. Malhotra R, Chan A, Ostbye T (2010) Prevalence and correlates of clinically significant depressive symptoms among elderly people in sri lanka: Findings from a national survey. Int Psychogeriatr 22: 227–236.
17. Seplaki CL, Goldman N, Weinstein M, Lin YH (2006) Before and after the 1999 chi-chi earthquake: Traumatic events and depressive symptoms in an older population. Soc Sci Med 62: 3121–3132.
18. Galea S, Ahern J, Resnick H, Kilpatrick D, Bucuvalas M, et al. (2002) Psychological sequelae of the september 11 terrorist attacks in new york city. N Engl J Med 346: 982–987.
19. Akiyama T, Win T, Maung C, Ray P, Sakisaka K, et al. (2013) Mental health status among burmese adolescent students living in boarding houses in thailand: A cross-sectional study. BMC Public Health 13: 337-2458-13-337.
20. Yu X, Stewart SM, Wong PT, Lam TH (2011) Screening for depression with the patient health questionnaire-2 (PHQ-2) among the general population in hong kong. J Affect Disord 134: 444–447.
21. Lowe B, Kroenke K, Grafe K (2005) Detecting and monitoring depression with a two-item questionnaire (PHQ-2). J Psychosom Res 58: 163–171.
22. Zhang YL, Liang W, Chen ZM, Zhang HM, Zhang JH, et al. (2013) Validity and reliability of patient health questionnaire-9 and patient health questionnaire-2 to screen for depression among college students in china. Asia Pac Psychiatry.
23. Monahan PO, Shacham E, Reece M, Kroenke K, Ong'or WO, et al. (2009) Validity/reliability of PHQ-9 and PHQ-2 depression scales among adults living with HIV/AIDS in western kenya. J Gen Intern Med 24: 189–197.
24. Inagaki M, Ohtsuki T, Yonemoto N, Kawashima Y, Saitoh A, et al. (2013) Validity of the patient health questionnaire (PHQ)-9 and PHQ-2 in general internal medicine primary care at a japanese rural hospital: A cross-sectional study. Gen Hosp Psychiatry 35: 592–597.
25. The American Psychiatric Association (1994) Diagnostic and statistical manual of mental disorders, fourth edition; DSM-IV.
26. Spitzer RL, Kroenke K, Williams JB (1999) Validation and utility of a self-report version of PRIME-MD: The PHQ primary care study. primary care evaluation of mental disorders. patient health questionnaire. JAMA 282: 1737–1744.
27. World Health Organization (2010) Definition of an older or elderly person. 2013. Available at: http://www.who.int/healthinfo/survey/ageingdefnolder/en/. Accessed 2014 March 28.
28. Tani K (2012) Distribution of the number of deaths and the death rate on the great east japan earthquake. Occasional paper of Department of Geography, Saitama University: 1–26.
29. Kawakami N, Takeshima T, Ono Y, Uda H, Hata Y, et al. (2005) Twelve-month prevalence, severity, and treatment of common mental disorders in communities in japan: Preliminary finding from the world mental health japan survey 2002–2003. Psychiatry Clin Neurosci 59: 441–452.
30. Frankenberg E, Friedman J, Gillespie T, Ingwersen N, Pynoos R, et al. (2008) Mental health in sumatra after the tsunami. Am J Public Health 98: 1671–1677.
31. Chen YL, Lai CS, Chen WT, Hsu WY, Wu YC, et al. (2011) Risk factors for PTSD after typhoon morakot among elderly people in taiwanese aboriginal communities. Int Psychogeriatr 23: 1686–1691.
32. Fan F, Zhang Y, Yang Y, Mo L, Liu X (2011) Symptoms of posttraumatic stress disorder, depression, and anxiety among adolescents following the 2008 wenchuan earthquake in china. J Trauma Stress 24: 44–53.
33. Goenjian AK, Molina L, Steinberg AM, Fairbanks LA, Alvarez ML, et al. (2001) Posttraumatic stress and depressive reactions among nicaraguan adolescents after hurricane mitch. Am J Psychiatry 158: 788–794.
34. The Japan Research Institute (2011) Impact on employment of catastrophe and countermeasures. 2013. Available at: http://www.jri.co.jp/MediaLibrary/file/report/other/pdf/5491.pdf. Accessed 2014 March 28.
35. Nakagawa H (2011) Current situation and problems of support systems and employment measures for disaster victims. Reference (in Japanese) 61: 29; 29–49; 49.
36. Fullerton CS, Ursano RJ, Kao TC, Bharitya VR (1999) Disaster-related bereavement: Acute symptoms and subsequent depression. Aviat Space Environ Med 70: 902–909.
37. Schoen R (1997) Why do americans want children? Population and development review 23: 333; 333–358; 358.
38. The Japan Research Institute (2008) Towards the social capital of our country policy development. 2013. Available at: http://www.osipp.osaka-u.ac.jp/npocenter/scarchive/sc/file/004/document4_1.pdf. Accessed 2014 March 28.
39. Noujima N (2011) Overview of the great east japan earthquake recovery lifeline (edited chronological order) (ver.1 until 31 march, 2011). 2013. Available at: http://www.jsce.or.jp/committee/eec2/eq_report/201103tohoku/nojima1.pdf. Accessed 2013 April 8.
40. Mizuho Information & Research Institute (2012) Study on the stable supply of LP gas in future that takes into consideration of the great east japan earthquake. 2013. Available at: http://www.meti.go.jp/press/2011/03/20120307002/20120307002-2.pdf. Accessed 2014 March 28.
41. Nishi D, Koido Y, Nakaya N, Sone T, Noguchi H, et al. (2012) Peritraumatic distress, watching television, and posttraumatic stress symptoms among rescue workers after the great east japan earthquake. PLoS One 7: e35248.
42. Adams RE, Boscarino JA (2011) Perievent panic attack and depression after the world trade center disaster: A structural equation model analysis. Int J Emerg Ment Health 13: 69–79.

Measuring the Bright Side of Being Blue: A New Tool for Assessing Analytical Rumination in Depression

Skye P. Barbic[1], Zachary Durisko[1], Paul W. Andrews[2]*

1 Social Aetiology of Mental Illness (SAMI) Canadian Institute of Health Research (CIHR) Training Program, Centre for Addiction and Mental Health, Toronto, Ontario, Canada, 2 Department of Psychology, Neuroscience & Behaviour, McMaster University, Hamilton, Canada

Abstract

Background: Diagnosis and management of depression occurs frequently in the primary care setting. Current diagnostic and management of treatment practices across clinical populations focus on eliminating signs and symptoms of depression. However, there is debate that some interventions may pathologize normal, adaptive responses to stressors. Analytical rumination (AR) is an example of an adaptive response of depression that is characterized by enhanced cognitive function to help an individual focus on, analyze, and solve problems. To date, research on AR has been hampered by the lack of theoretically-derived and psychometrically sound instruments. This study developed and tested a clinically meaningful measure of AR.

Methods: Using expert panels and an extensive literature review, we developed a conceptual framework for AR and 22 candidate items. Items were field tested to 579 young adults; 140 of whom completed the items at a second time point. We used Rasch measurement methods to construct and test the item set; and traditional psychometric analyses to compare items to existing rating scales.

Results: Data were high quality (<1% missing; high reliability: Cronbach's alpha $=0.92$, test-retest intraclass correlations >0.81; evidence for divergent validity). Evidence of misfit for 2 items suggested that a 20-item scale with 4-point response categories best captured the concept of AR, fitting the Rasch model ($\chi^2=95.26$; df $=76$, $p=0.07$), with high reliability ($r_p=0.86$), ordered response scale structure, and no item bias (gender, age, time).

Conclusion: Our study provides evidence for a 20-item Analytical Rumination Questionnaire (ARQ) that can be used to quantify AR in adults who experience symptoms of depression. The ARQ is psychometrically robust and a clinically useful tool for the assessment and improvement of depression in the primary care setting. Future work is needed to establish the validity of this measure in people with major depression.

Editor: Ali Montazeri, Iranian Institute for Health Sciences Research, ACECR, Islamic Republic of Iran

Funding: Funding from the Social Aetiology of Mental Illness Funding Program, Centre for Addiction and Mental Health, TGF-96115. The role of the funder was to provide salary support for the two post-doctoral students who participated in the study (SB, ZD). The authors report that the funder had no role in study design, data collection and analysis, decision to publish, or preparation of the manuscript.

Competing Interests: The authors have declared that no competing interests exist.

* Email: pandrews@mcmaster.ca

Introduction

Depression affects approximately 350 million people worldwide and is a leading cause of global disability [1,2]. Alleviating depression assumes ever increasing importance as the individual and societal costs associated with depression rise every day [3]. Depression is associated with factors that increase mortality risk such as poor adherence to medical treatment and self-care for diabetes and cardiovascular disease [4] [5], health behaviors such as smoking and lack of physical activity [6], cognitive impairment [7] and disability [8]. It is also a common consequence of changes in health status (i.e., cancer [9] & stroke [10]), and/or new life roles (i.e., caregiving [11], immigration [12], and loss of employment [13]).

Primary care is a frequent entry point into the health care system for depressed patients. Since the 1980's gaps in quality of depression care in primary care systems have been noted and continue to be highlighted today [3,14–16]. Studies show that only 25% to 50% of patients with depression are accurately diagnosed by primary care physicians and, among those who are accurately diagnosed, few receive the recommended dosage and duration of either pharmacotherapy or evidence-based psychotherapy [16,17]. Confusing the picture, the medical community receives conflicting accounts of subclinical symptoms. Some argue that subclinical and clinical episodes are part of a single pathological continuum that should often be treated with medication [18], while others argue subclinical symptoms are often a normal response to stress [19].

In short, greater understanding of both clinical and subclinical depression will help primary care physicians, who are often the first line of treatment for depression, improve the overall health and quality of life of their patients.

Why does depression exist?

Despite decades of research, the molecular and physiological mechanisms underlying depression are not fully understood [20–22]. In addition, there is ongoing debate about the safety and efficacy of pharmacological and psychological treatments [23–28]. While efforts continue to understand *how* people become depressed, research from an evolutionary perspective (so-called "Darwinian Psychiatry" or "Evolutionary Medicine") asks *why* depression exists. Evolutionary medicine seeks to understand the difference between healthy and disordered states and why humans are susceptible to disease [29,30]. This perspective has informed our understanding of a broad range of psychiatric conditions and has been reviewed in detail previously [31,32]. Evolutionary hypotheses of the aetiology of depression are numerous [33,34], but typically suggest that depression has evolved as an adaptation to help regulate energy use and navigate adverse situations. If depression can indeed be adaptive, primary health care providers and researchers may need to consider different approaches to treatment.

The Concept of Interest: Analytical Rumination

One leading hypothesis of the origin of depression proposes that many depressions are the result of an ancient defence mechanism designed by natural selection to promote analytical thinking in response to complex life stressors [35]. The *analytical rumination hypothesis* [35] states that the symptoms of depression result in extended bouts of persistent, distraction-resistant cognitive analysis, which can function to help individuals resolve challenges in their lives. This hypothesis recognizes that the resolution of exceptionally complex problems, such as those associated with adverse life events and major stressors, can require prolonged and in-depth bouts of analysis that lead to impairment and disengagement from everyday life. Problems can occur in a variety of contexts, but analysis will involve thinking through the components of the problem such as (1) its cause; (2) the aspects that need solving; (3) potential solutions; and (4) the costs and benefits associated with implementing various solutions.

While the ruminative thoughts associated with depression are commonly considered maladaptive [36–38], several authors have argued that depressive ruminations may be useful, or at least may begin as a useful means to focus and analyze problems in order to gain insight [39–41]. A substantial body of evidence indicates that depressed mood is associated with increased cognitive processing, improved accuracy on complex tasks, and enhanced detail-oriented judgement on tasks that require deliberate information processing [42–46]. Individuals with depression have also been shown to consistently outperform non-depressed controls when the experimental tasks involve cost-benefit analysis [47–52].

Clinical implications for understanding analytical rumination

Understanding analytical rumination has important clinical implications for how to assess and treat depression. Rather than viewing depression as an impairment or malfunction of the brain, the evolutionary perspective hypothesizes that it may sometimes occur as an adaptive response to promote the cognitive analysis required to understand and resolve current problems. Depressive episodes associated with high levels of analytical rumination may be most usefully treated by facilitating rumination and analysis rather than medications or psychotherapies that may treat rumination as unproductive.

The challenge to understanding analytical rumination

Research in this arena has been limited by the lack of a reliable and valid psychometric instrument for analytical rumination. Analytical rumination, similar to many other important health constructs (i.e, quality of life), is not directly measurable (i.e., it is *latent*). Primary health care providers must rely on patient-reported outcomes (PROs) to gain information about the patient that cannot be collected by means of traditional clinical metrics such as lab values. Recently, the use of PROs has been emphasized as a valuable means to enhance care management by helping providers to understand not just whether a clinical value is within range, but how patients' lives may be affected by the value [53]. In order to develop a PRO that can be integrated into routine care in a clinically meaningful way, development and testing needs to carefully consider the concept of interest, content of use, and measurement rigour (i.e., precision, standardization, and comparability of scores across studies and diseases) [53,54].

Based on a thorough review of the theoretical construct [35], we are unaware of any measure that captures the full range of analytical rumination in a clinically meaningful way. The objective of this study was to develop and test a conceptually and psychometrically sound measure of analytical rumination to inform fundamental decisions in primary care practice, health research, and treatment trials.

Methods

Measure design

We developed a conceptual model (Figure 1) based on an extensive review of published theory on analytical rumination and depression [35]. The analytical rumination hypothesis states that individuals with depression engage in analysis to understand at least four different parts (domains) of their problems: (1) understanding the cause (e.g., "I tried to understand why I had these problems"); (2) understanding the aspects of the problems that need to be solved (e.g., "I tried to understand what was wrong in my life"; (3) generating possible solutions (e.g., "I thought about all my options for dealing with my problems"); and (4) evaluating the advantages and disadvantages of possible solutions (e.g., "I thought about whether my options for dealing with one problem would make other problems worse"). From this model, we generated 22 candidate items to capture the full range of analytical rumination, which we refer to as the Analytical Rumination Questionnaire (ARQ).

As described below, each item of the ARQ candidate item pool was scored on a 5-point Likert scale. Scoring categories range from

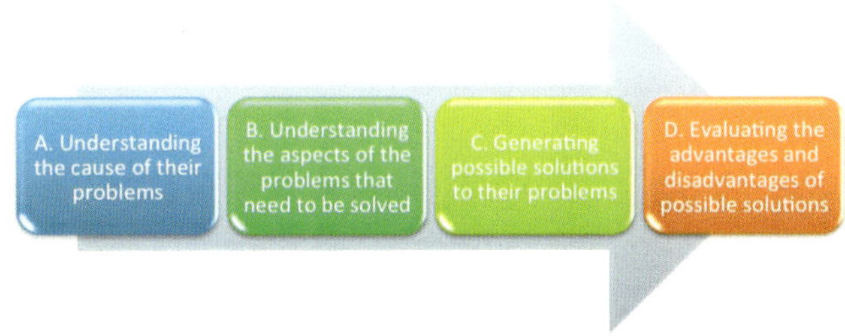

Figure 1. Working model describing the theoretical conceptualization of analytical rumination.

1 (none of the time) to 5 (all of the time). Possible scores ranged from 22–110, with a higher score indicating a higher level of analytical rumination (see Appendix S1 for candidate items in ARQ). We hypothesized that the four domains and the items themselves had a natural implicit ordering from low to high. Specifically, we hypothesized that people first attempt to understand why they have a problem (domain 1) and what needs to be solved (domain 2) before they attempt to generate (domain 3) and evaluate (domain 4) possible solutions.

Questionnaire administration

Participants, recruitment, and data collection. All participants were students at McMaster University taking undergraduate psychology courses. English-speaking adults aged 18 years and over were eligible to participate. We collected data in two studies. In the first, 439 participants filled out the ARQ at one time point, and in the second 140 participants filled it out at two time points. In order to encourage high response rates, we offered academic credit for participation. Both studies were approved by the McMaster Research Ethics Board and written informed consent was obtained prior to completing the ARQ.

Analysis Procedure

We used both traditional and Rasch psychometric analyses to evaluate the properties of the ARQ.

Traditional analyses

Traditional psychometric analyses have been described in detail elsewhere [55]. In brief, they use correlation and descriptive analyses to evaluate scaling assumptions (legitimacy of summing items), reliability, and validity [56]. Accordingly, we examined data from the ARQ for quality (percent missing for each item), scaling assumptions, scale to sample targeting (score means; standard deviation (SD); floor and ceiling effects), and internal consistency and reliability(Cronbach's alphas) [57]. We determined convergent and discriminant construct validity by examining correlations between the ARQ and other 3 other measures and variables (age and sex). For discriminant validity testing, we used the Beck Depression Inventory (BDI) [58] and the Positive and Negative Affect Scale (PANAS) [59]. For convergent validity testing we used the reflective pondering subscale of the Ruminative Response Scale (RRS) [37,38]. We hypothesized that correlations would be the highest with the ARQ and the reflective pondering subscale of the RRS, and the correlations of the ARQ with other variables would be lower.

Rasch Measurement Psychometric Testing

Rasch measurement is a paradigm commonly used to guide the development and testing of rating scales. Many statistical techniques for evaluating psychometric instruments attempt to develop a model from data that describes how people use an instrument. In contrast, a fundamental goal of Rasch measurement is to develop a psychometric instrument that reflects an *a priori* specified conceptual model [60]. One component of this conceptual model is *specific objectivity* (i.e., the instrument objectively measures the latent trait in the same way that a yardstick is an instrument for objectively measuring length). A specifically objective psychometric instrument must have several properties. First, all the items of the instrument must be related to a single latent trait (i.e., the instrument must be unidimensional) [61]. Second, for each item, there must be a monotonic relationship between the ordering of the responses of that item and the ordering of the latent trait [56]. For instance, for item 1 of the ARQ, people who rank higher on the latent analytical rumination trait must be probabilistically more likely to endorse higher responses. Third, there must be local independence [62], which means that the answer to an item does not depend on the order in which items are presented. Finally, while a Rasch model allows items to differ in how diagnostic they are of the latent trait (i.e., some items indicate low levels of the latent trait while other items indicate high levels of the latent trait), the diagnostic ordering of items should not vary across the range of the latent trait [63]. For example, if a person who is low on the latent trait of analytical rumination is more likely to endorse item 1 of the ARQ than item 13, then this ordering must be preserved at higher levels of the latent trait. These assumptions are difficult to achieve in practice, so a psychometric instrument that fits the Rasch model has passed an important, rigorous test of measurement.

When a psychometric instrument satisfies the rigorous assumptions of the Rasch model, the sum of the scores of the individual items provides a complete description of the person's standing on the latent variable. An instrument that defines the full spectrum of the latent variable will range from -4 to +4 logits, corresponding to ±4 standard deviations of a standard normal distribution, and items will cover all levels of the latent distribution. Moreover, an instrument that fits the context of use is one that captures the full range of the latent distribution in a given population [64,65]. A range of parameters arising from the Rasch analysis can be used to judge the extent to which there is misfit between the items and people on this range, and as a result, the extent to which scoring and summing items is in fact, a valid and reliable approach [66].

For this analysis, we used all 22 candidate items. All assumptions were verified using the Masters' partial credit Rasch polytomous model [67], an appropriate mathematical derivation of the Rasch model suitable for investigating items with ordinal response options. All analyses were performed using RUMM 2030 [68].

Clinical Meaning. We examined the extent to which ARQ items were clinically cohesive and reflected our *a priori* hypothesis about how items covered the latent spectrum of low to high analytical rumination.

Thresholds for item response options. Each item of the ARQ was scored on a 5-point Likert scale, with five response categories (none of the time, some of the time, half of the time, most of the time, all of the time), and five integer scores assigned to each category (1, 2, 3, 4, and 5, respectively). The successive nature of the scores implies that there is a natural order to the assignment that reflects a continuum of increasing impact from less (i.e., 1 = not at all) to more (i.e., 5 = all of the time). We tested this assumption by statistical and graphical inspection of threshold locations and plots.

Item fit statistics. We tested the extent to which the participant's responses to an item fit the rigorous expectations of the Rasch model. Misfit of an item implies that the item is not working as intended and may not be measuring the intended construct. We used three indicators of fit: (1) log residuals (item-person interaction) (2) chi-square values (item-trait interaction), and (3) item characteristic curves. Rather than using absolute criteria for interpreting fit, these three indicators of fit were interpreted separately to understand the context of their use as a full item set capturing analytical rumination.

Item locations and targeting. We carefully looked at how items were distributed along the proposed latent analytical rumination continuum. We flagged items in similar locations as potentially redundant and warranting further investigation. We gauged the calibration of the instrument to the population by comparing graphically how closely the amount of analytical rumination displayed by the respondents was adequately measured by the items on the scale.

Person Separation Index (PSI) [69]. We used the PSI as a reliability statistic, analogous to Cronbach's alpha [57], to test the extent to which scale scores in the sample can be separated. Higher scores indicate higher reliability.

Differential Item Functioning (DIF). We determined whether each item's location on the latent analytical rumination construct was stable across groups using item characteristic curves and two-way analyses of variance with a Bonferroni correction of 0.05 for multiple comparisons. Groups included gender, age, ethnicity, and whether the individual reported a medical condition.

Unidimensionality. We tested the scale's ability to measure a single latent construct using a principal components analysis (PCA) of the residuals. We specifically tested the presence of a pattern of the residuals grouping into more than one subscale once the "Rasch factor" was extracted. We hypothesized that the response structure would be unidimensional and that, apart from a single variable and the item parameters mapped on this variable, the remaining variation was random. Depending on the factor loadings resulting from the PCA, we performed paired t-tests to assess whether person estimates derived from the subtests of items were significantly different from each other. If greater than 5% of t-tests were significant, explanation for the anomaly was put into question.

Dependency. We tested to see whether the responses to any of the items in the scale directly influenced the response to other items by examining item residual correlations.

Results

The sample consisted of 308 women (53%) and 271 men (47%) at enrollment with a mean age of 19 years (SD: 1.9). Thirty percent reported being of white-European descent, followed by 16% Asian, 9% East Asian, 5% African, 2% Aboriginal, and 14% reporting "Other". Thirty-three percent of the sample reported taking medication, with 28% of this sub-sample reporting contraceptive medication, and 7% reporting a form of anti-depressant medication.

Traditional Psychometric Results

Data satisfied criteria for all evaluated traditional psychometric properties. Missing data from all items ranged from <1%–2%. Scale scores were computable for 99% of respondents. Scale scores spanned the range of the scale and were not notably skewed. We did not observe any ceiling and floor effects.

Reliability and Validity. Internal consistency reliability was high (Cronbach alphas = 0.91), and the mean inter-item correlation was 0.83, supporting scale reliability. Scale validity was supported by the high Cronbach alpha coefficient and interscale correlations. Table 1 shows the results of the convergent and discriminant construct validity testing of the ARQ. Patterns of correlations were consistent with our predictions. Mean ARQ scores were correlated highest with the RRS subscale ($r = 0.40$), followed by the BDI and PANAS. As expected, the mean scores for men and women did not differ, nor did age impact ARQ scores.

Rasch Measurement Results

Clinical Meaning. The hierarchy of the items was clinically meaningful. Most (20/22) items mapped back to the *a priori* hypothesized analytical rumination continuum, with the expected order of item difficulty capturing a theoretical distribution of low to high. Table 2 shows the ordering of the items from least to most difficult.

Threshold Response options. The item response options for 13/22 (59%) items were disordered. As shown in Figure 2b, we rescored disordered items by collapsing the middle category "half of the time" with the second category "some of the time". After rescoring, statistical and graphical evidence of misfit remained for only two items: "*I thought about all the bad things that could happen to me because of the situation I am in*" (item 13: fit residual = 5.95; $\chi^2 = 48.09$, df = 9, $p<0.01$); and "*I thought about how others were likely to respond to some of the actions I could take*" (item 9: fit residual = 4.33; $\chi^2 = 29.42$, df = 9, $p<0.01$). Both items had ICCs well below the theoretical curve, providing evidence of poor discrimination ability. After consultation with two content experts and two clinicians, and revision of conceptual model, the two items were removed.

Fit and targeting. Figure 2a shows the distribution of participants along the measurement continuum, ranging from −4.31.to +3.09, reflecting a broad, even spread. As shown in Table 3, overall person fit (i.e., mean person fit residual) was near the targeted level of 0 (mean location = 0.273, SD = 1.05) indicating the sample was representative of an expected population distribution. Person locations ranged from −4.50 to +3.20, with only 3 individuals lying outside of the individual fit residual range of −2.5 to +2.5. Item locations and their standard errors are reported in Table 2. Fit of the items was good. Figure 2c illustrates the item threshold range from −3.6 to +2.3 logits which covered 74% of the measurement continuum. Overall item fit was good with a mean (SD) of 0.28 (1.53) as shown in Table 2. Item residuals, χ^2 fit statistic, and the F-test after Bonferroni correction also were consistent with a reasonable fit.

Figures 2a and 2c show the targeting of the sample to the 20 remaining items, offering evidence of the strong targeting of our sample for evaluating ARQ performance. Scores spanned the range of the scale and were not notably skewed with little evidence of ceiling and floor effects. Of note was that a gap of items was observed >2.3, suggesting that individuals above this range are not as precisely measured as the remainder of the sample ($n = 9$, < 2% of the sample).

Person Separation Index. Scale reliability was high (PSI = 0.87), indicating the items adequately separated this sample along measurement continuum.

Unidimensionality. Examination of the eigenvalues from the principal component analysis suggested the presence of two or more subscales. This was also supported by the loadings in the first principle component that showed clear patterns of residuals on successive components, with 5 items with large positive correlations, and 5 others with negative loadings. The first set of items queried the first domain of our conceptual model (understanding the problem), whereas the second set queried the third domain (generating possible solutions to the problem). Evidence from grouping these items together in subtests provided some evidence of multi-dimensionality of borderline relevance, with 8% of the subtests ($n = 55$) showing significant differences in the estimated differences generated ($t = 3.21$, $p = 0.04$).This was a mild deviation from the 5% expected value, warranting further consideration and caution in future testing.

Differential Item Functioning. Both graphical and statistical evidence showed the difficulty level of the items was uniform across age, sex, ethnic background, self-report medication use, and time.

Table 1. Traditional psychometric methods: convergent and discriminant construct validity and group differences validity.

Instrument/variable	Scale/Variable	Correlation to the ARQ
RRS- Reflective Pondering	Sub Score	0.40*
RRS- Brooding	Sub Score	0.22
BDI	Total Score	0.25
PANAS	Total Score	0.20
Demographic variables		
	Age	0.13
	Sex	0.03
	Medication	0.15

*Significant <0.05; ARQ: Analytical Rumination Questionnaire, high scores indicate greater analytical rumination; RRS: Ruminative Response Scale, high scores indicate greater rumination; BDI: Beck Depression Scale, high scores indicate greater depression; PANAS: Positive and negative affect scale.

Discussion

The objective of this study was to provide evidence for the conceptual and measurement properties of a new concept of interest in health called *analytical rumination*. Our preliminary results support a set of 20 items, collectively called the Analytical Rumination Questionnaire (ARQ), that cover the full range of our conceptual model of analytical rumination[35]. By application of traditional psychometric and Rasch measurement testing, we have demonstrated that the ARQ is reliable, unidimensional, and meets the criteria for objective rigorous measurement as outlined by the Rasch model. The Rasch model specifically confirmed the presence of a higher-order scale that consisted of 20 items reflecting each of the four theoretical domains previously mapped to the analytical rumination construct (see Figure 1) [35]. From a clinical perspective, our findings support a set of items that suggest a meaningful story of what it may mean to move from "low" analytical rumination to "high" analytical rumination (a fundamental prerequisite of measurement) [60,63]. For example, Table 1 shows that items on the lower end ask about problem

Table 2. Measures of fit and location (SE) of ARQ items.

Item	Item label	Location	SE	Fit Resid.	$\chi^{2\dagger}$	Prob*
22	I tried to think through my difficulties	−0.642	0.059	0.509	4.991	0.288
16	I tried to learn from my mistakes	−0.550	0.057	1.719	1.354	0.852
17	I tried to find a goal or purpose that was meaningful to me	−0.511	0.057	1.539	1.112	0.892
20	I tried to find a way to resolve an important issue	−0.405	0.059	−1.498	7.203	0.126
7	I tried to figure out the best option for dealing with my dilemma	−0.309	0.060	−0.929	7.268	0.122
19	I tried to figure out how to stick to my goals	−0.292	0.058	−1.577	9.721	0.050
18	I tried to find an answer to my problems	−0.273	0.055	1.077	1.362	0.850
6	I thought about all the options for dealing with my problems	−0.269	0.062	−1.169	10.407	0.034
12	I tried to figure out how to make the best out of a bad situation	−0.137	0.054	**−2.621**	12.412	0.023
8	I tried to figure out which of the problems I was facing were the most important and which I should do first	−0.006	0.056	−0.224	1.572	0.813
21	I tried to understand the past and the present	0.036	0.073	0.811	0.575	0.966
5	I thought about all the aspects of the problems I was facing that needed to be solved	0.053	0.057	−1.116	4.979	0.297
3	I thought about what I may have done to avoid these problems	0.081	0.054	0.116	1.583	0.812
1	I tried to understand why I had these problems	0.122	0.057	−0.468	4.708	0.319
2	I tried to figure out what I had done wrong	0.230	0.055	1.440	6.227	0.183
14	I tried to figure out how to best avoid future problems	0.278	0.057	1.027	0.388	0.983
10	I thought about whether some of the options I could take were likely to solve my problems or make things worse.	0.425	0.052	2.283	9.427	0.051
4	I thought about all the ways my life had become more difficult	0.496	0.052	2.048	12.494	0.015
15	I tried to figure out what was wrong in my life	0.509	0.052	1.474	2.426	0.658
11	I thought about whether my options for dealing with one problem would make other problems worse	1.028	0.055	1.277	8.768	0.067

Items are located in order of difficulty (from high AR to low AR). † degrees of freedom (620,4); *Bonferroni adjustment with a probability base of 0.01 (p = 0.005 for 20 items); note item 12 of borderline misfit. Included in the model because graphical fit was good and fit conceptual model.

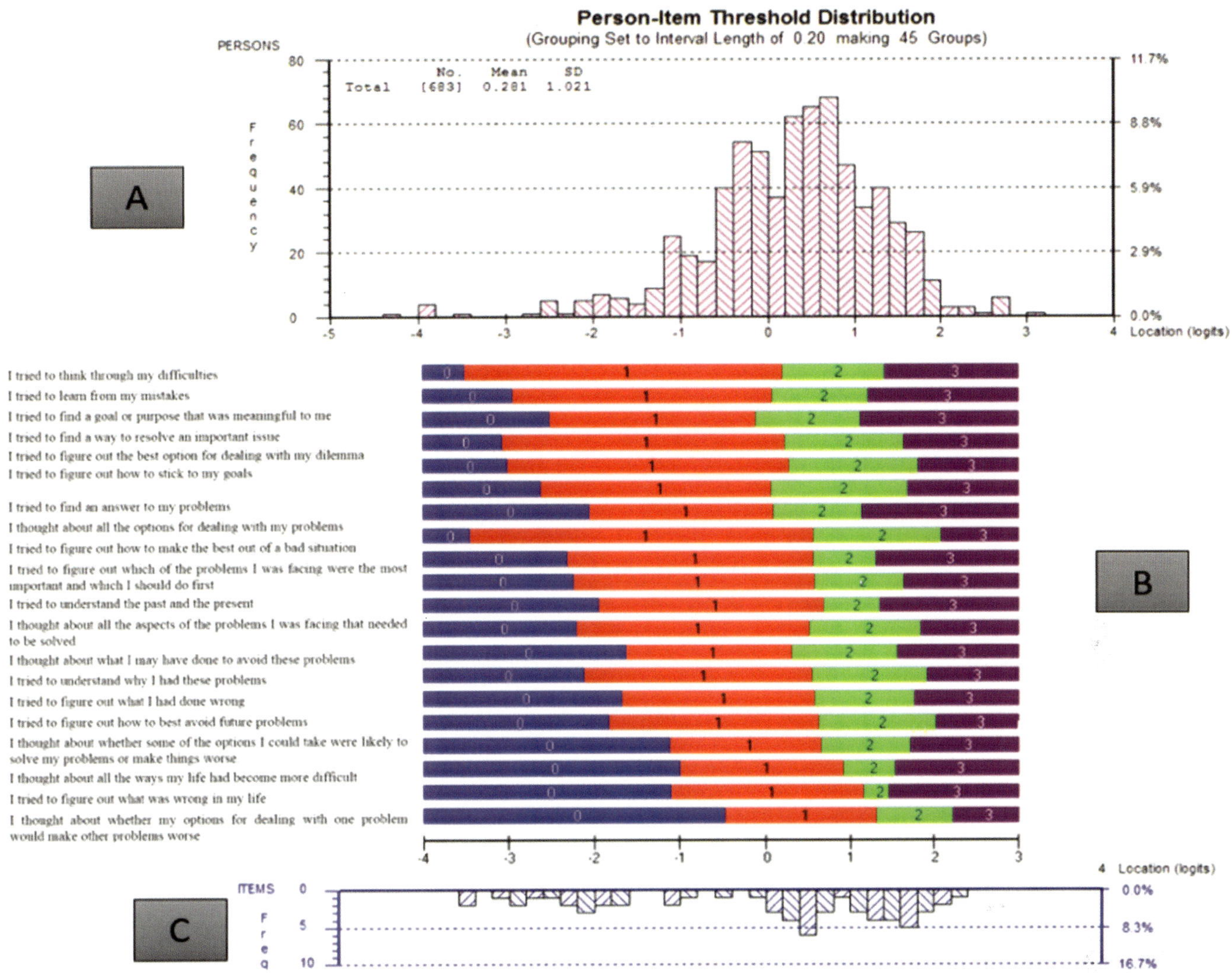

Figure 2. Summary of targeting to the sample of 20 items included in the Analytical Rumination Questionnaire. A. Distribution of items across the measurement continuum in the prototype analytical rumination questionnaire (ARQ). B. Item map showing expected score to each item, with items shown in order of difficulty. C. The location of the 20 items, relative to each other, on an interval scale.

Table 3. Indices of fit to a Rasch model.

ITEM-TRAIT INTERACTION	
Total Item χ	95.26
Total degrees of Freedom	76
Total χ^2 Probability	0.07
ITEM-PERSON INTERACTION	
ITEM	
Difficulty	0.00 ± 0.43
Fit Residual	0.28 ± 1.30
PERSON	
Measure	0.27 ± 1.05
Fit Residual	-0.49 ± 1.91

identification ("I tried to think about my difficulties"). As difficulty increases, items capture domains hypothesized to reflect higher analytical rumination such as: identifying and understanding problems, generating possible solutions, evaluating the possible solutions, and learning how to prevent problem recurrence.

Given that recent meta-analyses indicate similar treatment efficacy for cognitive therapies (i.e., psychotherapy) and antidepressant medications [23,28], the development of the ARQ is timely. The ordering of the items supports the construct validity of analytical rumination, and could possibly be used as a guide to understand how individuals progress from problem identification to the problem resolution. At the level of primary care, family physicians or other health professionals may be able to use this information to engage in a dialogue with patients who experience depressive symptoms. We suggest that the effective assessment and treatment of depression could include helping patients (1) identify of a problems/stressor, (2) prioritize aspects that need solving, (3) identify potential solutions and plans for implementation, and (4) develop a plan to prevent further recurrence of the triggering problem. We hope that clinicians will use this perspective of the potentially adaptive aspects of depression in order to inform treatment. The evolutionary perspective suggests that there are many different aetiological pathways to the diagnostic symptoms of depression, each of which may be best suited to a different treatment strategy. One pathway is the functioning of adaptations designed to promote analytical rumination. The ARQ may be used to identify such cases, and to design personalized interventions that help patients make progress toward the resolution of their triggering problem.

The ARQ currently offers a quick and easy way to assess the stage and progress of a patient's problem-solving analysis. Interventions may therefore be tailored and personalized according to a patient's practical needs to resolve precipitating problems, rather than solely to treat symptoms. For example, psychiatrists and psychologists have developed several treatment strategies that may be effective at the low end of the ARQ spectrum, where patients have not yet identified aspects of their problems or the best solution. Current evidence-based interventions such as "exposure-based" therapies, mindfulness, and problem-solving therapy [70–75], that work to increase awareness of problems and reduce avoidance of stressors, may provide an alternative option for care for a population that is difficult to treat with medication alone. At the higher end of the spectrum, there may be more of a role for allied health professionals (e.g., occupational therapy) with expertise in goal-orientated cognitive therapies to help individuals who have identified the problem and goal, but are having difficulty implementing their plan of action. The ARQ developed in the present study will be an invaluable tool for future research to understand the effectiveness of these types of interventions.

From the original 22 candidate items, we found that 2 of the items functioned poorly. Further investigation of the anomalies revealed that each item consisted of more than one question per item (items 9 and 13). We removed these two items since the item locations were close to other items on the scale, and were conceptually redundant. Rasch analysis also revealed inherent problems in the initial 5 option response scale. Upon reflection, we propose two possible explanations for the aberrant behaviour of this scoring structure. First, there may have been too many response options for the target population. A second possibility is that the scoring options were confusing because the categories included both qualitative (all the time, some of the time, etc.) and quantitative (half of the time) response options. Examination of the category frequencies and provided evidence that an optimal scoring structure for this scale would favour four response categories. The anomaly revealed in the scoring structure was resolved upon collapsing the middle category "half of the time", with the preceding category "some of the time."

Limitations of our study

The intended context of use for this scale is adults who experience depressive symptoms. For exploratory purposes, we began our conceptual and measurement testing with young adults in a university setting. Our preliminary results show that the ARQ targets this population very well and has excellent person separation. This sample may not generalise to patients who meet formal diagnostic criteria for clinical syndromes. However, as it currently stands, the ARQ may be useful in a primary care setting, where subclinical symptoms are often encountered. Future work in understanding this concept further in people with depression should include an iterative process of both qualitative and quantitative work to ensure the ARQ items are fit for purpose and measure what they purport to measure.

Conclusion

Our study provides preliminary results for a set of 20 items (Analytical Rumination Questionnaire) that collectively can be used as a reliable and valid instrument for the quantification of analytical rumination. The ARQ provides a starting point to provide insight into the conceptual underpinnings and measurement of analytical rumination for potential application in the self-management and clinical treatment of depression. Future analyses will further assess the construct validity of the scale by assessing the performance of the items in a clinical population of people with depression.

Supporting Information

Appendix S1 Candidate items for the Analytical Rumination Questionnaire.

Author Contributions

Conceived and designed the experiments: SB ZD PA. Performed the experiments: PA ZD. Analyzed the data: SB. Contributed reagents/materials/analysis tools: SB. Wrote the paper: SB ZD PA.

References

1. Mathers C, Boerma T, Fat DM (2008) The global burden of disease: 2004 update. World Health Organization.
2. Ferrari AJ, Somerville AJ, Baxter AJ, Norman R, Patten SB, et al. (2013) Global variation in the prevalence and incidence of major depressive disorder: a systematic review of the epidemiological literature. 43Psychological Medicine.
3. Pickett YR, Ghosh SC, Rohs A, Kennedy GJ, Bruce ML, et al. (2014) Healthcare use among older primary care patients with minor depression. American Journal of Geriatric Psychiatry 22: 207–210.
4. Ciechanowski PS, W.J K, Russo JE (2000) Depression and diabetes: impact of depressive symptoms on adherence, function, and costs. Archives of Internal Medicine 160: 3278–3285.
5. Whooley MA, Wong JM Depression and Cardiovascular Disorders. Annual Review of Clinical Psychology 9: 327–354.
6. Freedland KE, Carney RM, Skala JA (2005) Depression and smoking in coronary heart disease. Psychosomatic Medicine 67: S42–46.
7. Alexopoulos GS, Meyers BS, Young RC, Kalayam B, Kakuma T (2000) Executive dysfunction and long-term outcomes of geriatric depression. Archives of General Psychiatry 57: 285–290.
8. Murray CLJ, Lopez AD (1996) The global burden of disease: a comprehensive assessment of mortality and disability from diseases, injuries, and risk factors in 1990 and projected to 2020. Boston, MA: Harvard University Press.

9. Krebber AMH, Buffart LM, Kleijn G, Riepman IC, de Bree R, et al. (2014) Prevalence of depression in cancer patients: a meta-analysis of diagnostic interviews and self-report instruments. Psycho-Oncology 23: 221–230.
10. Rochette A, Bravo G, Desrosier J, St.Cyr D, Bourget A (2007) Adaptation process, participation and depression over six months in first-stroke individuals and spouses. Clinical Rehabilitation 21: 554–562.
11. Cameron JI, Cheung AM, Streiner D, Coyte PC, Stewart DE (2011) Stroke Survivor Depressive Symptoms Are Associated With Family Caregiver Depression During the First 2 Years Poststroke. Stroke 42: 302–306.
12. Wong E, Miles JNV (2014) Prevalence and Correlates of Depression Among New U.S. Immigrants. Journal of Immigrant and Minority Health 16: 422–428
13. Olesen SC, Beutterworth P, Leach LS, LKelaher M, Pirkis J Mental health affects future employment as job loss affects mental health: findings from a longitudinal population study. BMC Psychiatry.
14. Whitebird RR, Solberg LI, Margolis KL, Asche SE, Trangle MA, et al. (2013) Barriers to Improving Primary Care of Depression: perspectives of Medical Group Leaders. Qualitative Health Research 23: 805–814
15. Katzelnick DJ, Kobak KA, Greist JH, Jefferson JW, Henk HJ (1997) Effect of primary care treatment of depression on service use by patients with high medical expenditures. Psychiatric Services 48: 59–64.
16. Katon W, Von Korff M, Lin E (1995) Collaborative management to achieve treatment guidelines. Impact on depression in primary care. JAMA 273: 1026–1031.
17. Mojtabai R, Olfson M (2011) Proportion Of Antidepressants Prescribed Without A Psychiatric Diagnosis Is Growing. Health Affairs 30: 1434–1442.
18. Pies R (2014) Grief and major depression. British Medical Journal 348: g179.
19. Dorwick C, Frances A (2013) Medicalising unhappiness: new classification of depression risks more patients being put on drug treatment from which they will not benefit. British Medical Journal 347: f7140.
20. Hamilton JP, Etkin A, Furman DJ, Lemus MG, Johnson RF, et al. (2012) Functional neuroimaging of major depressive disorder: A meta-analysis and new integration of baseline activation and neural response data. American Journal of Psychiatry 169: 693–703.
21. Krishnan V, Nestler EJ (2008) The molecular neurobiology of depression. Nature 455: 894–902.
22. Valenstein ES (1998) Blaming the brain: The truth about drugs and mental health. New York, NY: The Free Press.
23. Andrews PW, Thomson JA, Jr., Amstadter A, Neale MC (2012) Primum non nocere: An evolutionary analysis of whether antidepressants do more harm than good. Frontiers in Psychology 3: 117.
24. Barlow DH (2010) Negative effects from psychological treatments: A perspective. American Psychologist 65: 13–20.
25. Fournier JC, DeRubeis RJ, Hollon SD, Dimidjian S, Amsterdam JD, et al. (2010) Antidepressant drug effects and depression severity: A patient-level meta-analysis. Jama-Journal of the American Medical Association 303: 47–53.
26. Hollon SD, Thase ME, Markowitz JC (2002) Treatment and prevention of depression. Psychological Science in the Public Interest 3: 39–77.
27. Kirsch I, Deacon BJ, Huedo-Medina TB, Scoboria A, Moore TJ, et al. (2008) Initial severity and antidepressant benefits: A meta-analysis of data submitted to the Food and Drug Administration. Plos Medicine 5: 260–268.
28. Cuijpers P, Turner EH, Mohr DS, Hofmann SG, Andersoon G, et al. (2014) Comparison of psychotherapies for adult depression to pill placebo control groups: a meta-analysis. Psychological Medicine 44: 685–695.
29. Williams G, Nesse R (1991) The dawn of Darwinian medicine. Quarterly Review of Biology 66: 1–22.
30. Gluckman P, Beedle A, Hanson M (2009) Principles of evolutionary medicine. Oxford, UK: Oxford University Press.
31. Stevens A, Price J (2000) Evolutionary Psychiatry: A New Beginning: Routledge.
32. Brüne M (2008) Textbook of Evolutionary Psychiatry: The origins of psychopathology. New York: Oxford University Press.
33. Nesse RM (2000) Is depression an adaptation? Archives of General Psychiatry 57: 14–20.
34. Hagen EH (2011) Evolutionary theories of depression: a critical review. Canadian Journal of Psychiatry - Revue Canadienne de Psychiatrie 56: 716–726.
35. Andrews PW, Thomson JA (2009) The bright side of being blue: depression as an adaptation for analyzing complex problems. Psychological Review 116: 620–654.
36. Lyubomirsky S, Nolen-Hoeksema S (1993) Self-perpetuating properties of dysphoric rumination. Journal of Personality and Social Psychology 65: 339–349.
37. Nolen-Hoeksema S, Morrow J (1991) A prospective study of depression and posttraumatic stress symptoms after a natural disaster: the 1989 Loma Prieta Earthquake. Journal of Personality and Social Psychology 61: 115–121.
38. Nolen-Hoeksema S, Parker LE, Larson J (1994) Ruminative coping with depressed mood following loss. Journal of Personality and Social Psychology 67: 92–104.
39. Gut E (1985) Productive and Unproductive Depression: Interference in the Adaptive function of the Basic Depressed Response. British Journal of Psychotherapy 2: 95–113.
40. Martin L, Tesser A (1996) Some ruminative thoughts. In: Wyer J, Robert S, editors. Ruminative Thoughts Advances in Social Cognition. Hillsdale, New Jersey, England: Lawrence Erlbaum Associates. pp.1–47.
41. Papageorgiou C, Wells A (2001) Metacognitive beliefs about rumination in recurrent major depression. Cognitive and Behavioral Practice: 160–164.
42. Forgas J (1998) On being happy and mistaken: mood effects on the fundamental attribution error. Journal of Personality and Social Psychology 75.
43. Sinclair R (1998) Mood, categorization breadth, and performance appraisal: The effects of order of information acquisition and affective state on halo, accuracy, information retrieval. Organizational Behavior and Human Decision Processes 42: 22–46.
44. Sinclair RC, Mark MM (1995) The effects of mood state on judgemental accuracy: Processing strategy as a mechanism. Cognition and Emotion 9: 417–438.
45. Braverman J (2005) The effect of mood on detection of covariation. Personality & Social Psychology Bulletin 31: 1487–1497.
46. Storbeck J, Clore GL (2005) With sadness comes accuracy; with happiness, false memory: mood and the false memory effect. Psychological Science 16: 785–791.
47. Pietromonaco PR, Rook KS (1987) Decision style in depression: The contribution of perceived risks versus benefits. Journal of Personality and Social Psychology 52: 399–408.
48. Hertel G, Neuhof J, Theuer T, Kerr NL (2000) Mood effects on cooperation in small groups: Does positive mood simply lead to more cooperation? Cognition and Emotion 14: 441–472.
49. Au K, Chan G, Wang D, Vertinsky I (2003) Mood in foreign exchange trading: Cognitive processes and performance. Organizational Behavior and Human Decision Processes, 91: 322–338.
50. Smoski MJ, Lynch TR, Rosenthal MZ, Cheavens JS, Chapman AL, et al. (2008) Decision-making and risk aversion among depressive adults. Journal of Behavior Therapy and Experimental Psychiatry 39: 567–576.
51. Overall NC, Hammond MD (2013) Biased and accurate: depressive symptoms and daily perceptions within intimate relationships. Personality & Social Psychology Bulletin 39: 636–650.
52. von Helversen B, Wilke A, Johnson T, Schmid G, Klapp B (2011) Performance benefits of depression: sequential decision making in a healthy sample and a clinically depressed sample. Journal of Abnormal Psychology: 962–968.
53. Food and Drug Administration (2009) Patient reported outcome measure: use in medical product development to support labelling claims.
54. Mokkink LB, Terweea CB, Patrick D, Alonso J, Stratford JW, et al. (2010) The COSMIN study reached international consensus on taxonomy, terminology, and definitions of measurement properties for health-related patient-reported outcomes. Journal of Clinical Epidemiology 63: 737–745.
55. Streiner D, Norman G (2007) Health measurement scales: a practical guide to their development and use. Oxford: Oxford University Press.
56. Hobart JC, Cano SJ, Zajicek JP, Thompson AA (2007) Rating scales as outcome measures for clinical trials in neurology: problems, solutions, and recommendations. Lancet Neurology 6: 1094–1105.
57. Cronbach LJ (1951) Coefficient alpha and the internal structure of tests. Psychometrika 16: 297–334.
58. Beck AT, Ward CH, Mendelson M, Mock J, Erbaugh J (1961) An inventory for measuring depression. Archives of General Psychiatry 4: 561–571.
59. Watson D, Clark LA, Tellegen A (1988) Development and validation of brief measures of positive and negative affect: The PANAS scale. Journal of Personality and Social Psychology 54: 1063–1070.
60. Stone MH, Wright BD, Stenner AJ (1999) Mapping variables. Journal of Outcome Measurement 3: 308–322.
61. Marais I, Andrich D (2008) Effects of varying magnitude and patterns of response dependence in the unidimensional Rasch model. Journal of Applied Measurement 9: 105–124.
62. Sideridis GD (2011) The effects of local item dependence on estimates of ability in the Rasch Model. Rasch Measurement Transactions 25: 1334–1336.
63. Stenner AJ, Stone M, Burdick D (2011) How to model and test for the mechanisms that make measurement systems tick. Joint International IMEKO Jena, Germany.
64. Andrich D (2011) Rating Scales and Rasch Measurement. Expert Review of Pharmacoeconomics and Outcomes Research 11: 571–585.
65. Andrich D (1988) Rasch models for measurement. Beverly Hills: Sage Publications.
66. Andrich D, Sheridan B, Luo G RUMM 2030. 4.0 for windows (upgrade 4600.0109) edn Perth, WA. RUMM laboratory Pty Ltd 1997–2010.
67. Masters G (1982) A Rasch model for partial credit scoring. Psychometrika 47: 149–174.
68. Andrich D, Sheridan B, Luo G (2007) RUMM2020. Rasch unidimensional measurement models software. Perth, Western Australia: RUMM laboratory.
69. Andrich D (1982) An index of person separation in latent trait theory, the traditional KR20 index, and the Guttman scale response pattern. Educational Psychology Research 9: 95–104.
70. Nezu A (1986) Efficacy of a social problem-solving therapy approach for unipolar depression. Journal of Consulting and Clinical Psychology 54: 196–202.
71. Nezu A, Nezu C (2001) Problem solving therapy. Journal of Psychotherapy Integration 11.
72. Teasdale JD, Scott J, Moore R, Hayhurst H, Pope M, et al. (2001) How does cognitive therapy prevent relapse in residual depression? Evidence from a controlled trial. Journal of Consulting and Clinical Psychology 69: 347–357.
73. Hayes AM, Beevers CG, Feldman GC, Laurenceau J-P, Perlman C (2005) Avoidance and processing as predictors of symptom change and positive growth

in an integrative therapy for depression. International Journal of Behavioral Medicine 12.
74. Hayes AM, Feldman GC, Beevers CG, Laurenceau J-P, Cardaciotto L, et al. (2007) Discontinuities and cognitive changes in an exposure-based cognitive therapy for depression. Journal of Consulting and Clinical Psychology 75: 409–421.
75. Krpan KM, Kross E, Berman MG, Deldin PJ, Askren MK, et al. (2013) An everyday activity as a treatment for depression: the benefits of expressive writing for people diagnosed with major depressive disorder. Journal of Affective Disorders 150: 1148–1151.

11

Predictors of the Onset of Manic Symptoms and a (Hypo)Manic Episode in Patients with Major Depressive Disorder

Lynn Boschloo[1,2*], Annet T. Spijker[3], Erik Hoencamp[4,5], Ralph Kupka[2], Willem A. Nolen[1], Robert A. Schoevers[1], Brenda W. J. H. Penninx[1,2,6]

1 University of Groningen, University Medical Center Groningen (UMCG), Interdisciplinary Center Psychopathology and Emotion Regulation (ICPE)/University Center Psychiatry (UCP), Groningen, The Netherlands, **2** Vrije University Medical Center (VUMC), Department of Psychiatry and Extramuraal Geneeskundig Onderzoek (EMGO) Institute for Health and Care Research, Amsterdam, The Netherlands, **3** PsyQ, Department of Mood Disorders, The Hague, The Netherlands, **4** Parnassia Group, The Hague, The Netherlands, **5** Leiden University, Institute of Psychology, Leiden, The Netherlands, **6** Leiden University Medical Center, Department of Psychiatry, Leiden, The Netherlands

Abstract

Objective: One third of patients with a major depressive episode also experience manic symptoms or, even, a (hypo)manic episode. Retrospective studies on the temporal sequencing of symptomatology suggest that the majority of these patients report depressive symptoms before the onset of manic symptoms. However, prospective studies are scarce and this study will, therefore, prospectively examine the onset of either manic symptoms or a (hypo)manic episode in patients with a major depressive disorder. In addition, we will consider the impact of a large set of potential risk factors on both outcomes.

Methodology: Four-year follow-up data were used to determine the onset of manic symptoms as well as a CIDI-based (hypo)manic episode in a large sample (n = 889, age: 18–65 years) of outpatients with a major depressive disorder and without manic symptoms at baseline. Baseline vulnerability (i.e., sociodemographics, family history of depression, childhood trauma, life-events) and clinical (i.e., isolated manic symptoms, depression characteristics, and psychiatric comorbidity) factors were considered as potential risk factors.

Results: In our sample of depressed patients, 15.9% developed manic symptoms and an additional 4.7% developed a (hypo)manic episode during four years. Baseline isolated manic symptoms and comorbid alcohol dependence predicted both the onset of manic symptoms and a (hypo)manic episode. Low education only predicted the onset of manic symptoms, whereas male gender, childhood trauma and severity of depressive symptoms showed strong associations with, especially, the onset of (hypo)manic episodes.

Conclusions: A substantial proportion (20.6%) of patients with a major depressive disorder later developed manic symptoms or a (hypo)manic episode. Interestingly, some identified risk factors differed for the two outcomes, which may indicate that pathways leading to the onset of manic symptoms or a (hypo)manic episode might be different. Our findings indirectly support a clinical staging model.

Editor: James Bennett Potash, University of Iowa Hospitals & Clinics, United States of America

Funding: This study was supported by the Geestkracht program of the Netherlands Organization for Health Research and Development (A.T.F. Beekman; grant number 10-000-1002; www.zonmw.nl/en) and Astra Zeneca Nederland (ATS and EH; www.astrazeneca.nl). There was no additional funding for this specific study. LB and ATS were supported by Astra Zeneca; EH was supported by Astra Zeneca and Parnassia Group; RK was supported by Astra Zeneca, Lundbeck and Bristol Myers Squibb; WAN was supported by the Netherlands Organization for Health Research and Development, the European Union, the Stanley Medical Research Institute, Astra Zeneca, GlaxoSmithKline and Wyeth; BWJHP was supported by the Netherlands Organization for Health Research and Development; and, RAS did not report any funding. The funders had no role in study design, data collection and analysis, decision to publish, or preparation of the manuscript.

Competing Interests: LB and AS have received speaking fees and unrestricted grants from Astra Zeneca. EH has received an unrestricted grant from Astra Zeneca and is currently supported by Parnassia Group. RK has received unrestricted grants from Astra Zeneca and honoraria from Astra Zeneca, Lundbeck and Bristol Myers Squibb. WN has received unrestricted grants from the Netherlands Organization for Health Research and Development, the European Union, the Stanley Medical Research Institute, Astra Zeneca, GlaxoSmithKline and Wyeth; and has received honoraria/speaker's fees from Astra Zeneca and Lundbeck. BWJHP has received unrestricted grants from the Netherlands Organization for Health Research and Development.

* Email: L.Boschloo@umcg.nl

Introduction

Converging evidence from community and clinical studies support the high prevalence of manic symptoms as well as (hypo)manic episodes in patients with a major depressive episode [1–2]. For example, Angst et al. [2] showed that 35% of depressed patients reported manic symptoms and an additional 12% met criteria for a (hypo)manic episode. The clinical relevance of bipolarity has motivated the DSM-5 work group to not only include bipolar disorders but also a mixed features specifier for major depressive disorder in the new version of the DSM [3]. As bipolar disorder often starts with depressive episodes [4], this implies that the initial presence of a major depressive episode in the absence of manic symptoms or a (hypo)manic episode may be a critical phase and could therefore be a potential target for early intervention strategies.

As much is still unclear about the underlying processes, an essential next step would be to identify risk factors for the onset of manic symptoms as well as a (hypo)manic episode in depressed patients. Sociodemographics (e.g., male gender [5–6]) and other vulnerability factors (e.g., childhood trauma [7]) have shown to be more strongly related to bipolar disorder than to major depressive disorder. In addition, manic symptoms [1,8], depression characteristics (e.g., severity [10–11]) and psychiatric comorbidity (e.g., anxiety disorders or alcohol dependence [6]) are clinical factors that have been associated with bipolarity in depressed patients. As only few prospective studies have considered both the onset of manic symptoms and the onset of a (hypo)manic, it is still unclear whether risk factors differ for these outcomes.

Therefore, the present study focuses on the onset of manic symptoms as well as a (hypo)manic episode during four years of follow-up in a large sample of patients with a lifetime major depressive disorder and so far without significant lifetime manic symptoms at baseline (n = 889). We will examine whether several vulnerability and clinical factors *independently* predict the onset of manic symptoms or a (hypo)manic episode and it was, additionally, tested whether risk factors differ for these two outcomes.

Methods

Study sample

Data were derived from the Netherlands Study of Depression and Anxiety (NESDA), an ongoing cohort study aimed at examining the long-term course and consequences of depressive and anxiety disorders in the adult (18–65 years) population. A total of 2,981 persons were included at the baseline assessment in 2004–2007, consisting of healthy controls (22%) and patients with a lifetime depressive and/or anxiety disorder (78%). To represent various settings and stages of psychopathology, persons were recruited from the community (19%), primary care (54%) and outpatient mental health care services (27%). Community-based participants had previously been identified in a population-based study; primary care participants were identified through a three-stage screening procedure (involving the Kessler-10 [11] and the short-form Composite International Diagnostic Interview [CIDI] psychiatric interview by phone) conducted among a random sample of patients of 65 General Practitioners; and mental health care participants were recruited consecutively when newly enrolled at one of the 17 participating mental health organization locations. Persons with insufficient command of the Dutch language or a primary clinical diagnosis of bipolar disorder, obsessive compulsive disorder, severe substance use disorder, psychotic disorder or organic psychiatric disorder, as reported by them or their (mental) health practitioner, were excluded. A detailed description of the NESDA study design and sampling procedures can be found elsewhere [12]. The research protocol was approved by the Ethical Committee of participating universities and all participants provided written informed consent.

The baseline assessment consisted of an extended face-to-face interview, including a standardized diagnostic psychiatric interview, and paper-and-pencil questionnaires. For the present study, we selected patients with a lifetime DSM-IV major depressive disorder (n = 1,925), as assessed with the CIDI (version 2.1) at baseline. The CIDI is highly reliable and valid [13] and was administered by specially trained research staff. To examine the onset of manic symptoms as well as a (hypo)manic episode, we aimed to exclude all patients with significant lifetime manic symptoms at baseline. Unfortunately, the CIDI section on bipolar disorders was not conducted at baseline and, consequently, it was not possible to determine whether patients met criteria for a DSM-IV bipolar disorder at baseline. However, patients with a self-reported or health care professional-reported primary clinical diagnosis of bipolar disorder had already been excluded for the initial participation in NESDA. In addition, we excluded all patients with lifetime manic symptoms (n = 581) as assessed with the Mood Disorder Questionnaire (MDQ [14–15]) or with missing data on this measure (n = 274) at baseline. The MDQ is a fifteen-item self-report questionnaire comprising thirteen dichotomous items on the lifetime presence or absence of manic symptoms as well as two additional questions regarding the clustering of symptoms in time and severity of related problems. We considered lifetime manic symptoms to be present when a patient reported at least seven positive answers from the thirteen items, irrespective of the answers on the two additional questions. Our group [16] recently showed that this cut-off is especially adequate in detecting a recent (i.e. past two years) (hypo)manic episode (sensitivity = 0.83 and specificity = 0.82).

In addition to the baseline assessment, follow-up assessments were conducted after two years (overall response rate: 87.1% [17]) and four years (overall response rate: 80.6%). In the subsample of 1,070 participants with a lifetime MDD and without lifetime manic symptoms at baseline, 181 (16.9%) did not provide complete data at the two-year or four-year follow-up assessments, resulting in a sample of 889 patients for the current analyses. Non-responders were significantly less educated (11.7 versus 12.4 years of education, p = 0.01) compared to responders, whereas gender (p = 0.47) and age (p = 0.45) were not associated with non-response.

Measures

Outcome variables. In our sample, we considered the onset of manic symptoms as well as a (hypo)manic episode during four years of follow-up. The onset of manic symptoms was based on the presence of seven or more positive answers on the MDQ at the two-year or four-year follow-up assessment, in the absence of a (hypo)manic episode. The onset of a (hypo)manic episode was based on the presence of a DSM-IV hypomanic or manic episode as assessed with the CIDI section on bipolar disorders at the two- or four-year follow-up assessment.

Baseline predictors. On the basis of previously reported associations with manic symptoms or a (hypo)manic episode, an extensive set of potential predictors (i.e., vulnerability and clinical factors) was selected.

1. Vulnerability factors included sociodemographics, family history of depressive disorder, childhood trauma and life-events at baseline.

a. Sociodemographics included gender, age (in years) and education (in years).
b. Family history of a unipolar or bipolar depressive episode was assessed with the family tree method [18], which obtains information on the presence of psychiatric disorders among first-degree relatives (not including offspring of the patient).
c. Based on the Childhood Trauma Inventory, a cumulative childhood trauma index (range: 0–8) was constructed considering the frequency (never = 0, once/sometimes = 1, often or more = 2) of emotional neglect, psychological abuse, physical abuse and sexual abuse before the age of 16 years [19].
d. A total count of twelve negative life events in the past year was constructed using Brugha's List of Threatening Experiences [20].

2. Clinical factors included isolated manic symptoms, various depression characteristics and psychiatric comorbidity at baseline.

a. The number of isolated manic symptoms was defined as the count of the thirteen dichotomous MDQ items on the lifetime presence or absence of manic symptoms. As patients with a total score of seven or higher were already excluded (see sample description), the number of isolated manic symptoms ranged from zero to six.
b. From the depression characteristics, we first considered the age (in years) of onset of major depressive disorder as based on CIDI questions regarding the onset of a lifetime diagnosis at the baseline assessment. We also considered whether patients had experienced recurrent episodes versus a single episode during their life. The severity of depressive symptoms in the week prior to baseline was defined as the total score on the 30-item self-report Inventory of Depressive Symptomatology (IDS) [21]. We also determined whether the disorder had atypical features as assessed by specific IDS items. The atypical subtype was defined as having mood reactivity and at least three of the following: increased appetite, hypersomnia, leaden paralysis, and interpersonal rejection sensitivity [22]. Sleep duration was based on the average number of hours of sleep per night during the month prior to baseline by distinguishing short (≤6 hours) versus normal (>6 hours) duration.
c. Psychiatric comorbidity was assessed by the CIDI interview separately considering lifetime diagnoses of any anxiety disorder (i.e., generalized anxiety disorder, social phobia, panic disorder, and agoraphobia) and alcohol dependence.

Statistical analyses

Analyses were conducted using SPSS version 20 statistical software (SPSS Inc, Chicago, Illinois). In our sample of patients with major depressive disorder and without significant lifetime manic symptoms, we first determined the onset of manic symptoms and a (hypo)manic episode. Then, descriptive statistics were used to summarize the sample characteristics across these groups. To identify independent risk factors (i.e., vulnerability and clinical factors) of each outcome, multinomial logistic regression analyses were performed in which predictors with a p≤0.05 in univariable analyses were entered into one multivariable analysis. To provide insight into the nature of these associations, results of the univariable as well as multivariable analyses were shown. Additional logistic regression analyses were performed to test whether predictors showed differential associations with the onset of manic symptoms versus a (hypo)manic episode. To be able to compare odds ratios across all continuous factors, odds ratios with 95% confidence intervals were expressed per standard deviation increase.

Results

Sample characteristics

In our sample of patients with lifetime major depressive disorder and without significant lifetime manic symptoms at baseline (n = 889), the mean age was 43.0 (SD = 12.4; range = 18–65) years and 26.9% were men. Figure 1 shows that the onset was 15.9% (n = 141) for manic symptoms (i.e., at least seven positive items on the MDQ) and 4.7% (n = 42) for a DSM-IV hypomanic (n = 17) or manic (n = 25) episode during four years of follow-up. To provide more information about prodromal stages of bipolar disorder patients with a (hypo)manic episode during follow-up were asked about their age during which they first developed several manic symptoms. The onset of manic symptoms preceded the onset of a (hypo)manic episode with an average of 12.7 (SD = 13.9) years. This also implies that the majority (69%) of patients with a (hypo)manic episode reported the onset of first manic symptoms before the baseline assessment. Among patients with only manic symptoms but no (hypo)manic episodes during follow-up, no information about the age of onset of their first manic symptoms was available as this was not considered in the MDQ.

Predictors of the onset of manic symptoms or a (hypo)manic episode

Descriptive statistics (Table 1) are presented in order to explore the role of vulnerability and clinical factors as predictors of the onset of manic symptoms and a (hypo)manic episode, respectively. To identify independent risk factors, a multivariable multinomial logistic regression analysis was performed including all predictors with a p≤0.05 in the univariable analyses (both results are presented in Table 2).

Vulnerability factors. From the sociodemographics, male gender was a significant risk factor for the onset of both manic

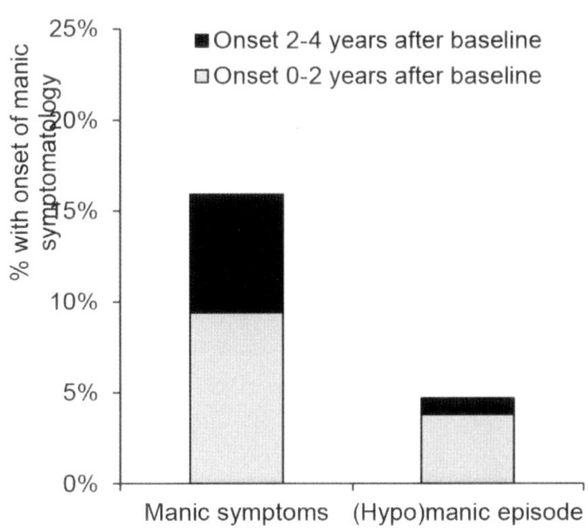

Figure 1. The onset of manic symptoms as well as a (hypo)manic episode during four years of follow-up.

Table 1. Sample characteristics.

		Onset of manic symptomatology	
		Manic	(Hypo)manic
	Unipolar depression	symptoms	episode
	(n = 706)	(n = 141)	(n = 42)
	Mean (sd)/%	Mean (sd)/%	Mean (sd)/%
Vulnerability factors			
Gender (male)	23.8%	35.5%	57.1%
Age in years	43.1 (12.6)	42.3 (11.9)	43.5 (11.2)
Education in years	12.6 (3.2)	11.4 (3.1)	11.8 (3.5)
Family history of depressive disorder (yes)	71.7%	78.7%	78.6%
Severity of childhood trauma	1.6 (2.0)	1.8 (2.2)	2.9 (2.3)
Number of life events	0.8 (1.0)	0.8 (1.0)	0.9 (1.2)
Clinical factors			
Number of manic symptoms	3.0 (1.9)	4.3 (1.7)	4.2 (1.6)
Age of onset of MDD	28.5 (12.6)	28.2 (12.2)	28.2 (12.3)
Recurrent MDD (yes)	53.4%	50.4%	45.2%
Severity of depressive symptoms	21.7 (12.9)	26.2 (13.0)	33.4 (11.7)
Atypical depression subtype (yes)	9.6%	12.1%	26.2%
Short sleep duration (yes)	30.9%	30.5%	50.0%
Anxiety disorder (yes)	65.0%	69.5%	71.4%
Alcohol dependence (yes)	11.8%	19.9%	26.2%

symptoms and a (hypo)manic episode, even after adjustment for other important vulnerability and clinical factors. Logistic regression analyses additionally showed that this association was stronger for a (hypo)manic episode than for manic symptoms. Low education was only independently related with manic symptoms, whereas childhood trauma was only independently associated with a (hypo)manic episode. None of the other vulnerability factors predicted the onset of manic symptomatology.

Clinical factors. The total number of isolated manic symptoms (i.e., no more than six positive items on the MDQ) was a strong and independent predictor of the onset of manic symptoms as well as a (hypo)manic episode. These associations were similar for both outcomes, which was also illustrated in Figure 2 showing comparable dose-response relationships. In addition, severity of depressive symptoms was an independent predictor of both manic symptoms and (hypo)manic episodes. However, logistic regression analyses additionally showed that this association was stronger for the onset of a (hypo)manic episode compared to manic symptoms (see also Figure 3). Atypical features of depression and a short sleep duration were related to the onset of a (hypo)manic episode in the univariable but not the multivariable analyses, whereas none of the other depression characteristics showed a significant association with the onset of manic symptomatology. Comorbid alcohol dependence, but not a comorbid anxiety disorder, was a significant predictor of both outcomes in the univariable analyses. Although this association remained significant for the onset of manic symptoms in the multivariable analyses, the association with the onset of a (hypo)manic episode only reached a borderline significance level.

Discussion

Main findings

The present study aimed to improve our knowledge about the onset of manic symptoms as well as (hypo)manic episodes in patients with a lifetime major depressive disorder and without significant lifetime manic symptoms at baseline. During the subsequent four years, 15.9% of patients had developed manic symptoms and an additional 4.7% had developed a DSM-IV hypomanic or manic episode. Our study also identified several independent risk factors for the onset of manic symptoms and a (hypo)manic episode and showed that some of these factors played differential roles for the two outcomes.

Clinical staging models for bipolar disorders

Our study showed that a substantial proportion (i.e., 20.6%) of patients with a diagnosis of major depressive disorder developed manic symptoms or a (hypo)manic episode during the subsequent four years. The presence of isolated manic symptoms was the most important risk factor for both outcomes, which is in line with a recent study demonstrating that these symptoms are a precursor of a later (hypo)manic episode [8]. In addition, patients who had developed a (hypo)manic episode during follow-up retrospectively reported that the presence of manic symptoms had preceded the onset of the full-blown episode with an average of thirteen years. These findings support a clinical staging model in which manic symptoms may increase over time and eventually result in a (hypo)manic episode [23–26].

Our findings further showed that depression severity was an important risk factor for the onset of manic symptoms and,

Table 2. Vulnerability and clinical factors predicting the onset of manic symptoms as well as a (hypo)manic episode during four-year follow-up.

	Unadjusted[a]						Adjusted[b]						
	Manic symptoms			(Hypo)manic episode			Manic symptoms			(Hypo)manic episode			
	OR	95%CI	p	OR	95%CI	p	OR	95%CI	p	OR	95%CI	p	p[c]
Vulnerability factors													
Gender (male)	1.76	1.20–2.59	0.004	4.27	2.26–8.06	<0.001	1.54	1.01–2.34	0.04	5.17	2.52–10.59	<0.001	0.01
Age in years[d]	0.94	0.79–1.13	0.50	1.03	0.76–1.41	0.83	-	-	-	-	-	-	-
Education in years[d]	0.68	0.56–0.82	<0.001	0.79	0.57–1.08	0.13	0.77	0.62–0.94	0.01	1.00	0.72–1.41	0.98	0.13
FH of depressive disorder (yes)	1.46	0.95–2.26	0.09	1.45	0.68–3.08	0.34	-	-	-	-	-	-	-
Severity of childhood trauma[d]	1.09	0.91–1.31	0.33	1.74	1.33–2.28	<0.001	0.99	0.81–1.20	0.88	1.53	1.13–2.08	0.005	0.03
No. of life events[d]	1.02	0.86–1.23	0.80	1.10	0.82–1.48	0.52	-	-	-	-	-	-	
Clinical factors													
No. of isolated manic symptoms[d]	2.13	1.72–2.63	<0.001	2.06	1.44–2.95	<0.001	1.98	1.60–2.48	<0.001	1.74	1.17–2.60	0.006	0.90
Age of onset of MDD	0.97	0.81–1.17	0.76	0.97	0.71–1.33	0.86	-	-	-	-	-	-	
Recurrent MDD (yes)	0.89	0.62–1.27	0.51	0.72	0.39–1.35	0.31	-	-	-	-	-	-	
Severity of depressive symptoms[d]	1.42	1.18–1.69	<0.001	2.34	1.72–3.18	<0.001	1.33	1.06–1.68	0.01	1.85	1.24–2.74	0.002	0.048
Atypical subtype (yes)	1.29	0.73–2.26	0.38	3.33	1.60–6.92	0.001	0.73	0.38–1.42	0.35	1.60	0.63–4.04	0.32	0.34
Short sleep duration (yes)	0.98	0.66–1.45	0.93	2.24	1.20–4.19	0.01	0.70	0.45–1.08	0.11	1.15	0.57–2.33	0.70	0.28
Anxiety disorder (yes)	1.23	0.83–1.81	0.31	1.35	0.68–2.67	0.40	-	-	-	-	-	-	-
Alcohol dependence (yes)	1.86	1.16–2.98	0.01	2.66	1.29–5.50	0.008	1.74	1.05–2.90	0.03	1.80	0.81–4.01	0.15	0.94

[a]= Unadjusted analyses, based on univariable multinomial logistic regression analyses.
[b]= Adjusted analyses, based on multivariable multinomial logistic regression analyses including all variables that had $p \leq 0.05$ in the univariable analyses.
[c]= Based on multivariable logistic regression analyses directly comparing patients developing manic symptoms with patients developing a (hypo)manic episode, including all variables that had $p \leq 0.05$ in the univariable analyses.
[d]= For continuous variables, ORs are presented per SD increase.

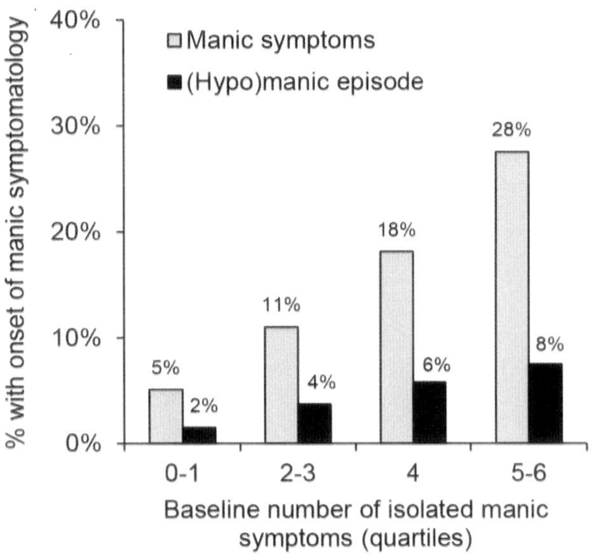

Figure 2. Baseline number of isolated manic symptoms predicting the onset of manic symptoms as well as a (hypo)manic episode during four years of follow-up.

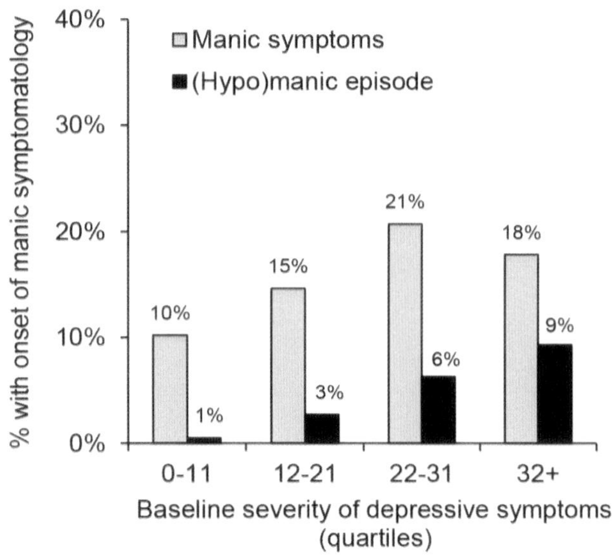

Figure 3. Baseline severity of depressive symptoms predicting the onset of manic symptomatology during four years of follow-up.

especially, a (hypo)manic episode. This is in line with previous studies on bipolar disorders [2,9–10] and, again, supports a clinical staging model in which patients with a major depressive disorder, and especially those who have progressed to a more severe subtype, have an increased risk of developing manic symptoms or a (hypo)manic episode [23–26]. This was also indirectly supported by our finding that comorbid alcohol dependence was a risk factor for both outcomes. The presence of alcohol dependence is known to be especially high in severe subtypes of major depressive disorder [27] and, as expected, reported associations with manic symptoms or a (hypo)manic episode decreased substantially after adjustment for baseline depression severity. Nonetheless, comorbid alcohol dependence could be an important indicator for both outcomes and screening instruments, such as the Alcohol Use Disorders Identification Test [28–29], may help to identify these high risk patients.

Onset rates of (hypo)manic episodes

In our sample of depressed outpatients, an average of 1.2% had developed a (hypo)manic episode per year during follow-up. This annual onset rate is smaller than, for example, the 2.8% that was observed in depressed outpatients in Finland [10] and the 3.1% in hospitalized inpatients in the United States [30]. These contrasting findings may be explained by methodological differences. Our study, for example, excluded all patients with significant manic symptoms at baseline, as assessed with a screening instrument for manic symptoms. In contrast, the two previous studies excluded patients with a (hypo)manic episode, as assessed with a clinical interview, but did not consider baseline manic symptoms [10,30]. Consequently, these samples may have included some patients with subthreshold manic symptoms, which could have resulted in higher onset rates of (hypo)manic episodes.

In addition, primary diagnoses of obsessive compulsive disorder, severe substance use disorder or psychotic disorder were all exclusion criteria for our study, but not for the two previous studies. As some of these factors might be risk factors for the onset of manic symptoms or a (hypo)manic episode [8,30], onset rates in these studies are likely to be higher. An additional methodological difference is that our sample consisted of adults with a mean age of 43.0 years, which is comparable to the 40.2 years in the study of Holma et al. [10] but is much older than the 23.0 years in the sample of Goldberg et al. [30]. Although the majority of bipolar disorders typically develops earlier in life (i.e., before the age of 30 years), an additional peak of onset rates has been observed between 35 and 45 years of age [31]. The development of a (hypo)manic episode in our study should therefore be considered as a late-onset (hypo)manic episode and may be different from (hypo)manic episodes that develop earlier in life [31–32] (see also the 'Risk factors' section).

Risk factors

Our study is unique in simultaneously examining the independent effects of several clinical as well as vulnerability factors on the onset of manic symptoms versus a (hypo)manic episode. From the clinical factors, the number of isolated manic symptoms and comorbid alcohol dependence tend to show similar associations with the onset of manic symptoms and a (hypo)manic episode, which may indicate that these factors play similar roles. However, the severity of depressive symptoms may be more important for the onset of a (hypo)manic episode compared to manic symptoms as the association with the first was stronger than with the latter. A similar pattern was found for male gender, as a vulnerability factor, which was an independent risk factor for the onset of manic symptoms and, especially, for a (hypo)manic episode. This is in line with previous studies showing that patients with increasing manic symptomatology were more often male [1,5–6,33]. We also found that childhood trauma independently predicted the onset of a (hypo)manic episode, which corroborates previous cross-sectional findings [7], but not the onset of manic symptoms. In contrast, low education predicted the onset of manic symptoms, but not a (hypo)manic episode. Although more research is needed, these findings are intriguing as they may indicate that processes underlying the onset of manic symptoms or the onset of a (hypo)manic episode might be different.

Our study also showed that family history of depressive disorders as well as an early onset of MDD were not related to the onset of manic symptoms or a (hypo)manic episode. This contradicts the findings of previous studies showing strong associations between these factors and bipolar disorder [8–10]. As genetic vulnerability may be more important for early-onset compared to late-onset bipolarity [31–32], this may explain the non-significant findings of our study mainly focussing on late-onset manic symptoms or a (hypo)manic episode. Future studies including both younger and older patients are necessary to determine whether etiological pathways for the development of early- versus late-onset manic symptoms or a (hypo)manic episode indeed differ.

Strengths and limitations

Our study has both strengths and limitations. Methodological strengths are that we were one of the first studies that could prospectively examine the onset of manic symptoms as well as a (hypo)manic episode. In addition, we included a large sample (n = 889) of patients with a DSM-IV diagnosis of major depressive disorder without lifetime manic symptoms at baseline and tested the independent effects of several potential risk factors. Although we assessed various potential predictors of manic symptomatology, we did not have information about some well-known risk factors such as a family history of bipolar disorder [8–9] or psychotic symptoms [8,30]. Although these factors may be less important for late-onset manic symptoms or (hypo)manic episodes (i.e. focus of our study) [31–32], we would like to encourage future researchers to gather this information, also in older samples of depressed patients.

Another important limitation is that the CIDI section on bipolar disorders was not conducted at baseline and, consequently, information about DSM-IV (hypo)manic episodes was not available at that time. However, patients with a baseline self-reported or health care professional-reported diagnosis of bipolar disorder were excluded from the study as well as patients with significant lifetime manic symptoms as assessed with the MDQ. Previous studies have shown mixed results regarding the validity of the MDQ (see [34] for a thorough review of the literature) and these inconsistencies might have resulted from recall bias (a patient's recall of recent symptoms is likely to be more reliable than recall of symptoms earlier in life). This was also demonstrated by a recent study of our group, in which we showed that the MDQ was adequate for detecting recent (hypo)manic episodes but not for lifetime episodes [16]. Consequently, our sample may have included some patients with a history of manic symptoms or, even, a (hypo)manic episode and this might have impacted our results. On the other hand, our sample may be similar to depressed patients in clinical practice as a history of manic symptoms or a (hypo)manic episode is often not recognized by patients or health care professionals [35–36]. The time lag between initial help seeking and the correct diagnosis is often more than ten years [37,38] and, therefore, misdiagnosis of bipolar disorder is a major problem for both clinicians and researchers.

Conclusions

In conclusion, 15.9% of patients with a major depressive disorder had developed manic symptoms and an additional 4.7% had developed a (hypo)manic episode during four years of follow-up. The number of isolated manic symptoms at baseline was an important, independent predictor of both stages in the development of bipolar disorder. This study also identified several other independent risk factors and demonstrated that some risk factors were different for the two outcomes.

Acknowledgments

We appreciate and would like to thank the Netherlands Organization for Health Research and Development that funded the Netherlands Study of Depression and Anxiety (NESDA), and all the participating universities and mental health care organizations. We are grateful to all participants who gave their time and support to participate in the study.

Author Contributions

Conceived and designed the experiments: LB AS EH RK WN RS BP. Performed the experiments: LB RS BP. Analyzed the data: LB. Contributed reagents/materials/analysis tools: LB. Wrote the paper: LB AS EH RK WN RS BP.

References

1. Zimmermann P, Brückl T, Nocon A, Pfister H, Lieb R, et al. (2009) Heterogeneity of DSM-IV major depressive disorder as a consequence of subthreshold bipolarity. Archives of General Psychiatry 66: 1341–1352.
2. Angst J, Cui L, Swendsen J, Rothen S, Cravchik A, et al. (2010) Major depressive disorder with subthreshold bipolarity in the National Comorbidity Survey Replication. American Journal of Psychiatry 67: 1194–1201.
3. American Psychiatric Association (2013) Diagnostic and Statistical Manual of mental disorders, 5th edition. Washington: American Psychiatric Association.
4. Mesman E, Nolen WA, Reichart CG, Wals M, Hillegers MH (2013) The Dutch Offspring Study: 12-year follow-up. American Journal of Psychiatry 170: 542–549.
5. Mantere O, Melartin TK, Suominen K, Rytsälä HJ, Valtonen HM, et al. (2006) Differences in Axis I and II comorbidity between bipolar I and II disorders and major depressive disorder. Journal of Clinical Psychiatry 67: 584–593.
6. Jabben N, Penninx BW, Beekman AT, Smit JH, Nolen WA (2011) Co-occurring manic symptomatology as a dimension which may help explaining heterogeneity of depression. Journal of Affective Disorders 131: 224–232.
7. Hyun M, Friedman SD, Dunner L (2000) Relationship of childhood physical and sexual abuse to adult bipolar disorder. Bipolar Disorders 2: 131–135.
8. Fiedorowicz JG, Endicott J, Leon AC, Solomon DA, Keller MB, et al. (2011) Subthreshold hypomanic symptoms in progression from unipolar major depression to bipolar disorder. American Journal of Psychiatry 168: 40–48.
9. Akiskal HS, Maser JD, Zeller PJ, Endicott J, Coryell W, et al. (1995) Switching from 'unipolar' to bipolar II. An 11-year prospective study of clinical and temperamental predictors in 559 patients. Archives of General Psychiatry 52: 114–123.
10. Holma KM, Melartin TK, Holma IAK, Isometsä ET (2008) Predictors for switch from unipolar major depressive disorder to bipolar disorder type I or II: A 5-year prospective study. Journal of Clinical Psychiatry 69: 1267–1275.
11. Kessler RC, Berglund P, Demler O, Jin R, Merikangas KR, et al. (2005) Lifetime prevalence and age-of-onset distributions of DSM-IV Disorders in the National Comorbidity Survey Replication. Archives of General Psychiatry 62: 593–602.
12. Penninx BW, Beekman AT, Smit JH, Zitman FG, Nolen WA, et al. (2008) The Netherlands Study of Depression and Anxiety (NESDA): rationale, objectives and methods. International Journal of Methods in Psychiatric Research 17: 121–140.
13. Wittchen HU, Robins LN, Cottler LB, Sartorius N, Burke JD, et al. (1991) Cross-cultural feasibility, reliability and sources of variance of the Composite International Diagnostic Interview (CIDI). The Multicentre WHO/ADAMHA Field Trials. The British Journal of Psychiatry 159: 645–653, 658.
14. Hirschfeld RM, Williams JB, Spitzer RL, Calabrese JR, Flynn L, et al. (2000) Development and validation of a screening instrument for bipolar spectrum disorder: the Mood Disorder Questionnaire. American Journal of Psychiatry 157: 1873–1875.
15. Hirschfeld RM (2002) The Mood Disorder Questionnaire: a simple, patient-rated screening instrument for bipolar disorder. Primary care companion to the Journal of Clinical Psychiatry 4: 9–11.
16. Boschloo L, Nolen WA, Spijker AT, Hoencamp E, Kupka R, et al. (2013) The Mood Disorder Questionnaire (MDQ) for detecting (hypo)manic episodes: Its validity an impact of recall bias. Journal of Affective Disorders 151: 203–208.
17. Lamers F, Hoogendoorn AW, Smit JH, Van Dyck R, Zitman FG, et al. (2012) Sociodemographic and psychiatric determinants of attrition in the Netherlands Study of Depression and Anxiety (NESDA). Comprehensive Psychiatry 53, 63–70.
18. Fyer AJ, Weissman MM (1999) Genetic linkage study of panic: clinical methodology and description of pedigrees. American Journal on Medical Genetics 88: 173–181.
19. Wiersma JE, Hovens JG, Van Oppen P, Giltay EJ, Van Schaik DJ, et al. (2009) The importance of childhood trauma and childhood life events for chronicity of depression in adults. Journal of Clinical Psychiatry 70: 983–989.

20. Brugha T, Bebbington P, Tennant C, Hurry J (1985) The List of Threatening Experiences: a subset of 12 life event categories with considerable long-term contextual threat. Psychological Medicine 15: 189–194.
21. Rush AJ, Gullion CM, Basco MR, Jarrett RB, Trivedi MH (1996) The Inventory of Depressive Symptomatology (IDS): psychometric properties. Psychological Medicine 26: 477–486.
22. Novick JS, Stewart JW, Wisniewski SR, Cook IA, Manev R, et al. (2005) Clinical and demographic features of atypical depression in outpatients with major depressive disorder: preliminary findings from STAR*D. Journal of Clinical Psychiatry 66, 1002–1011.
23. Berk M, Conus P, Lucas N, Hallam K, Malhi GS, et al. (2007) Setting the stage: from prodrome to treatment resistance in bipolar disorder. Bipolar Disorders 9: 671–678.
24. Conus P, Ward J, Hallam KT, Lucas N, Macneil C, et al. (2008) The proximal prodrome to first episode mania – a new target for early intervention. Bipolar Disorders 10: 555–565.
25. Kapczinski F, Dias VV, Kauer-Sant'Anna M, Brietzke E, Vázquez GH, et al. (2009) The potential use of biomarkers as an adjunctive tool for staging bipolar disorder. Prog Neuropsychopharmacol Biol Psychiatry 33: 1366–1371.
26. Scott J, Leboyer M, Hickie I, Berk M, Kapczinski F, et al. (2013) Clinical staging in psychiatry: a cross-cutting model of diagnosis with heuristic and practical value. The British Journal of Psychiatry 202: 243–245.
27. Boschloo L, Vogelzangs N, Van den Brink W, Smit JH, Veltman DJ, et al. (2013) Depressive and anxiety disorders predicting first incidence of alcohol use disorders: results of the Netherlands Study of Depression and Anxiety. Journal of Clinical Psychiatry 74: 1233–1240.
28. Babor TF, Fuente JRDI, Saunders J, Grant M (1992) The Alcohol Use Disorders Identification Test: Guidelines for Use in Primary Health Care. Geneva, World Health Organization.
29. Boschloo L, Vogelzangs N, Smit JH, Van den Brink W, Veltman DJ, et al. (2010) The performance of the Alcohol Use Disorder Identification Test (AUDIT) in detecting alcohol abuse and dependence in a population of depressed or anxious persons. Journal of Affective Disorders 126: 441–446.
30. Goldberg JF, Harrow M, Whiteside JE (2001) Risk for bipolar illness in patients initially hospitalized for unipolar depression. American Journal of Psychiatry 158: 1265–1270.
31. Schürhoff F, Bellivier F, Jouvent R, Mouren-Siméoni M, Bouvard M, et al. (2000) Early and late onset bipolar disorders: two different forms of manic-depressive illness. Journal of Affective Disorders 58: 215–221.
32. Hays JC, Krishnan KR, George LK, Blazer DG (1998) Age of first onset of bipolar disorder: demographic, family history, and psychosocial correlates. Depression and Anxiety 7: 76–82
33. Bowden CL (2005) A different depression: clinical distinctions between bipolar and unipolar depression. Journal of Affective Disorders 84: 117–125.
34. Zimmerman M, Galione JN (2011) Screening for bipolar disorder with the Mood Disorders Questionnaire: a review. Harvard Review of Psychiatry 19: 219–228.
35. Angst J (2006) Do many patients with depression suffer from bipolar disorder. Canadian Journal of Psychiatry 51: 3–5.
36. Angst J, Azorin JM, Bowden CL, Perugi G, Vieta E, et al. (2011) Prevalence and characteristics of undiagnosed bipolar disorders in patients with a major depressive episode: the BRIDGE study. Archives of General Psychiatry 68: 791–198.
37. Lish JD, Dime-Meenam S, Whybrow PC, Price RA, Hirschfeld RMA (1994) The National Depressive and Manic-Depressive Association (DMDA) survey of bipolar disorders. Journal of Affective Disorders 31: 281–294.
38. Hirschfeld RMA, Lewis L, Vornik LA (2003) Perceptions and impact of bipolar disorder: how far have we really come? Results of the National Depressive and Manic-Depressive Association 2000 Survey of Individuals With Bipolar Disorder. Journal of Clinical Psychiatry 64: 161–174.

Delineation of Early and Later Adult Onset Depression by Diffusion Tensor Imaging

Yuqi Cheng[1]*, Jian Xu[2]*, Hongjun Yu[3], Binbin Nie[4], Na Li[1], Chunrong Luo[3], Haijun Li[3], Fang Liu[1], Yan Bai[1], Baoci Shan[4], Lin Xu[5]*, Xiufeng Xu[1]*

1 Department of Psychiatry, First Affiliated Hospital of Kunming Medical University, Kunming, PR China, **2** Department of Internal Medicine, First Affiliated Hospital of Kunming Medical University, Kunming, PR China, **3** Magnetic Resonance Imaging Center, the First Hospital of Kunming City, Kunming, PR China, **4** Key Laboratory of Nuclear Analysis Techniques, Institute of High Energy Physics, Chinese Academy of Sciences, Beijing, PR China, **5** Key Laboratory of Animal Models and Human Disease Mechanisms, Chinese Academy of Sciences & Yunnan Province, Kunming Institute of Zoology, Kunming, PR China

Abstract

Background: Due to a lack of evidence, there is no consistent age of onset to define early onset (EO) versus later onset (LO) major depressive disorder (MDD). Fractional anisotropy (FA), derived from diffusion tensor imaging (DTI), has been widely used to study neuropsychiatric disorders by providing information about the brain circuitry, abnormalities of which might facilitate the delineation of EO versus LO MDD.

Method: In this study, 61 pairs of untreated, non-elderly, first-episode MDD patients and healthy controls (HCs) aged 18–45 years old received DTI scans. The voxel-based analysis method (VBM), classification analysis, using the Statistical Package for the Social Sciences (SPSS), and regression analyses were used to determine abnormal FA clusters and their correlations with age of onset and clinical symptoms.

Results: Classification analysis suggested in the best model that there were two subgroups of MDD patients, delineated by an age of onset of 30 years old, by which MDD patients could be divided into EO (18–29 years old) and LO (30–45 years old) groups. LO MDD was characterized by decreased FA, especially in the white matter (WM) of the fronto-occipital fasciculus and posterior limb of internal capsule, with a negative correlation with the severity of depressive symptoms; in marked contrast, EO MDD showed increased FA, especially in the WM of the corpus callosum, corticospinal midbrain and inferior fronto-occipital fasciculus, while FA of the WM near the midbrain had a positive correlation with the severity of depressive symptoms.

Conclusion: Specific abnormalities of the brain circuitry in EO vs. LO MDD were delineated by an age of onset of 30 years old, as demonstrated by distinct abnormal FA clusters with opposite correlations with clinical symptoms. This DTI study supported the evidence of an exact age for the delineation of MDD, which could have broad multidisciplinary importance.

Editor: Yiru Fang, Shanghai Mental Health Center, Shanghai Jiao Tong University School of Medicine, China

Funding: This work is supported by grants from National Natural Science Foundation of China (81101005, 81160379, 81160171, U1032605, and 81161120536), the 973 Program from the Ministry of Science and Technology of China (2009CB941300), Yunnan Provincial Health Science and Technology Plan (2011WS008), the NSFC-Yunnan Joint Foundation (U1032605), and the united founding of Yunnan Administration of Science & Technology and Kunming Medical University (2011FB167). The funders had no role in study design, data collection and analysis, decision to publish, or preparation of the manuscript.

Competing Interests: The authors have declared that no competing interests exist.

* Email: lxu@vip.163.com (LX); xfxu2004@sina.com (XX)

These authors contributed equally to this work.

Introduction

Major depressive disorder (MDD) is well known for its clinical heterogeneity, including variability in the age of onset, constellations of depressive symptoms, and disease severity and course [1]. This heterogeneity has been believed to be one of the greatest barriers to successful treatment of MDD because it has been assumed to be attributable to different etiologies and pathophysiologies [2], for which MDD patients would require different treatments, and based on which patients would have different responses to the same treatment. Unfortunately, evidence is still lacking for defining the heterogeneity of MDD.

Genetic studies might have provided molecular evidence for the heterogeneity of MDD. Twin studies have estimated the average heritability of MDD at approximately 40% [3], but it this rate increased to 47% in early onset (EO, <30 years old), while it decreased to only 10% in later onset (LO, >30 years old) [4]. Furthermore, the heritability of MDD was found to be significantly lower as a function of the age of onset, at 50% in first-degree relatives when the proband's age of onset was younger than

20 years old but 36% when probands were in their 20 s, 25% when they were in their 30 s and 16% when they were older than 40 years old [5]. These genetic studies suggested that EO (<30 years old) and LO (>30 years old) MDD possibly have different etiologies. Moreover, a large-scale genetic association study recruited MDD patients with age of onset younger than 30 years old as EO patients vs. LO, and EO was found to be associated with disease severity and the chronicity of depressive symptoms [6]. Nevertheless, the delineative age of onset for EO vs. LO has been highly inconsistently reported in different studies, in which an ages of onset younger than18 [7], 25 [8], 30 [9] or 45 [10] years old have all been used to define EO vs. LO MDD. Thus far, due to a lack of evidence, there is no generally agreed upon age of onset to define EO vs. LO MDD.

An increasing number of studies have supported the theory of dysfunction of the whole brain network in MDD. The brain circuitry might be a good candidate for delineating EO from LO MDD because it is believed to be an intermediate step between molecular and behavioral levels. The white matter (WM) contains neuronal fibers that connect neurons in the network of the brain. MDD patients showed reduced density and number of glial cells in the anterior cingulate cortex [11]. Altered density and ultrastructure of oligodendrocytes were also detected in the prefrontal cortex and amygdala of MDD patients [12]. Nonintrusive brain imaging techniques have been widely used to study neuropsychiatric disorders clinically [13]. In particular, fractional anisotropy (FA), derived from diffusion tensor imaging (DTI), has been widely used to quantify neural tracts [14], abnormalities of which could cause EO or LO MDD, based on specific information about the brain circuitry [15], which could connect evidence on the molecular and behavioral levels.

Imaging studies have revealed global or regional WM abnormalities in depression, but significant differences between EO and LO depression suggest different etiological mechanisms [16]. Widespread FA abnormalities, especially in the frontal and temporal lobes, have been found to be associated with late-life MDD [17–19] and with disease outcomes [20]. These abnormalities might also present in non-elderly patients or in the early course of MDD [21], and they have been associated with special executive dysfunction [22] and poor response to antidepressant treatment [23]. However, highly variable location of clusters with FA abnormalities in MDD patients has been reported, and both increased and decreased FA have been reported following treatment with antidepressants [23,24]. Perhaps these inconsistencies could be at least partially attributed to the heterogeneity of MDD. Recently, a DTI study was conducted to differentiate bipolar depression from unipolar depression [25], raising the possibility of classifying MDD via a DTI technique. Because the sensitivity of dendrites to stress [26] and age-dependent FA changes were discovered [27], FA value could be developed as good indicators, reflecting the possible differences between MDD patients with different ages of onset. Nevertheless, as variable constellations of depressive symptoms, differences in responses to antidepressants, in age of onset and in severity of course could compromise the study of and individual medication treatment for MDD, so the classification of MDD, based on both clinical data and biomarkers, such as regional FA values, should be a useful method for these purposes. To examine this possibility, we recruited sixty-one pairs of untreated non-elderly, first-episode MDD patients and healthy controls (HCs) aged 18–45 years old to exclude possible interferences, such as drug treatment, recurrent episodes and vascular problems in older age (>45 years old).

Materials and Methods

Subjects

This research was approved by the Institutional Review Board of Kunming Medical University, Yunnan Province, P. R. China (ClinicalTrials.gov: NCT00703742). The protocol for this trial and supporting checklist are available as supporting information; see Checklist S1 and Protocol S1. Each participant was required to sign a written informed consent form after receiving a complete description of the study. All of the participants were recruited from June 2008 to July 2011.

The diagnosis of MDD was independently made by two experienced psychiatrists in accordance with the Diagnostic and Statistical Manual of Mental Disorders, Fourth Edition (DSM-IV, American Psychiatric Association, 1994). A total of 77 right-handed MDD patients were recruited from among the out/inpatients of the Department of Psychiatry, the First Affiliated Hospital of Kunming Medical University. Two MDD patients refused to sign written informed consent forms, and another two MDD patients signed written informed consent form but did not participate in the study. Thus, 73 MDD patients underwent clinical screening (Figure S1 in File S1). These MDD patients were Han Chinese people between 18 and 45 years old, and had scores of 17 or greater on the 17-item Hamilton Depression Rating Scale (HDRS), and were untreated and in their first episodes. Data on age, age of onset, duration of disease, sex and years of education were collected. The duration of disease was less than 2 years, defined as the initial manifestation clearly attributable to MDD until the day of acquisition of magnetic resonance imaging (MRI).

The exclusion criteria included the following items: (1) another diagnosed axis I psychiatric disorder; (2) organic brain disorders or neurological disorders; (3) obvious psychiatric symptoms, such as delusions or hallucinations; (4) any physical illness as assessed by personal history; (5) clinical conditions that could cause cerebral atrophy (such as a history of arterial hypertension, diabetes mellitus, stroke); and (6) inability to undergo an MRI scan, including subjects with metal implants. Of these MDD patients who participated in clinical screening, only 68 MDD patients met the exclusion criteria and thus underwent MRI scans.

Matched by sex, age and years of education with the MDD patients on one-to-one basis, 65 right-handed Han Chinese healthy controls (HCs) were recruited by an advertisement in the local community. All of the HCs were free of histories of any psychiatric, neurological or organic diseases according to the exclusion criteria and were without known histories of any psychiatric illnesses in first-degree relatives.

The depressive symptoms and anxiety of all of the participants were assessed by an experienced psychiatrist using the 17-item Hamilton Depression Rating Scale (HDRS, Hamilton 1960) and the 14-item Hamilton Anxiety Scale (HAMA).

Image acquisition

MRI sequences were performed by a skilled radiological technician on a 1.5-T clinical GE MRI scanner (Twinspeed, Milwaukee, WI, USA) equipped with a birdcage head coil. Restraining foam pads were used to minimize head motion. All of the participants underwent a normal T1 scan to detect obvious structural abnormalities, and the parameters were as follows: repetition time (TR)/echo time (TE) = 1800/8.9 ms; matrix size = 256×256; slice thickness = 5 mm; gap = 1 mm; and field of view = 240 mm.

Diffusion tensor imaging (DTI) was acquired using a diffusion tensor echo planar pulse sequence, and the parameters were as follows: TR/TE = 12,000/89 ms; matrix size = 128×128; slice thickness = 6 mm with no interslice gap; field of view = 240 mm; and number of excitations = 5. The diffusion sensitizing gradients were applied in 13 non-collinear directions ($b = 1000\ s/mm^2$), together with acquisition without diffusion weighting ($b = 0$). Twenty-four contiguous slices were acquired to cover the entire brain. All of the sections were acquired parallel to the anterior-posterior commissure line.

Data preprocessing

All of the images were transferred to an IBM workstation in DICOM format. For each participant, all of their DTI images with b0 images were analyzed using DTI-Studio software (https://www.dtistudio.org/, version 2.3; H. Jiang, S. Mori; the Johns Hopkins University, Baltimore, MD, USA), and parametric images with FA were generated. The FA images and b0 images were saved in ANALYZE format. Statistical Parametric Mapping software (SPM5, Wellcome Department of Cognitive Neurology, London, UK) was used to normalize the b0 images to the standard Montreal Neurological Institute (MNI) space and to resample them at a final voxel size of $1\times1\times1\ mm^3$. The transformation matrix was applied to the FA map to normalize the FA map to the standard MNI space. Before statistical analysis, the normalized FA maps were smoothed by using an 8-mm full-width half-maximum Gaussian kernel.

Identification of differences between MDD patients and HC

The two-sample t test was performed in a voxel-by-voxel manner using SPM5, to detect abnormal FA clusters from the whole brain between the MDD patients and HCs. A threshold of $p<0.05$ after small volume correction was considered to be statistically significant.

FA value retrieval and classification analysis

The abnormal FA clusters, identified using SPM5, were set as the regions of interest (ROIs), and the mean FA value of each ROI was calculated for each individual. Using classification analysis in the Statistical Package for the Social Sciences 17.0 (SPSS, Inc., Chicago, IL, USA), the mean FA value of each ROI and the age of onset were analyzed as follows: (1) two-step cluster analysis identified the best numbers of category of subgroups using the Schwarz Bayesian Criterion (BIC); and (2) K-means cluster analysis identified each individual in the subgroups. All the FA data of these ROIs were standardized before clustering.

Characterization of different subgroups

According to the results revealed by classification analysis in SPSS, the MDD patients and their paired HCs were divided into 2 subgroups. Then, the two-sample t test (SPM5) was used to determine abnormal FA clusters from the whole brain between the MDD patients and HCs in each subgroup, and multiple regression analysis (SPM5) was used to detect the associations between FA map and HDRS scores. All of the results were considered to be statistically significant at a level of $p<0.05$ after the corrections described above.

Results

Clinical data

Sixty-eight MDD patients who met the inclusion and exclusion criteria received DTI scans. Seven cases were discarded because of brain structural abnormalities detected by T1 weighted MRI (4 cases with focal ischemia in the frontal lobe or basal ganglia, 2 cases with focal infarctions in the left parietal lobe and 1 case with a brain cyst in the right occipital lobe). Sixty-five healthy controls (HCs) also received DTI scans. Four cases were discarded for similar reasons (3 cases with focal ischemia in the frontal lobe and 1 case with a brain cyst in the basal ganglia). In total, sixty-one pairs of MDD patients and HCs were used for further analyses (Figure S1 in File S1).

There were no group differences in age, years of education and sex ratio (17 men and 44 women) between the sixty-one pairs of MDD patients and the HCs (Table S1 in File S1). The sixty-one MDD patients showed a mean duration of disease of 12.34 ± 8.40 months, and the total scores on the HDRS and HAMA were 22.43 ± 3.86 and 17.03 ± 6.36, respectively (Table 1).

MDD subgroups

A voxel-based analysis method (VBM) for diffusion tensor imaging (DTI) was used to identify abnormal FA clusters in MDD patients vs. HCs. When sixty-one pairs of participants between 18 and 45 years old were collected, we found a pattern of two clusters with decreased FA located in the right temporal lobe (RTEMP) and right middle frontal lobe (RMFG), while one cluster with increased FA was in the left occipital lobe (LOCG) (Figure 1A). We suspected that this result might have been only the average effect of MDD without considering different ages of onset in the effects on different patterns of significant FA clusters.

To address this possibility, the clusters RTEMP, RMFG and LOCG were set as the regions of interest (ROIs), and their FA values were retrieved from each individual. Using the FA value of these three ROIs, two-step classification analysis in SPSS17.0 software revealed that the best number of categories (subgroup) for MDD patients was two (Table S1 in File S1), and K-mean cluster analysis categorized each individual into one of the two subgroups. We found that the age ranges of the onset for the two subgroups were 18–29 and 30–45 years old (Table S2 in File S1), which was surprisingly consistent with the definition of EO vs. LO in certain genetic association studies. Due to the relatively short durations of depression in the present samples, the age (actual age when patients received the MRI scans) ranges for the 2 subgroups were 18–29 and 30–45 years old also (Table S2 in File S1). To understand this best model further, we created a scatter plot of FA values for RTEMP against age (Figure 1B), in which a clear borderline at 30 years old for these two groups was found.

Abnormal FA clusters

Accordingly, the sixty-one pairs of participants were divided into two subgroups, of which the EO group consisted of thirty-two pairs aged 18–29 years old, and the LO group had twenty-nine pairs aged 30–45 years old. The EO and LO MDD patients had no differences in mean score on the HDRS ($t = 0.042$, $p = 0.967$) or mean duration of disease ($t = 0.090$, $p = 0.928$). However, we found that EO and LO MDD patients indeed were the major contributors of abnormal clusters with increased and decreased FA, respectively.

In EO MDD patients, compared with their paired HCs, decreased FA values were found only in the left inferior longitudinal fasciculus (near the parahippocampal gyrus and superior temporal gyrus), wherever increased FA was identified in vast areas, including the bilateral corpus callosum (near the posterior cingulate gyrus), left inferior fronto-occipital fasciculus (superior occipital gyrus), right forceps major and optical radiation (cuneus, middle occipital gyrus) and right corticospinal midbrain (near the substantia nigra) (Figure 2; Table S3 in File S1).

In marked contrast, in LO MDD patients, compared with their paired HCs, all seven of the clusters showed decreased FA, and

Table 1. Demographic data and FA value of three clusters with difference between MDD and HCs.

Variable	*HCs (n = 61) Mean (SD)*	*MDD (n = 61) Mean (SD)*		*t/χ²*	*P value*
Sex (male/female)	**17/44**	**17/44**		–	–
Age (year)	**29.56 (7.06)**	**29.02 (7.97)**		**0.397**	**0.692**
Education (year)	**13.16 (2.79)**	**12.93 (3.00)**		**0.437**	**0.663**
HDRS score	**2.38 (2.18)**	**22.70 (3.80)**		**−36.249**	**0.000**
HAMA score	**2.37 (2.27)**	**17.00 (6.39)**		**−16.832**	**0.000**
FA value of RTEMP	**0.3196 (0.0251)**	**0.3032 (0.0288)**		**3.344**	**0.001**
FA value of RMFG	**0.2212 (0.0287)**	**0.2074 (0.0219)**		**2.997**	**0.003**
FA value of LOCG	**0.2042 (0.0236)**	**0.2173 (0.0232)**		**−3.087**	**0.003**
		EO (n = 32)	*LO (n = 29)*		
Sex (male/female)	–	**10/22**	**7/22**	**0.383**	**0.536**
Age (year)	–	**22.38 (3.60)**	**36.35 (3.96)**	**−14.457**	**0.000**
Age of onset (year)	–	**21.22 (3.61)**	**35.14 (3.87)**	**−14.537**	**0.000**
Education (year)	–	**12.78 (2.85)**	**13.10 (3.20)**	**−0.416**	**0.679**
HDRS score	–	**22.97 (4.21)**	**22.41 (3.34)**	**0.577**	**0.573**
HAMA score	–	**17.38 (7.23)**	**16.59 (5.42)**	**0.478**	**0.634**
Duration (month)	–	**12.35 (9.56)**	**11.62 (6.95)**	**0.338**	**0.736**
FA value of RTEMP		**0.3037 (0.0299)**	**0.3026 (0.0281)**	**0.140**	**0.889**
FA value of RMFG		**0.2043 (0.0195)**	**0.2109 (0.0241)**	**−0.281**	**0.246**
FA value of LOCG		**0.2157 (0.0229)**	**0.2190 (0.0238)**	**−0.861**	**0.586**

RTEMP, RMFG and LOCG represent significant clusters in MDD differed from HCs (showed in Figure S2 in File S1). Abbreviations: MDD, major depressive disorder; HCs, healthy control; HDRS, Hamilton depression rating scale; HAMA, Hamilton anxiety scale; EO, early onset depression; LO, later onset depression. RTEMP, right temporal lobe; RMFG, right middle frontal lobe; LOCG, left occipital lobe.

their locations were much different from those of the clusters in the EO MDD patients. The seven clusters were in the white matter in the bilateral inferior fronto-occipital fasciculus (near the bilateral orbitales gyrus), left posterior limb of the internal capsule (near the caudate), right posterior corona radiate (near the precunus), right inferior longitudinal fasciculus (inferior temporal gyrus), right superior thalamic radiation (near the cingulated gyrus) and inferior fronto-occipital fasciculus (near the middle occipital lobe) (Figure 2; Table S3 in File S1).

To confirm further whether EO and LO MDD were the major contributors to increased and decreased FA clusters, respectively, we hypothesized that there was a transient period, such as 26–29 years old, between EO and LO, and if the samples within this period were removed, the increased and decreased FA clusters for EO and LO MDD, respectively, would become clear-cut. Remarkably, after removal of MDD patients with ages of onset 26–29 years old (7 subjects), as well as the paired HCs, we found that EO MDD patients (18–25 years old, 25 subjects) now had abnormal clusters all with increased FA only (Table S4 and Figure S2 in File S1), which was in marked contrast to the LO MDD patients (30–45 years old), who showed abnormal clusters, all with decreased FA only. Thus, the delineation of EO and LO MDD at the age of onset of 30 years old, with 26–29 years old as a transient period, revealed distinct characteristics of the brain circuitry consistent with the assumption that EO and LO MD are attributable to different etiologies and pathophysiologies.

Correlation with clinical symptoms

It is believed that the brain circuitry, as an intermediate step, can be used as a substitute for both molecular and clinical meaningful observations. Because EO and LO MDD < delineated by the age of onset on 30 years old, have different heritability, we expected that this delineation of EO and LO MDD would also have distinct correlations with clinical symptoms, such as HDRS scores. Using multiple regression analyses of SPM5, we found that EO and LO MDD patients indeed showed distinct correlations with HDRS scores.

In EO MDD patients, both positive and negative correlations were identified between the total HDRS score and the FA values of some regions. Positive correlations were found in the left corticospinal/corticopontine tract in midbrain (near the substantia nigra) and inferior longitudinal fasciculus (near the fusiform gyrus and parahippocampal gyrus) (red color in Figure 3; see also Table S5 in File S1). Negative correlations were found in the left inferior longitudinal fasciculus (near the middle temporal gyrus), superior longitudinal fasciculus (near the inferior parietal lobule) and right superior longitudinal fasciculus (near the middle frontal gyrus) (Figure 3; Table S5 in File S1).

In marked contrast, in the LO MDD patients, only negative correlations were found between all nine clusters and HDRS scores. These regions were the left inferior fronto-occipital fasciculus (near the orbitales gyrus), right uncinate fasciculus/inferior fronto-occipital fasciculus (near the orbitales gyrus), right anterior corona radiata/superior fronto-occipital fasciculus (near the inferior frontal gyrus), left eternal capsule/inferior fronto-occipital fasciculus (near the insula), right superior longitudinal fasciculus (near the precentral gyrus), left fornix (near the thalamus), right anterior limb of internal capsule (near the caudate), right cingulum (near the parahippocampal gyrus) and

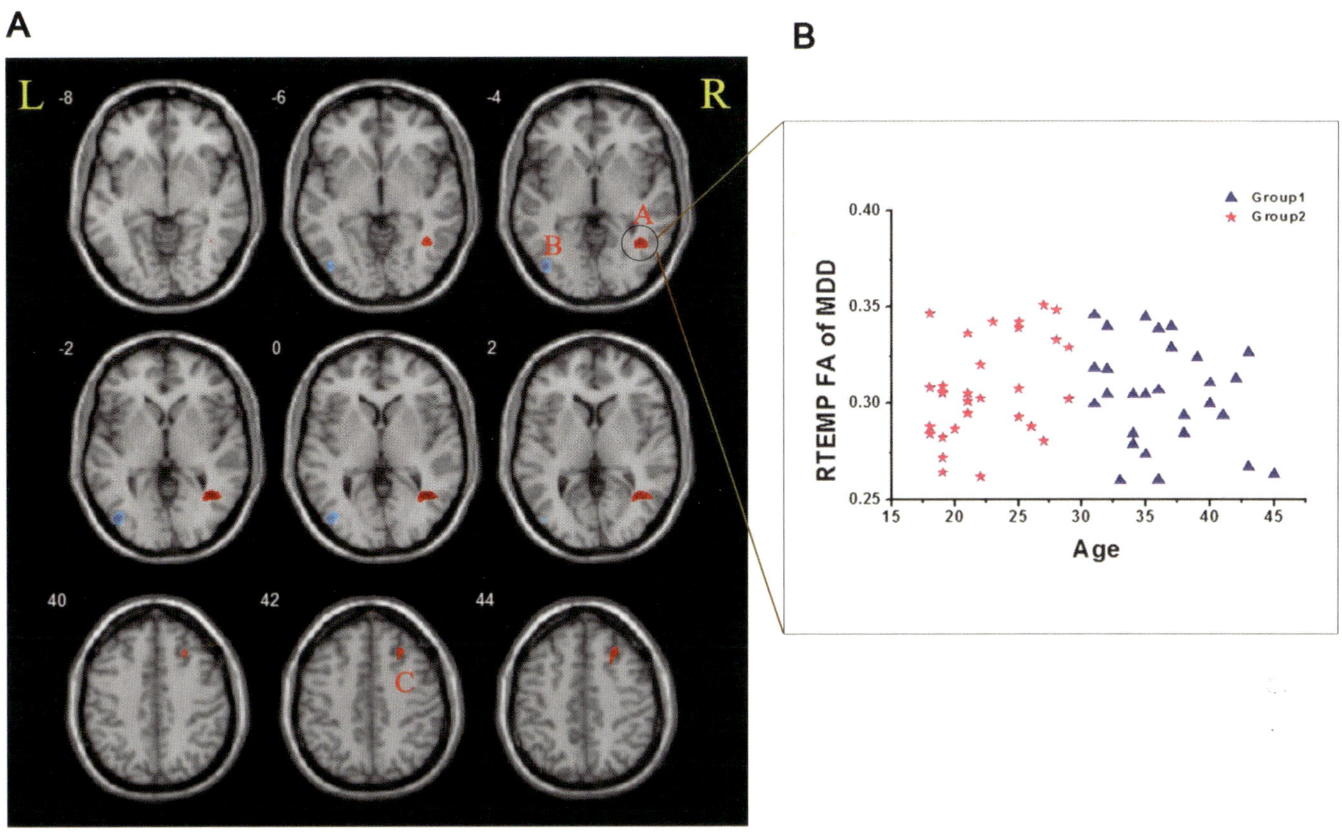

Figure 1. Classification analysis based on the differences in FA between MDD patients and HCs. A. Clusters of red color indicate significant increases in FA values, while those of blue color show decreases in FA values in MDD patients, compared with HCs. B. FA values of the cluster in each individual were classified into two groups, indicated by red (EO) and blue (LO) points plotted against age. L, left side; R, right side; a, cluster near right temporal lobe; b, cluster near left occipital lobe; c, cluster near right middle frontal lobe; MDD, major depressive disorder; HCs, healthy controls; RTEMP, right temporal lobe.

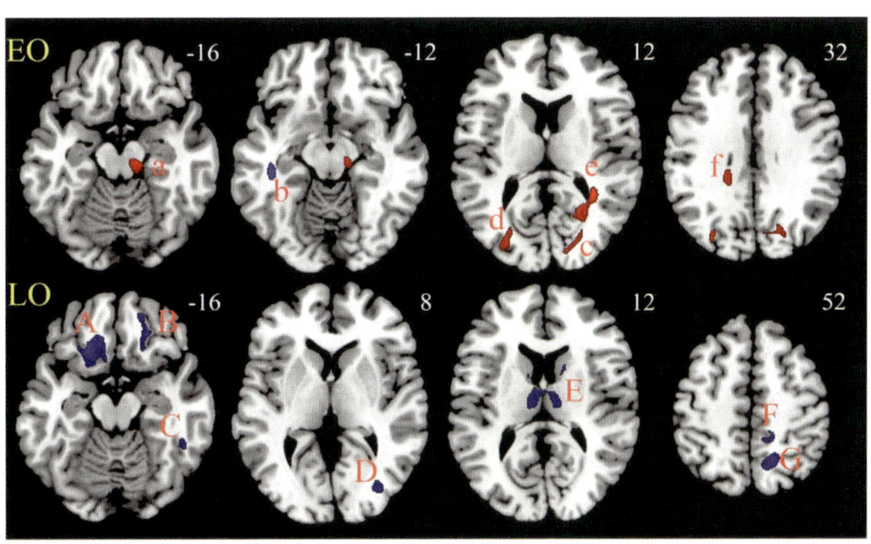

Figure 2. FA clusters for EO vs. LO MDD. Upper panel (EO): Five clusters (a, c–f) with increased FA (red color) but one cluster (b) with decreased FA (blue color) was found in EO patients, compared with the paired HCs. Lower panel (LO): seven clusters (A–G), all with decreased FA (blue color), were found in LO patients compared with the paired HCs. EO, early onset; LO, later onset; MDD, major depressive disorder; HCs, healthy controls.

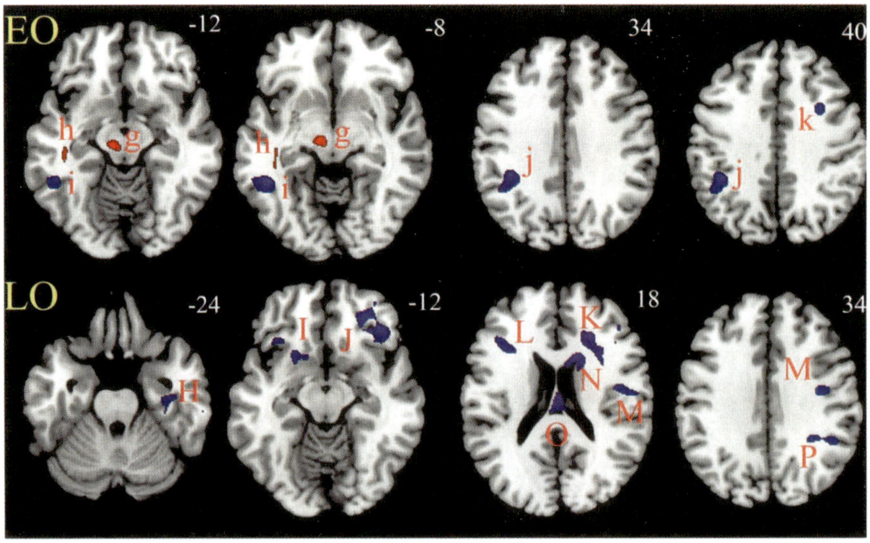

Figure 3. FA clusters with correlations with HDRS scores for EO vs. LO MDD. Upper panel (EO): two FA clusters (g, h) with positive correlations (red color) and three FA clusters (i, j, k) with negative correlations (blue color) with HDRS scores. Lower panel (LO): nine FA clusters (H-P), all with negative correlations (blue) with HDRS scores. EO, early onset; LO, later onset; MDD, major depressive disorder; HDRS, Hamilton Depression Rating Scale.

right posterior corona radiata/superior longitudinal fasciculus (near the precuneus) (Figure 3; Table S5 in File S1).

Finally, when we considered the clusters with both abnormal FA and correlations with clinical symptoms, the characteristics of the brain circuitry for EO and LO MDD patients became more clear. In LO MDD, some regions with decreased FA values overlapped with regions correlated with the depressive severity. FA values in the cluster in the bilateral uncinate fasciculus/inferior fronto-occipital fasciculus near the orbital frontal lobe decreased obviously wherever they were negatively correlated with HDRS score. For the fornix/posterior limb of the internal capsule near the posterior cingulate gyrus, FA values also decreased obviously in MDD patients and were negatively correlated with HDRS scores. In EO MDD, the FA values of the cluster in the left inferior longitudinal fasciculus near the parahippocampal gyrus decreased obviously wherever they were positively correlated with HDRS scores (Figure S3 in File S1).

Discussion

In the present study, we demonstrated the novel finding that specific DTI evidence about information regarding the brain circuitry, with distinct correlations with clinical symptoms, supported the delineation of EO versus LO MDD in non-elderly patients, based on an age of onset of 30 years old. This finding was consistent with the distinct heritability of EO (<30 years old) vs. LO MDD (>30 years old) reported in certain genetic association studies. Thus, there might be at least two different groups in non-elderly MDD: one with a younger age of onset and characterized by stronger WM connectivity; and another with an older age of onset but characterized by WM microstructural deficits. Even with similar clinical manifestations, these two groups might have different neurological pathologies.

The regions with decreased FA for LO were mainly located in the WM near the orbital frontal cortex (OFC) and thalamus. The FA values of these regions were also negatively correlated with severity of depression, suggesting that the WM deficits of these areas constituted the main pathophysiology of LO MDD. Alterations in the functional balance between the OFC and the circuits it forms with related areas of the temporal lobe, striatum, thalamus, and brain stem might underlie the pathophysiology of MDD [28]. As a key structure inducing the stress response in the body, the thalamus has been believed to underlie emotional distress in humans [29] and was found to be related to depression [30]. A study in animals also confirmed that older adults responded to stress with greater increases in plasma levels of adrenocorticotropic hormone and modest reductions in glucocorticoid feedback sensitivity, compared to young adults [31]. Thus, these results might reflect the possibility of greater stress effects in the LO MDD group than in the EO MDD group.

Unlike in LO MDD, the FA values increased in brain regions near the frontal, parietal and cingulate areas in the EO group. Although most articles have reported decreased FA in MDD patients, contrary results were also reported recently. MDD patients who did not remit after sertraline treatment exhibit higher FA values in the superior frontal gyri and anterior cingulate cortices [24]. Wildly increased FA has also been reported in obsessive compulsive disorder patients, including in the regions near the subinsular cortex [32], the cingulum and the anterior limb of the internal capsule [33], and the corpus callosum [34]. These increased regional FA values could be restored by antidepressants [34]. Until now, the essential association of FA with mental disorders has not been fully understood yet. However, it has been suggested that the higher FA might be related to an increase in the connectivity of WM bundles [35]. In schizophrenia, higher FA in the anterior corpus callosum was found in individuals with symptoms of hallucinations [36]. These results suggested that higher FA in some regions might have reflected strengthened connectivity and might have been related to special characteristics, such as recurrence, in the EO group [37]. However, for the LO group, the main pathology might be deficits in WM microstructural integrity.

The present finding that specific DTI abnormalities with distinct correlations with clinical symptoms supported the delineation of EO and LO MDD based on the age of onset of 30 years old could have significant impact on multidisciplinary treatment for MDD. First, due to a lack of evidence, there is no generally agreed upon age of onset to define EO and LO MDD. Second, a recent report suggested that DTI abnormalities could reflect genetic effects because the S-allele carriers of serotonin transporter polymorphisms had lower FA in the frontolimbic areas than L-allele homozygotes [38]. Thus, the present finding of a delineation of EO and LO MD based on the age of onset of 30 years old might also reflect genetic effects. Third, because the heritability of MDD is different for EO and LO patients [4], it is possible that DTI abnormalities for EO and LO of MDD might be attributable to differences in genetic effects and environmental factors [39,40]. Fourth, a large-scale study of DSM-IV disorders found that the lifetime prevalence of MDD was variable with different ages of onset, e.g., 15.4% for EO (18–29 years old) and 19.8% for LO (30–44 years old) [41]. Thus, the delineation of EO and LO MDD by an age of onset of 30 years old was supported by the present DTI evidence and also the evidence from previous molecular and clinical studies.

Because MDD is highly heterogeneous, it is difficult to find "common" clusters with abnormal FA in all individuals, particularly when the sample size is large and the range of ages or ages of onset is broad. As variable constellations of depressive symptoms, differences in responses to antidepressants, age of onset and severity of course could compromise the study of and individual medication treatment for MDD, so the classification of subtypes, based on both clinical data and biomarkers, such as regional FA values, could constitute a useful method for these purposes.

Supporting Information

Checklist S1 TREND checklist.

File S1 Supporting files. Figure S1, Procedure of recruiting and data collection. **Figure S2**, Only increased FA was found in MDD patients at the age of 18–25 years old compared with paired HCs. **Figure S3**, Clusters correlated to HDRS (Hamilton depression rating scale). **Table S1**, Results of Two-step classification using the FA value of three ROIs of RTEMP, RMFG and LOCG. **Table S2**, Result of K-mean cluster classify analysis in MDD. **Table S3**, Abnormal FA clusters in EO and LO subgroups of MDD. **Table S4**, Abnormal FA clusters in MDD patients at the age of 18–25 years old compared with paired HCs. **Table S5**, FA Clusters correlated with HDRS scores in EO and LO subgroups of MDD.

Protocol S1 Trial protocol.

Acknowledgments

We thank all the volunteers of this study. We thank Jing Lu, Chuanyuan Kang and Fang Liu of Psychiatry Department of The First Affiliated Hospital of Kunming Medical University for recruiting the volunteer; thank Qixin Zhou of Kunming Institute of Zoology the Chinese Academy of Sciences for the assistance in statistical analyses.

Author Contributions

Conceived and designed the experiments: LX XX BS. Performed the experiments: YC HY CL. Analyzed the data: JX BN HL. Contributed reagents/materials/analysis tools: BN. Wrote the paper: YC JX. Recruited patients: NL FL YB.

References

1. Merikangas KR, Wicki W, Angst J (1994) Heterogeneity of depression. Classification of depressive subtypes by longitudinal course. Br J Psychiatry 164: 342–348.
2. Belmaker RH, Agam G (2008) Major depressive disorder. N Engl J Med 358: 55–68.
3. Sullivan PF, Neale MC, Kendler KS (2000) Genetic epidemiology of major depression: review and meta-analysis. Am J Psychiatry 157: 1552–1562.
4. Lyons MJ, Eisen SA, Goldberg J, True W, Lin N, et al. (1998) A registry-based twin study of depression in men. Arch Gen Psychiatry 55: 468–472.
5. Weissman MM, Wickramaratne P, Merikangas KR, Leckman JF, Prusoff BA, et al. (1984) Onset of major depression in early adulthood. Increased familial loading and specificity. Arch Gen Psychiatry 41: 1136–1143.
6. Mondimore FM, Zandi PP, Mackinnon DF, McInnis MG, Miller EB, et al. (2006) Familial aggregation of illness chronicity in recurrent, early-onset major depression pedigrees. Am J Psychiatry 163: 1554–1560.
7. MacMaster FP, Kusumakar V (2004) Hippocampal volume in early onset depression. BMC Med 2: 2.
8. Marazita ML, Neiswanger K, Cooper M, Zubenko GS, Giles DE, et al. (1997) Genetic segregation analysis of early-onset recurrent unipolar depression. Am J Hum Genet 61: 1370–1378.
9. Price RA, Kidd KK, Weissman MM (1987) Early onset (under age 30 years) and panic disorder as markers for etiologic homogeneity in major depression. Arch Gen Psychiatry 44: 434–440.
10. Janssen J, Hulshoff Pol HE, Lampe IK, Schnack HG, de Leeuw FE, et al. (2004) Hippocampal changes and white matter lesions in early-onset depression. Biol Psychiatry 56: 825–831.
11. Cotter D, Mackay D, Landau S, Kerwin R, Everall I (2001) Reduced glial cell density and neuronal size in the anterior cingulate cortex in major depressive disorder. Arch Gen Psychiatry 58: 545–553.
12. Rajkowska G, Miguel-Hidalgo JJ (2007) Gliogenesis and glial pathology in depression. CNS Neurol Disord Drug Targets 6: 219–233.
13. Linden DE, Fallgatter AJ (2009) Neuroimaging in psychiatry: from bench to bedside. Front Hum Neurosci 3: 49.
14. Thomason ME, Thompson PM (2010) Diffusion Imaging, White Matter, and Psychopathology. Annu Rev Clin Psychol.
15. Blood AJ, Iosifescu DV, Makris N, Perlis RH, Kennedy DN, et al. (2010) Microstructural abnormalities in subcortical reward circuitry of subjects with major depressive disorder. PLoS One 5: e13945.
16. Herrmann LL, Le Masurier M, Ebmeier KP (2008) White matter hyperintensities in late life depression: a systematic review. J Neurol Neurosurg Psychiatry 79: 619–624.
17. Taylor WD, MacFall JR, Payne ME, McQuoid DR, Provenzale JM, et al. (2004) Late-life depression and microstructural abnormalities in dorsolateral prefrontal cortex white matter. Am J Psychiatry 161: 1293–1296.
18. Nobuhara K, Okugawa G, Minami T, Takase K, Yoshida T, et al. (2004) Effects of electroconvulsive therapy on frontal white matter in late-life depression: a diffusion tensor imaging study. Neuropsychobiology 50: 48–53.
19. Bae JN, MacFall JR, Krishnan KR, Payne ME, Steffens DC, et al. (2006) Dorsolateral prefrontal cortex and anterior cingulate cortex white matter alterations in late-life depression. Biol Psychiatry 60: 1356–1363.
20. Alexopoulos GS, Kiosses DN, Choi SJ, Murphy CF, Lim KO (2002) Frontal white matter microstructure and treatment response of late-life depression: a preliminary study. Am J Psychiatry 159: 1929–1932.
21. Ma N, Li L, Shu N, Liu J, Gong G, et al. (2007) White matter abnormalities in first-episode, treatment-naive young adults with major depressive disorder. Am J Psychiatry 164: 823–826.
22. Murphy CF, Gunning-Dixon FM, Hoptman MJ, Lim KO, Ardekani B, et al. (2007) White-matter integrity predicts stroop performance in patients with geriatric depression. Biol Psychiatry 61: 1007–1010.
23. Alexopoulos GS, Murphy CF, Gunning-Dixon FM, Latoussakis V, Kanellopoulos D, et al. (2008) Microstructural white matter abnormalities and remission of geriatric depression. Am J Psychiatry 165: 238–244.
24. Taylor WD, Kuchibhatla M, Payne ME, Macfall JR, Sheline YI, et al. (2008) Frontal white matter anisotropy and antidepressant remission in late-life depression. PLoS One 3: e3267.
25. Versace A, Almeida JR, Quevedo K, Thompson WK, Terwilliger RA, et al. (2010) Right orbitofrontal corticolimbic and left corticocortical white matter connectivity differentiate bipolar and unipolar depression. Biol Psychiatry 68: 560–567.
26. Watanabe Y, Gould E, McEwen BS (1992) Stress induces atrophy of apical dendrites of hippocampal CA3 pyramidal neurons. Brain Res 588: 341–345.
27. Pfefferbaum A, Sullivan EV, Hedehus M, Lim KO, Adalsteinsson E, et al. (2000) Age-related decline in brain white matter anisotropy measured with spatially corrected echo-planar diffusion tensor imaging. Magn Reson Med 44: 259–268.
28. Drevets WC (2007) Orbitofrontal cortex function and structure in depression. Ann N Y Acad Sci 1121: 499–527.

29. Sinha R, Lacadie C, Skudlarski P, Wexler BE (2004) Neural circuits underlying emotional distress in humans. Ann N Y Acad Sci 1032: 254–257.
30. Drevets WC (2001) Neuroimaging and neuropathological studies of depression: implications for the cognitive-emotional features of mood disorders. Curr Opin Neurobiol 11: 240–249.
31. Lyons DM, Yang C, Eliez S, Reiss AL, Schatzberg AF (2004) Cognitive correlates of white matter growth and stress hormones in female squirrel monkey adults. J Neurosci 24: 3655–3662.
32. Nakamae T, Narumoto J, Shibata K, Matsumoto R, Kitabayashi Y, et al. (2008) Alteration of fractional anisotropy and apparent diffusion coefficient in obsessive-compulsive disorder: a diffusion tensor imaging study. Prog Neuropsychopharmacol Biol Psychiatry 32: 1221–1226.
33. Cannistraro PA, Makris N, Howard JD, Wedig MM, Hodge SM, et al. (2007) A diffusion tensor imaging study of white matter in obsessive-compulsive disorder. Depress Anxiety 24: 440–446.
34. Yoo SY, Jang JH, Shin YW, Kim DJ, Park HJ, et al. (2007) White matter abnormalities in drug-naive patients with obsessive-compulsive disorder: a diffusion tensor study before and after citalopram treatment. Acta Psychiatr Scand 116: 211–219.
35. Dong Q, Welsh RC, Chenevert TL, Carlos RC, Maly-Sundgren P, et al. (2004) Clinical applications of diffusion tensor imaging. J Magn Reson Imaging 19: 6–18.
36. Hubl D, Koenig T, Strik W, Federspiel A, Kreis R, et al. (2004) Pathways that make voices: white matter changes in auditory hallucinations. Arch Gen Psychiatry 61: 658–668.
37. Giles DE, Jarrett RB, Biggs MM, Guzick DS (1989) Clinical predictors of recurrence in depression. Am J Psychiatry.
38. Alexopoulos GS, Murphy CF, Gunning-Dixon FM, Glatt CE, Latoussakis V, et al. (2009) Serotonin transporter polymorphisms, microstructural white matter abnormalities and remission of geriatric depression. J Affect Disord 119: 132–141.
39. Levinson DF (2006) The genetics of depression: a review. Biol Psychiatry 60: 84–92.
40. Mendlewicz J, Baron M (1981) Morbidity risks in subtypes of unipolar depressive illness: differences between early and late onset forms. Br J Psychiatry 139: 463–466.
41. Kessler RC, Berglund P, Demler O, Jin R, Merikangas KR, et al. (2005) Lifetime prevalence and age-of-onset distributions of DSM-IV disorders in the National Comorbidity Survey Replication. Arch Gen Psychiatry 62: 593–602.

13

The Scars of Childhood Adversity: Minor Stress Sensitivity and Depressive Symptoms in Remitted Recurrently Depressed Adult Patients

Gemma Kok[1¶], Gerard van Rijsbergen[1¶], Huibert Burger[2,3], Hermien Elgersma[1], Heleen Riper[4,5], Pim Cuijpers[4,5], Jack Dekker[6,7], Filip Smit[4,8,9], Claudi Bockting[1]*

1 Department of Clinical Psychology, University of Groningen, Groningen, The Netherlands, **2** Department of General Practice, University of Groningen, University Medical Center Groningen, Groningen, The Netherlands, **3** Interdisciplinary Center for Psychiatric Epidemiology, University of Groningen, University Medical Center Groningen, Groningen, The Netherlands, **4** Department of Clinical Psychology and EMGO + Institute for Health and Care Research, VU University and VU University Medical Centre, Amsterdam, the Netherlands, **5** Leuphana University, Lüneburg, Germany, **6** Research Department, Arkin Mental Health Institute, Amsterdam, The Netherlands, **7** Department of Clinical Psychology, VU University, Amsterdam, The Netherlands, **8** Department of Epidemiology and Biostatistics, EMGO + Institute for Health and Care Research, VU University Medical Centre, Amsterdam, the Netherlands, **9** Trimbos Institute (Netherlands Institute of Mental Health and Addiction), Utrecht, the Netherlands

Abstract

Background: Childhood adversity may lead to depressive relapse through its long-lasting influence on stress sensitivity. In line with the stress sensitization hypothesis, minor (daily) stress is associated with depressive relapse. Therefore, we examine the impact of childhood adversity on daily stress and its predictive value on prospectively assessed depressive symptoms in recurrently depressed patients.

Method: Daily stress was assessed in recurrently depressed adult patients, enrolled into two randomized trials while remitted. The reported intensity and frequency of dependent and independent daily stress was assessed at baseline. Independent stress is externally generated, for example an accident happening to a friend, while dependent stress is internally generated, for example getting into a fight with a neighbor. Hierarchical regression analyses were performed with childhood adversity, independent and dependent daily stress as predictor variables of prospectively measured depressive symptoms after three months of follow-up ($n = 138$).

Results: We found that childhood adversity was not significantly associated with a higher frequency and intensity of daily stress. The intensity of both independent and dependent daily stress was predictive of depressive symptom levels at follow-up (unadjusted models respectively: $B = 0.47$, $t = 2.05$, $p = 0.041$, 95% CI = 0.02–0.92; $B = 0.29$, $t = 2.20$, $p = 0.028$, 95% CI = 0.03–0.55). No associations were found between childhood adversity and depressive symptoms at follow-up.

Conclusion: No evidence was found supporting stress sensitization due to the experience of childhood adversity in this recurrently depressed but remitted patient group. Nevertheless, our research indicates that daily stress might be a target for preventive treatment.

Editor: Yutaka Matsuoka, National Center of Neurology and Psychiatry, Japan

Funding: This research is funded by ZonMW: The Netherlands association for health research and development. ZonMW Doelmatigheid, Kosten en Effecten grant number 171002401 (to Prof. dr. C.L.H. Bockting), ZonMW OOG Geestkracht grant number 100002035 (to Drs. H.J. Elgersma and Prof. dr. C.L.H. Bockting) and ZonMW Disease management Chronische Ziekten grant number 300020014 (to Prof. dr. C.L.H. Bockting). Funding sources did not play any role in the collection, analysis, and interpretation of the data; writing the manuscript or the decision to submit for publication.

Competing Interests: C.L.H. Bockting still serves as an editor for this journal.

* Email: C.L.H.Bockting@uu.nl

¶ These authors are shared first authors on this work.

Introduction

Major Depressive Disorder (MDD) is a highly recurrent disease with reported relapse and recurrence rates that range from 50–90% [1,2]. Each depressive episode heightens the risk of additional relapses and recurrences [1,3–5]. For readability we refer to the more conservative term relapse in case of relapse and recurrence [6]. There is ample evidence that the experience of childhood adversity is related to the persistence of depression and depressive relapse, even after successful treatment [7–9]. More specifically, sexual abuse and emotional neglect seem to be associated with a poor prognosis of depression, and appear as independent determinants of chronicity of the disorder [10–13]. Knowledge on how childhood adversity leads to a poor prognosis of depression would provide insight into the causal processes and might help tailor treatment.

Vulnerability-stress

An explanation of childhood adversity influencing the prognosis of depression, might be found in vulnerability-stress models [14–17]. Vulnerabilities, such as exposure to childhood adversity, are suggested to predispose someone to develop psychopathology after stress. Possibly, vulnerabilities cause heightened sensitivity to stress on the long-term. Indeed associations are found between childhood adversities and an increased sensitivity to daily stressors in adult life [18–20]. This is supported by neurobiological studies as well, where a link between childhood adversities and epigenetic modifications to sensitivity to stress has been demonstrated [21].

Stress sensitivity. Stress, such as life events or daily stressors, is known as one of the most consistent predictors of respectively onset and relapse in MDD [22–24]. According to the *stress sensitivity* or *kindling* hypothesis [25], with increasing numbers of previous depressive episodes, the role of major life stress diminishes and minor life stress is considered as a more important predictor of depressive relapse [22,26,27]. There is indeed evidence that minor life stress, such as the loss of personal belongings, plays a role in initiating the return of depressive symptoms and depressive episodes [22,23,28–30]. So far, of the three studies that examined the impact of childhood adversities on stress and subsequent depression, two demonstrated that the experience of childhood adversity was associated with higher sensitivity to stress, which successively heightened the risk of depression onset in adulthood [31,32]. Conversely, the third study found that childhood adversity did not lead to increases in stress in adulthood and therefore depression in an elderly cohort (55+n = 1887) [18]. Apart from the mere exposure to stress, McLaughlin and colleagues [31] demonstrated that exposure to childhood adversity was related to a higher perceived intensity of adult daily stress. They suggest that a higher perceived intensity of stress could lead to negative mental health consequences after stress exposure.

Stress generation. According to the potentially modifiable *stress generation* hypothesis of Hammen [33], characteristics and behaviors of persons themselves may lead to higher generation of stress. In this hypothesis, stress influenced by a person, such as having a disagreement, is defined as dependent stress and is considered to be more related to depression than externally generated independent stress, such as the loss of a friend (i.e. stress generation; [33]. In a recent study by Liu and colleagues [34] the experience of childhood emotional neglect came forward as a unique predictor of dependent stress generation in participants with a history of depression, while independent stress was not a predictor. Depression itself is related to a heightened stress generation, even during remission [33,35]. The influence of childhood adversity on stress could therefore eventually be overtaken by the influence of depression itself. Whether childhood adversity is associated to stress, irrespective of previous episodes, is unknown.

Current study

In the current study we examine if an association between childhood adversity and the return of depressive symptoms exists in a currently remitted but recurrently depressed patient sample and if this is mediated by daily stress. We first studied whether childhood adversity was related to 1) the return of depressive symptoms assessed at three month follow-up, and 2) whether this relationship was partially mediated by the reported frequency and intensity of dependent and independent daily stress. Finally, additionally and aside from the mediation analysis, we examined 3) whether the reported frequency and intensity of dependent and independent daily stress, was predictive of depressive symptoms at follow-up in recurrently depressed remitted patients. In line with Monroe et al. [30], dependent and independent daily stress were examined separately to test for the *stress generation* hypothesis. We expected only dependent stress to be predictive of depressive symptoms after remission.

Method

The protocol for these trials and supporting CONSORT checklist are available as supporting information; see Checklist S1 and Protocol S1 (trial B) and Protocol S2 (trial A).

Participants

The total sample consisted of 309 recurrently depressed patients that entered the study while remitted. They were recruited as part of two Randomized Controlled Trials (RCT) evaluating the effectiveness of Preventive Cognitive Therapy (PCT) to prevent relapse in depression. Trial A included remitted recurrently depressed patients that used antidepressants (n = 112), recruited from July 2009 till August 2012, and examines the effectiveness of face to face PCT in addition to or as alternative for antidepressant medication (ADM) versus ADM alone [36]. Trial B included remitted recurrently depressed patients (n = 197), recruited from March 2010 till August 2012, to examine the effectiveness of an online version of PCT in addition to Treatment as Usual (TAU) versus TAU alone [37]. There were no restrictions regarding the type or frequency of current TAU and TAU could consist of ADM treatment, primary care, secondary care or no treatment at all.

All participants were currently in remission at study start, for minimally two months but no longer than two years and experienced at least two depressive episodes in the past, assessed by the Structured Clinical Interview based on the Diagnostic and Statistical Manual of Mental Disorders (SCID-I; DSM-IV) [38], and a score of 10 or below on the 17-item Hamilton Rating Scale for Depression ($HRSD_{17}$) [39]. The SCID-I, administered by trained researchers over the telephone, was used to assess the number of previous Major Depressive Episodes (MDE), their timing and duration. The two most recent episodes of depression were assessed at symptom level in the SCID-I interview, in which the severity of an episode was established by assigning severity scores based on the number of symptoms (5 symptoms corresponds to mild, 6–7 symptoms corresponds to moderate, whereas 8–9 symptoms corresponds to severe depression). All other episodes were assessed by the core DSM-IV-TR criteria depressed mood (A1), or loss of interest (A2). The SCID-I was also used to exclude participants with: a) current or past mania or hypomania, b) current or past psychosis, c) current alcohol- or drug abuse, d) predominant anxiety disorder. Further exclusion criteria were recent electroconvulsive therapy and organic brain damage. All baseline data were acquired using online questionnaires before PCT took place. Both studies were approved by the Medical Ethical Committee and the participants provided written informed consent. All participants were above 18 years of age and able to consent. The authors confirm that all ongoing and related trials for this intervention are registered.

Measures

Childhood adversities. Adversities before the age of 16 were assessed retrospectively by the Dutch version of the Life Events Questionnaire (LEQ) [40]. Previous research rated the predictive validity of the LEQ as good [40]. Emotional neglect and emotional abuse were not assessed by the LEQ. We assessed information with questions 5a, 12 and 13, respectively concerning the occurrence of a) death of a parent, b) being the victim of sexual abuse or, c) being the victim of physical abuse. Questions could be answered with yes (score = 1) or no (score = 0). Although there is a variety of adverse events, many studies in this field focus on these specific events, which is why these were selected [12,13,41–43]. A dichotomous variable was made, in which the presence of one or more of the adversities assessed with questions 5a, 12, and 13 were coded as 1, and the absence of all three was coded as 0.

Daily stress. The Dutch version of the Everyday Problem Checklist was used to assess the occurrence of 114 daily stressors in the three months preceding the baseline measurement (EPCL) [44]. The items were assigned to the subscales dependent stress (28 items) or independent stress (21 items) based on the manual of the EPCL [44]. A subdivision into these subscales is useful because dependent stress is said to be more related to recurrent depression [45]. An example of a dependent event is *you got into a conflict with a colleague*, and an independent event is *you had to wait long at an appointment*. Additionally, the subscales total frequency and total intensity of dependent and independent stress were calculated in accordance to the manual of the EPCL. The intensity of daily stress describes how the impact of stressors is experienced and the score could range from 0 (no impact) to 3 (very much impact). The reliability of all the 114 EPCL items was $\alpha = .97$, this was $\alpha = .79$ for the dependent subscale (28 items) and $\alpha = .71$ for the independent subscale (21 items).

Depressive symptoms. The Dutch translation of the Inventory of Depressive Symptomatology was used to measure depressive symptoms at baseline and three month follow-up (IDS-SR) [46]. The inventory contains 30 items which can be answered on a 4-point scale, ranging from 0 (no symptom) to 3 (almost always troubled by symptom). The overall score is calculated by adding up all scores and ranges from 0–90. A score of 0–13 is categorized as no symptoms, 14–25 as mild symptoms, 26–38 moderate symptoms, 39–48 as severe symptoms and above 49 as very severe symptoms. The reliability of this measure according to Rush et al. [46] was good (α. = .79–.85). In this study the reliability was good as well ($\alpha = .77$).

Statistical analyses

All analyses were performed using SPSS version 20.0 and we considered two-sided p-values <.05 to be statistically significant. The characteristics of the study populations of the two trials were compared. Chi square tests were used to test differences in dichotomous variables and independent sample T-Tests were applied to normally-distributed continuous variables, for non-normally distributed variables the non-parametric Mann-Whitney U statistic was used.

In order to account for missing data on depressive symptoms, prospectively measured at three month follow-up, we used multiple imputation by chained equations. Multiple imputation is a state-of-the art technique, because it reduces the chance of systematic bias due to non-random missing data [47]. Forty imputations were performed and were combined according to Rubin's rules [48]. We restricted the analyses to the group that was randomized to the control conditions of both trials (continuation of ADM and TAU), because the experimental treatment (PCT) could have interacted with the effect of childhood adversity or daily stress on depressive symptoms. Separate linear regression analyses were performed with either childhood adversity or daily stress included as the only independent variable in the first step of the model. In step two we adjusted for gender, treatment group (TAU or continuation of ADM) and in step three for the number of previous depressive episodes.

Female gender was adjusted for because it is positively associated with both stress and depression and is no intermediary variable [49]. The number of previous episodes of depression is one of the most important predictors of future depression [1] and could be considered a confounder. However, previous episodes may be part of the causal chain between childhood adversity and present depression and including previous episodes could imply overcorrection. Therefore, this variable was only included in the final supplementary step to investigate whether adversity was related to current depression independent of previous episodes. We were interested in the association between daily stress and depressive symptom levels at follow-up. Therefore, we did not control for baseline depressive symptoms, or equivalently partial them out, because this would result in examining the extent to which daily stress predicts future depressive symptoms on top of current depressive symptoms, i.e. daily stress as a predictor of three month change in depressive symptoms.

If an overall association was found between childhood adversity and depression [50], we performed another regression analysis with presence of childhood adversity entered in the first step and daily stress in the second step to examine if daily stress was a mediator of the possible relation between childhood adversity and depressive symptoms. The relative change in the regression coefficient for childhood adversity when daily stress was added as an independent variable was assumed to be a measure of mediation and was expressed as a percentage. The regression analyses were performed separately for dependent and independent daily stress and also for the daily stress intensity and frequency. Not all daily life stressors are related to poor depression outcomes, and differentiating between the broad category of daily life stress is advised [30]. Therefore, the four daily stress subscales were treated as four distinct categories, as we expected them to be differentially related to depressive symptoms.

Results

Figure 1 provides an overview of the number of all the participants that were assessed and randomized to the trial conditions. Of the total group, n = 138 participants were assigned to the TAU group (n = 82, Trial B) and continuation of ADM group (n = 56, Trial A), of which n = 36 (26%) participants suffered at least one childhood adversity. Table 1 shows that most participants were female (68.1%) and had a mean age of 48.16 years (SD = 10.4). Participants experienced a median of four previous depressive episodes (IQR = 3.0). The baseline level of depressive symptoms was low, with a mean score of 3.53 (SD = 2.8) on the $HDRS_{17}$ [39], and a mean of 17.61 (SD = 10.2) on the $IDS\text{-}SR_{30}$ [46]. The trials did not differ on any of the demographic and clinical characteristics, except for ADM use ($p <$ .001).

Because participants in trial A had to use antidepressants continuously in the last six months to be included in the study, this led to significant differences with regard to ADM use and the rate of visiting a general practitioner between trial A and B. ADM use was not related to any of the daily stress subscales, and depressive symptoms at three month follow-up (all p's>.05). However, ADM use was related to a higher level of baseline depressive symptoms (p<.001). We controlled for these baseline differences by including

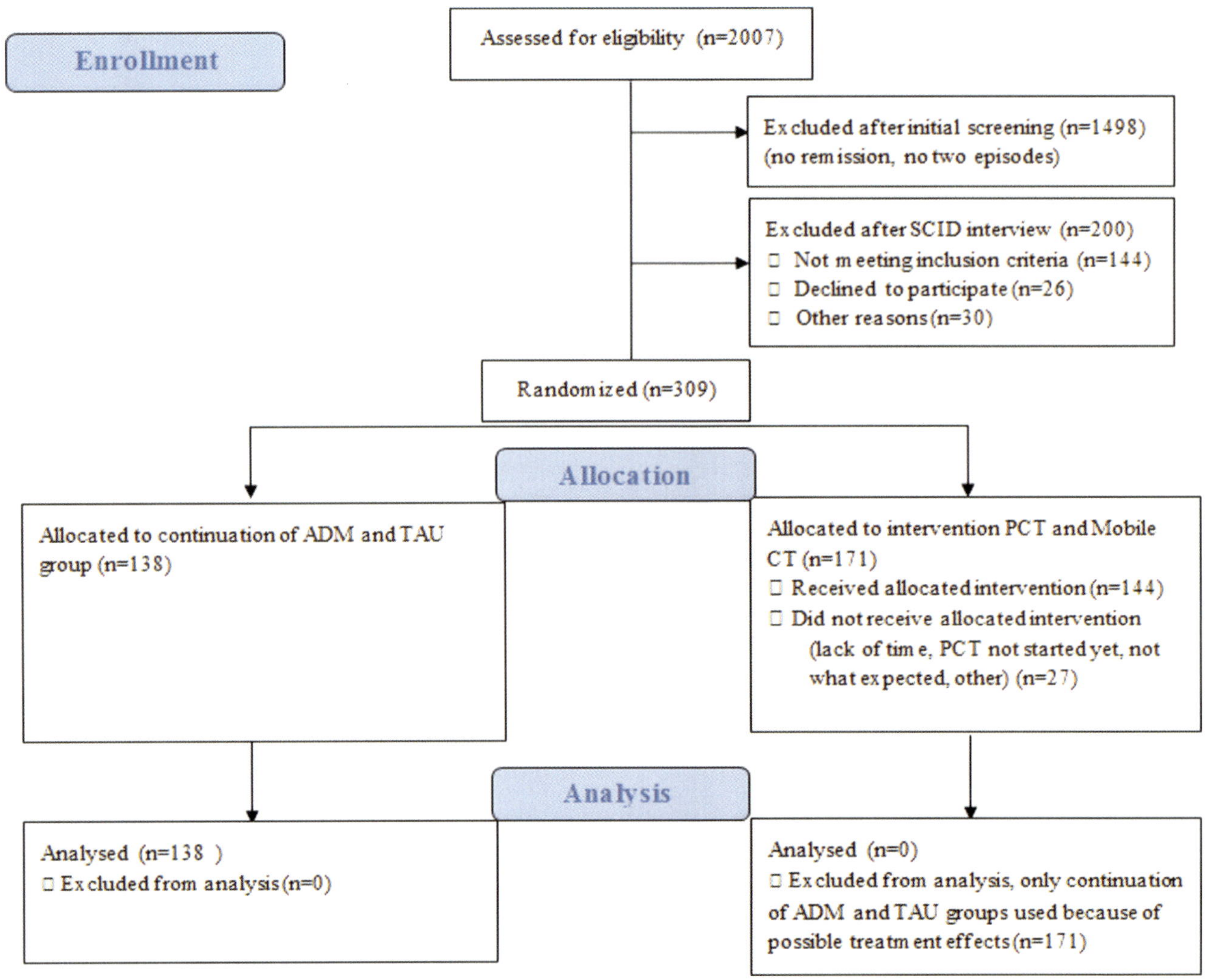

Figure 1. Consort Flow Diagram of participant flow.

the treatment group (continuation of ADM or TAU), as a variable in the regression analysis.

The data of the continuation of ADM condition of trial A and the TAU condition of trial B were merged. In the combined TAU and continuation of ADM group we estimated the pooled standard deviation (SD) of the IDS-SR_{30} to be 13. Given this SD, it was possible to detect moderate or larger effects ($d = 0.53$ or over) given 40 subjects with and 100 subjects without a history of childhood adversities, a two-sided alpha of 0.05 and a bèta of 0.8.

Regression analyses

Depressive symptoms at baseline and three month follow-up, did not significantly differ in participants with,-and without the experience of childhood adversity (Table 2). Childhood adversity did not significantly predict depressive symptoms at three months follow-up ($B = 4.073$, $t = 1.522$, $p = 0.128$, 95% CI $= -1.18$–9.33). Addition of any of the other variables in the next steps did not lead to any significant changes in this model. The R^2 and adjusted R^2 are small (respectively 0.048 and 0.019), indicating that only a small part in the variance of depressive symptoms is explained by the included variables.

The presence of childhood adversity was not related to any of the daily stress subscales($r = -.007$–.087), and the means and standard deviations of the four daily stress subscales did not significantly differ in participants with-, and without the experience of childhood adversity (all p's $>.05$) (Table 3) Therefore, we did not proceed to the analysis of a mediating role of daily stress.

Daily stress as a predictor of depressive symptoms at follow-up. All baseline daily stress subscales showed moderate to high correlations among themselves ($r = .414$–.819, $p<0.01$), and with baseline depressive symptoms ($r = .308$–.399, $p<0.01$). To prevent the loss of explained variance in depressive symptoms, four separate regression analyses were performed for each daily stress subscale (Tables 4–7). Both the reported intensity of independent- and dependent daily stress significantly predicted depressive symptoms at three months follow-up (respectively: $B = 0.470$, $t = 2.046$, $p = 0.041$, 95% CI $= 0.02$–0.92; $B = 0.291$, $t = 2.202$, $p = 0.028$, 95% CI $= 0.03$–0.55). After adjustments in the next steps, these results did not change significantly. Frequency of independent and dependent daily stress did not significantly predict depressive symptoms and again these results did not significantly change after adjustments. The R^2 of all the total models was small (0.044–0.073), as were the adjusted R^2 of the total models (0.015–0.045), meaning only a small part of the variation in prospectively depressive symptoms in remitted recurrently depressed patients was explained by the variables in

Table 1. Baseline demographic and clinical characteristics (n = 138).

Variable	Total (N = 138)	Trial A (N = 56)	Trial B (N = 82)	p[a]
Age, mean (SD)	48.16 (10.4) (n = 138)	48.32 (10.1) (n = 56)	48.05 (10.7) (n = 82)	.526
Female gender, no. (%)	92/138 (68.1)	35/56 (62.5)	57/82 (68.3)	.391
ADM at recruitment, no. (%)				
Yes ADM	102/138 (73.9)	56/56 (100.0)	46/82 (56.1)	.000
Current psychotherapy	47/138 (34.1)	20/56 (35.7)	27/82 (32.9)	.680
Age of first MDD episode, mean (SD)	30.10 (13.4) (n = 134)	30.27 (13.1) (n = 52)	29.79 (13.9) (n = 82)	.176
Previous episodes MDD, median (IQR)	4.0 (3.0)	4.0 (2.25)	4.0 (3.0)	.412
Depressive symptomatology $HDRS_{17}$	3.53 (2.8) (n = 138)	3.50 (2.6) (n = 56)	3.55 (2.9) (n = 82)	.416
Depressive symptomatology (IDS-SR)	17.61 (10.2) (n = 134)	19.90 (10.7) (n = 52)	16.16 (9.6) (n = 82)	.176
Severity last episode				
Minor (%)	21/138 (15.2)	5/56 (8.9)	16/82 (19.5)	.214
Moderate (%)	76/138 (55.1)	32/56 (57.1)	44/82 (53.7)	
Severe (%)	41/138 (29.7)	19/56 (33.9)	22/82 (26.8)	
Daily stress, mean (SD)	(n = 128)	(n = 48)	(n = 80)	
Dependent frequency	9.62 (5.0)	9.56 (4.9)	9.65 (5.0)	.881
Dependent intensity	12.61 (9.0)	11.65 (8.7)	13.19 (9.2)	.601
Independent frequency	6.00 (3.3)	5.58 (3.1)	6.18 (3.4)	..667
Independent intensity	7.27(5.2)	6.54 (4.4)	7.70 (5.6)	.137
Childhood adversity no. (%)				
Loss of a parent	11/131 (8.4)	4/51 (7.8)	7/80 (8.8)	.855
Physical abuse	16/131 (12.2)	4/51 (7.8)	12/80 (15.0)	.223
Sexual abuse	19/131(14.5)	8/51 (15.7)	11/80 (13.8)	.759

Note, [a] p-value based on chi-square statistic for categorical variables and analyses of variance for continuous variables and the Mann-Whitney U for previous episodes of MDD ADM = Antidepressant medication; MDD = Major Depressive Disorder; $HDRS_{17}$ = 17-item Hamilton Rating Scale for Depression; IDS = Inventory of Depressive Symptomatology

Table 2. Hierarchical regression model of the TAU and continuation of ADM group for the prediction of depressive symptoms at 3-month follow-up from childhood adversity (n = 138).

Variable		ö	t	95% CI	R^2 Change
Step 1					0.023
	(Constant)	19.535	14.044**	[16.81, 22.26]	
	CA presence	4.073	1.522	[−1.18, 9.33]	
Step 2					0.007
	(Constant)	19.727	4.967**	[11.94, 27.51]	
	CA presence	4.035	1.504	[−1.23, 9.30]	
	Female gender	1.553	0.629	[−3.29, 6.40]	
	Treatment group	−0.874	−0.371	[−5.50, 3.75]	
Step 3					0.002
	(Constant)	15.540	3.154**	[5.88, 25.20]	
	CA presence	4.046	1.515'	[−1.20, 9.29]	
	Female gender	1.029	0.417	[−3.81, 5.87]	
	Treatment group	−0.827	−0.353	[−5.42, 3.77]	
	Number of previous episodes	3.176	1.430	[−1.18, 7.53]	

Note, CA = Childhood adversity; R^2 final model = 0.048, Adjusted R^2 = 0.012.
* $p<0.05$.
** $p<0.01$.

Table 3. Depressive symptoms at baseline and three-month follow-up in participants with,-and without childhood adversity (n = 138).

Variable	With Childhood Adversity	Without Childhood Adversity	p^a
Depressive symptomatology (IDS-SR) baseline, mean (SD)	19.82 (10.3)	16.86 (9.8)	.132
Depressive symptomatology (IDS-SR) follow-up, mean (SD)	23.54 (12.4)	19.53 (13.2)	.136
Intensity dependent stress, mean (SD)	13.00 (9.9)	12.47 (8.7)	.233
Intensity independent stress, mean (SD)	7.82 (5.0)	7.07 (5.3)	.956
Frequency dependent stress, mean (SD)	9.42 (4.6)	9.68 (5.1)	.564
Frequency independent stress, mean (SD)	5.94 (3.2)	9.96 (3.3)	.923

Note, [a]p-value based on analyses of variance; IDS-SR = Inventory of Depressive Symptomatology.

the model. Performing the analyses in the original dataset did not lead to any substantial differences in results.

Discussion

Our first research aim was to investigate the influence of childhood adversity on the depressive symptoms three months after remission and whether adult daily stress was a mediator of this potential influence. We found no support for our hypothesis that childhood adversity predicts depressive symptoms. Additionally, in contrast to our hypothesis, childhood adversity was not related to daily stress in later life either. This is at odds with previous research where childhood adversity led to higher later life stress, which in turn predicted the onset of depression [31,32]. However, this is the first investigation of the effect of childhood adversity on daily stress and prospectively measured depressive symptoms in recurrently depressed patients while remitted. Importantly, these findings have to be interpreted in the context of our highly recurrent study sample. With a median of four previous depressive episodes (IQR = 3.0), a potential effect of childhood adversity on risk of relapse might have been overshadowed. Unfortunately, we cannot compare this to other related studies, because in comparable studies overall the information on the mean or median number of previous depressive episodes was not mentioned [51–54].

Alternatively, different pathways could lead from childhood adversity to depressive relapse. Cognitive variables, such as dysfunctional attitudes, may play a role given that they develop early in life and the occurrence of childhood adversities is presumed to negatively influence their development [55,56]. Evidence for this pathway was found in previous research in patients with a history of depression, where a negative cognitive style was a mediator in the relation between childhood adversity and stress generation [34]. More research is needed to specify this potential pathway in recurrent depression.

A final research aim was to examine if daily stress was predictive of depressive symptoms measured three months after baseline remission. In line with previous research [31], we found intensity of dependent and independent daily stress to be predictive of subsequent depressive symptoms after remission. Although we expected only dependent stress to be predictive, our finding is

Table 4. Hierarchical regression model of the TAU and continuation of ADM group for the prediction of depressive symptoms at 3-month follow-up from independent stress intensity (n = 138).

Variable		ö	t	95% CI	R^2 Change
Step 1					0.039**
	(Constant)	17.244	8.423**	[13.23, 21.26]	
	Independent stress, intensity	0.470	2.046*	[0.02, 0.92]	
Step 2					0.009
	(Constant)	16.185	3.609**	[7.39, 24.98]	
	Independent stress, intensity	0.488	2.086*	[0.03, 0.95]	
	Female gender	2.244	0.910	[−2.59, 7.08]	
	Treatment group	−0.415	−0.177	[−5.01, 4.18]	
Step 3					0.025
	(Constant)	10.768	1.967*	[0.33, 24.50]	
	Independent stress, intensity	0.533	2.279*	[0.07, 0.99]	
	Female gender	1.676	0.684	[−3.13, 6.48]	
	Treatment group	−0.315	−0.136	[−4.87, 4.24]	
	Number of previous episodes	3.785	1.711	[−0.55, 8.12]	

Note: R^2 final model = 0.073, Adjusted R^2 = 0.045.
* p <0.05.
** p <0.01.

Table 5. Hierarchical regression model of the TAU and continuation of ADM group for the prediction of depressive symptoms at 3-month follow-up from dependent stress intensity (n = 138).

Variable		ö	t	95% CI	R^2 Change
Step 1					0.044
	(Constant)	17.024	8.261**	[12.98, 21.07]	
	Dependent stress, intensity	0.291	2.202*	[0.03, 0.55]	
Step 2					0.005
	(Constant)	17.001	3.936**	[8.53, 25.47]	
	Dependent stress, intensity	0.284	2.138*	[0.02, 0.54]	
	Female gender	1.257	0.514	[−3.54, 6.05]	
	Treatment group	−0.525	−0.223	[−5.13, 4.08]	
Step 3					0.016
	(Constant)	13.218	2.542*	[3.02, 23.42]	
	Dependent stress, intensity	0.276	2.086*	[0.02, 0.54]	
	Female gender	0.781	0.319	[−4.02, 5.58]	
	Treatment group	−0.492	−0.210	[−5.08, 4.09]	
	Number of previous episodes	2.954	1.343	[−1.36, 7.27]	

Note: R^2 final model = 0.064, Adjusted R^2 = 0.036.
* $p<0.05$.
** $p<0.01$.

consistent with the study of Monroe et al. [30]. In their study, 126 recurrently depressed patients were followed over three years of maintenance treatment, where 'subject focused independent daily stress' (an event that happens to a person self instead of an acquaintance or relative), was predictive of depressive relapse. Abramson, Seligman & Teasdale [57], suggested that independent stress poses a risk for depressive relapse because of the lack of control on individual experiences when independent events occur which heightens the stress response.

Strengths and Limitations

While it is an advantage to study this high risk of relapse patient group to determine whether childhood adversity and daily stress influence the return of depression, the downside is that the experience of previous episodes could make the detection of pathways from childhood adversity to depressive relapse difficult. The following limitations have to be taken into account. First, the level of depressive symptoms at three-month follow-up is relatively low since patients were remitted at study start which could make

Table 6. Hierarchical regression model of the TAU and continuation of ADM group for the prediction of depressive symptoms at 3-month follow-up from independent stress frequency (n = 138).

Variable		ö	t	95% CI	R^2 Change
Step 1					0.022
	(Constant)	17.321	6.907**	[12.40, 22.24]	
	Independent stress, frequency	0.561	1.554	[−0.15, 1.27]	
Step 2					0.009
	(Constant)	16.569	3.459**	[7.17, 25.96]	
	Independent stress, frequency	0.591	1.609	[−0.13, 1.31]	
	Female gender	2.138	0.860	[−2.74, 7.01]	
	Treatment group	−0.617	−0.261	[−5.25, 4.01]	
Step 3					0.023
	(Constant)	11.292	1.960	[−0.01, 22.59]	
	Independent stress, frequency	0.659	1.800	[−0.06, 1.38]	
	Female gender	1.598	0.646	[−3.25, 6.45]	
	Treatment group	−0.531	−0.227	[−5.13, 4.06]	
	Number of previous episodes	3.631	1.631	[−0.74, 8.00]	

Note: R^2 final model = 0.054, Adjusted R^2 = 0.026.
* $p < 0.05$.
** $p < 0.01$.

Table 7. Hierarchical regression model of the TAU and continuation of ADM group for the prediction of depressive symptoms at 3-month follow-up from dependent stress frequency (n = 138).

Variable		ö	t	95% CI	R^2 Change
Step 1					0.018
	(Constant)	17.440	6.703**	[12.34, 22.54]	
	Dependent stress, frequency	0.337	1.427	[−0.13, 0.80]	
Step 2					0.007
	(Constant)	17.543	3.800**	[8.49, 26.60]	
	Dependent stress, frequency	0.339	1.428	[−0.13, 0.80]	
	Female gender	1.673	0.675	[−3.19, 6.53]	
	Treatment group	−0.888	−0.376	[−5.52, 3.74]	
Step 3					0.018
	(Constant)	13.361	2.430*	[2.58, 24.15]	
	Dependent stress, frequency	0.339	1.435	[−0.12, 0.80]	
	Female gender	1.150	0.465	[−3.70, 6.00]	
	Treatment group	−0.841	−0.358	[−5.45, 3.76]	
	Number of previous episodes	3.171	1.428	[−1.18, 7.53]	

Note: R^2 final model = 0.044, Adjusted R^2 = 0.015.
* $p < 0.05$.
** $p < 0.01$.

finding an effect difficult. Second, the limited follow-up time of three months and relatively small sample size may lower the chance of detecting an effect. However, based on the number of patients with-, versus without exposure to childhood adversity, detection of a moderate to large effect seemed possible. Although this standard deviation was derived out of our own study, it was comparable to other MDD populations [58]. Third, while retrospective assessment of childhood adversity is representative, irrespective of presence of mental illness even up to 20 years [59], self-report is said to lead to less strong associations than contextual measures [60]. Alloy, Liu and Bender [61], state that using a self-report checklist as assessment tool of stressful life events could lead to more interpretative biases by patients and the lack of contextual information makes it hard to differentiate between dependent and independent events. Furthermore, information about the intensity and frequency of childhood adversity is missing, but could be decisive with regard to long-lasting influences on stress and depression. Fourth, there is a wide variety of other types of childhood adversity that were not assessed but could be of importance. For example emotional neglect and emotional abuse were not assessed in our study, although they are potentially important to the prognosis of depression [10,12,13]. Additionally previous research in patients with a history of depression showed that specifically emotional neglect was the significant predictor of prospective negative dependent events [34]. Fifth, we used four separate regression analyses to examine the associations between the four daily stress subscales and depressive symptoms. However, these four hypotheses may not be completely independent. After a Bonferroni correction which is considered conservative, the intensity of dependent-, and independent daily stress would not be significant predictors of depressive symptoms at follow-up anymore. Bearing in mind that the use of adjustment procedures for multiple comparisons has been criticized for, amongst others, falsely reporting no significant associations [62], no adjustments are needed for multiple comparisons. Nevertheless, we stress the need for cautious interpretation of the results. Sixth, the participants in this study were recruited for two studies that differed with respect to ADM use and the mean severity of the previous depressive episode. Although we controlled for treatment group, these differences still may have influenced the results. Seventh, the low level of variance in depressive symptoms explained by intensity of daily stress suggests the existence of other predictors of depressive symptoms. Finally, it cannot be ruled out that the observed relationship between daily stress and depressive symptoms at follow-up is actually reverse, i.e. baseline depressive symptoms cause baseline daily stress and depressive symptoms at follow-up. However, in this study we were interested in the prediction of depressive symptoms from daily stress and we leave the possibility that the relationship is partially explained by baseline depressive symptoms as an intermediate variable open.

Conclusion and future directions

Our study suggests that the perceived intensity of daily stress is a predictor of depressive symptoms three months after remission, which heightens the risk of relapse in recurrently depressed patients. The intensity of daily stress is potentially modifiable and could therefore be a treatment aim in the prevention of depressive relapse, irrespective of experienced childhood adversity. There is an indication that PCT reduces the negative influence of daily stress on depressive relapse [22,23], but more information on the course of daily stress is required to examine long-term treatment effects on daily stress and relapse. Other studies, with a larger sample size and a longer follow-up time, are needed to replicate these findings and to examine other potential pathways of childhood adversity to depressive relapse, including cognitive variables.

Supporting Information

Checklist S1 CONSORT checklist.

Protocol S1 Trial protocol (trial B).

Protocol S2 Trial protocol (trial A).

Acknowledgments

We are very grateful to all participants for their participation in the study. Without them this study would not exist. Moreover, we would like to thank all recruitment sites for their efforts: Altrecht, Amsterdam Medical Center, Arkin, GGZ Centraal (Almere and Hilversum), GGZ Drenthe, GGZ Friesland, HSK, PsyQ (Amsterdam, Groningen and Rotterdam), Indigo/ Emergis Zeeland, RIAGG Maastricht, University Medical Center Groningen, participating General practitioners associated with Zorggroep Almere, the network General Practitioners VUmc, and all participating pharmacists associated with UPPER, University of Utrecht. We also thank all therapists for conducting the PCT and supporting the M-CT. Finally, we are grateful to all master students, honour's students, volunteers (specifically Isabel Schmidt), and research assistants (specifically Ellen Hendriks, Michelle van der Laan and Nicola Klein) for their help.

Author Contributions

Conceived and designed the experiments: CB. Performed the experiments: GK GR HE. Analyzed the data: GK GR HB. Wrote the paper: GK GR HB HE HR PC JD FS CB.

References

1. American Psychiatric Association (2000) Diagnostic and statistical manual of mental disorders. Washington DC: American Psychiatric Association.
2. Burcusa SL, Iacono WG (2007) Risk for recurrence in depression. Clin Psychol Rev 27: 959–985.
3. Consensus Development Panel NIMH/NIH (1985) Consensus development conference statement on mood disorders: Pharmacological prevention of recurrences. Am J Psychiatry 142: 469–476.
4. Kessing LV, Hansen MG, Andersen PK, Angst J (2004) The predictive effect of episodes on the risk of recurrence in depressive and bipolar disorders—A life-long perspective. Acta Psychiatr Scand 109: 339–344.
5. Solomon DA, Keller MB, Leon AC, Mueller TI, Lavori PW, et al. (2000) Multiple recurrences of major depressive disorder. Am J Psychiatry 157: 229–233.
6. Hollon SD, Stewart MO, Strunk D (2006) Enduring effects for cognitive behavior therapy in the treatment of depression and anxiety. Annu Rev Psychol 57: 285–315.
7. Hardeveld F, Spijker J, De Graaf R, Nolen WA, Beekman ATF (2013) Recurrence of major depressive disorder and its predictors in the general population: Results from the netherlands mental health survey and incidence study (NEMESIS). Psychol Med 43: 39–48.
8. Harkness KL, Bagby RM, Kennedy SH (2012) Childhood maltreatment and differential treatment response and recurrence in adult major depressive disorder. J Consult Clin Psychol 80: 342–353.
9. Nanni V, Uher R, Danese A (2012) Childhood maltreatment predicts unfavorable course of illness and treatment outcome in depression: A meta-analysis. Am J Psychiatry 169: 141–151.
10. Brown GW, Moran P (1994) Clinical and psychosocial origins of chronic depressive episodes: I. A community survey. The British Journal of Psychiatry 165: 447–456.
11. Klein DN, Arnow BA, Barkin JL, Dowling F, Kocsis JH, et al. (2009) Early adversity in chronic depression: Clinical correlates and response to pharmacotherapy. Depress Anxiety 26: 701–710.
12. Wiersma JE, Hovens JGFM, van Oppen P, Giltay EJ, van Schaik, Digna J F., et al. (2009) The importance of childhood trauma and childhood life events for chronicity of depression in adults. J Clin Psychiatry 70: 983–989.
13. Hovens JGFM, Wiersma JE, Giltay EJ, van Oppen P, Spinhoven P, et al. (2010) Childhood life events and childhood trauma in adult patients with depressive, anxiety and comorbid disorders vs. controls. Acta Psychiatr Scand 122: 66–74.
14. Bleuler M (1963) Conception of schizophrenia within the last fifty years and today [abridged]. Proc R Soc Med 56: 945–952.
15. Zubin J, Spring B (1977) Vulnerability: A new view of schizophrenia. J Abnorm Psychol 86: 103–126.
16. Rosenthal D (1963) A suggested conceptual framework. In: Rosenthal D, editor. New York, NY US: Basic Books. pp. 505–511.
17. Abramson LY, Metalsky GI, Alloy LB (1989) Hopelessness depression: A theory-based subtype of depression. Psychol Rev 96: 358–372.
18. Comijs HC, Beekman ATF, Smit F, Bremmer M, van Tilburg T, et al. (2007) Childhood adversity, recent life events and depression in late life. J Affect Disord 103: 243–246.
19. Glaser J, van Os J, Portegijs PJM, Myin-Germeys I (2006) Childhood trauma and emotional reactivity to daily life stress in adult frequent attenders of general practitioners. J Psychosom Res 61: 229–236.
20. Wichers M, Schrijvers D, Geschwind N, Jacobs N, Myin-Germeys I, et al. (2009) Mechanism of gene-environment interactions in depression: Evidence that genes potentiate multiple sources of adversity. Psychol Med 39: 1077–1086.
21. Tyrka AR, Price LH, Marsit C, Walters OC, Carpenter LL (2012) Childhood adversity and epigenetic modulation of the leukocyte glucocorticoid receptor: Preliminary findings in healthy adults. PLoS ONE 7.
22. Bockting CLH, Spinhoven P, Koeter MWJ, Wouters LF, Visser I, et al. (2006) Differential predictors of response to preventive cognitive therapy in recurrent depression: A 2-year prospective study. Psychother Psychosom 75: 229–236.
23. ten Doesschate MC, Bockting CLH, Koeter MWJ, Schene AH (2010) Prediction of recurrence in recurrent depression: A 5.5-year prospective study. J Clin Psychiatry 71: 984–991.
24. Kendler KS, Thornton LM, Gardner CO (2001) Genetic risk, number of previous depressive episodes, and stressful life events in predicting onset of major depression. Am J Psychiatry 158: 582–586.
25. Post RM (1992) Transduction of psychosocial stress into the neurobiology of recurrent affective disorder. Am J Psychiatry 149: 999–1010.
26. Monroe SM, Harkness KL (2005) Life stress, the 'kindling' hypothesis, and the recurrence of depression: Considerations from a life stress perspective. Psychol Rev 112: 417–445.
27. Mazure CM (1998) Life stressors as risk factors in depression. Clinical Psychology: Science and Practice 5: 291–313.
28. Ormel J, Oldehinkel AJ, Brilman EI (2001) The interplay and etiological continuity of neuroticism, difficulties, and life events in the etiology of major and subsyndromal, first and recurrent depressive episodes in later life. Am J Psychiatry 158: 885–891.
29. Monroe SM, Roberts JE, Kupfer DJ, Frank E (1996) Life stress and treatment course of recurrent depression: II. postrecovery associations with attrition, symptom course, and recurrence over 3 years. J Abnorm Psychol 105: 313–328.
30. Monroe SM, Torres LD, Guillaumot J, Harkness KL, Roberts JE, et al. (2006) Life stress and the long-term treatment course of recurrent depression: III. nonsevere life events predict recurrence for medicated patients over 3 years. J Consult Clin Psychol 74: 112–120.
31. McLaughlin KA, Conron KJ, Koenen KC, Gilman SE (2010) Childhood adversity, adult stressful life events, and risk of past-year psychiatric disorder: A test of the stress sensitization hypothesis in a population-based sample of adults. Psychological Medicine: A Journal of Research in Psychiatry and the Allied Sciences 40: 1647–1658.
32. LaNoue M, Graeber D, de Hernandez BU, Warner TD, Helitzer DL (2012) Direct and indirect effects of childhood adversity on adult depression. Community Ment Health J 48: 187–192.
33. Hammen C (1991) Generation of stress in the course of unipolar depression. J Abnorm Psychol 100: 555–561.
34. Liu RT, Choi JY, Boland EM, Mastin BM, Alloy LB (2013) Childhood abuse and stress generation: The mediational effect of depressogenic cognitive styles. Psychiatry Res 206: 217–222.
35. Hammen C (2006) Stress generation in depression: Reflections on origins, research, and future directions. J Clin Psychol 62: 1065–1082.
36. Bockting CLH, Elgersma HJ, van Rijsbergen GD, de Jonge P, Ormel J, et al. (2011) Disrupting the rhythm of depression: Design and protocol of a randomized controlled trial on preventing relapse using brief cognitive therapy with or without antidepressants. BMC Psychiatry 11.
37. Bockting CLH, Kok GD, van den Kamp L, Smit F, van Valen E, et al. (2011) Disrupting the rhythm of depression using mobile cognitive therapy for recurrent depression: Randomized controlled trial design and protocol. BMC Psychiatry 11.
38. First M, Spitzer RL, Gibbon M (2001) Structural clinical interview for DSM-IV-TR axis I disorders, research version patient edition with psychotic screen. New York: New York State Psychiatric Institute.
39. Hamilton M (1960) A rating scale for depression. J Neurol Neurosurg Psychiat 23: 56–61.
40. Kraaij V, de Wilde EJ (2001) Negative life events and depressive symptoms in the elderly: A life span perspective. Aging & Mental Health 5: 84–91.
41. Bockting CLH, Lok A, Visser I, Assies J, Koeter MW, et al. (2012) Lower cortisol levels predict recurrence in remitted patients with recurrent depression: A 5.5 year prospective study. Psychiatry Res 200: 281–287.
42. Nemeroff CB, Heim CM, Thase M, Klein DN, Rush AJ, et al. (2003) Differential responses to psychotherapy versus pharmacotherapy in patients with chronic forms of major depression and childhood trauma. Proc Natl Acad Sci U S A 100: 14293–14296.
43. Spinhoven P, Elzinga BM, Hovens JGFM, Roelofs K, Zitman FG, et al. (2010) The specificity of childhood adversities and negative life events across the life span to anxiety and depressive disorders. J Affect Disord 126: 103–112.
44. Vingerhoets AJJM, van Tilburg MAL (1994) Everyday problem checklist (EPCL): Lisse: Swets & Zeitlinger B.V.
45. Harkness KL, Bruce AE, Lumley MN (2006) The role of childhood abuse and neglect in the sensitization to stressful life events in adolescent depression. J Abnorm Psychol 115: 730–741.

46. Rush AJ, Giles DE, Schlesser MA, Fulton CL, Weissenburger J, et al. (1986) The inventory for depressive symptomatology (IDS): Preliminary findings. Psychiatry Res 18: 65–87.
47. Schafer JL, Graham JW (2002) Missing data: Our view of the state of the art. Psychol Methods 7: 147–177.
48. Rubin DB (1987) Multiple imputation for nonresponse in surveys. New York: J. Wiley & Sons.
49. Liu RT, Alloy LB (2010) Stress generation in depression: A systematic review of the empirical literature and recommendations for future study. Clin Psychol Rev 30: 582–593.
50. Baron RM, Kenny DA (1986) The moderator-mediator variable distinction in social psychological research: Conceptual, strategic, and statistical considerations. J Pers Soc Psychol 51: 1173–1182.
51. Collishaw S, Pickles A, Messer J, Rutter M, Shearer C, et al. (2007) Resilience to adult psychopathology following childhood maltreatment: Evidence from a community sample. Child Abuse Negl 31: 211–229.
52. Ritchie K, Jaussent I, Stewart R, Dupuy A, Courtet P, et al. (2009) Association of adverse childhood environment and 5-HTTLPR genotype with late-life depression. J Clin Psychiatry 70: 1281–1288.
53. Suija K, Aluoja A, Kalda R, Maaroos H (2011) Factors associated with recurrent depression: A prospective study in family practice. Fam Pract 28: 22–28.
54. Wainwright NWJ, Surtees PG (2002) Childhood adversity, gender and depression over the life-course. J Affect Disord 72: 33–44.
55. Beck AT (1967) Depression: Clinical, experimental, and theoretical aspects. New York: Hoeber.
56. Beck AT (1987) Cognitive models of depression. Journal of Cognitive Psychotherapy 1: 5–37.
57. Abramson LY, Seligman ME, Teasdale JD (1978) Learned helplessness in humans: Critique and reformulation. J Abnorm Psychol 87: 49–74.
58. Schulte-van Maaren YWM, Carlier IVE, Zitman FG, van Hemert AM, de Waal, Margot W M., et al. (2013) Reference values for major depression questionnaires: The leiden routine outcome monitoring study. J Affect Disord 149: 342–349.
59. Lizardi H, Klein DN (2005) Long-term stability of parental representations in depressed outpatients utilizing the parental bonding instrument. J Nerv Ment Dis 193: 183–188.
60. Kessler RC, Davis CG, Kendler KS (1997) Childhood adversity and adult psychiatric disorder in the US national comorbidity survey. Psychological Medicine: A Journal of Research in Psychiatry and the Allied Sciences 27: 1101–1119.
61. Alloy LB, Liu RT, Bender RE (2010) Stress generation research in depression: A commentary. International Journal of Cognitive Therapy 3: 380–388.
62. Rothman KJ (1990) No adjustments are needed for multiple comparisons. Epidemiology 1: 43–46.

14

Relationship of Temperament and Character in Remitted Depressed Patients with Suicidal Ideation and Suicide Attempts—Results from the CRESCEND Study

Young Sup Woo[1], Tae-Youn Jun[1]*, Yang-Hwan Jeon[1], Hoo Rim Song[1], Tae-Suk Kim[1], Jung-Bum Kim[2], Min-Soo Lee[3], Jae-Min Kim[4], Sun-Jin Jo[5]

1 Department of Psychiatry, The Catholic University of Korea School of Medicine, Seoul, Korea, **2** Department of Psychiatry, Keimyung University School of Medicine, Daegu, Korea, **3** Department of Psychiatry, College of Medicine, Korea University, Seoul, Korea, **4** Department of Psychiatry, Chonnam National University Medical School, Gwangju, Korea, **5** Department of Preventive Medicine, The Catholic University of Korea School of Medicine, Seoul, Korea

Abstract

The aim of this study was to evaluate the Temperament and Character Inventory (TCI) scores of a sample of Korean patients with remitted depression who had attempted suicide and reported suicidal ideation and to compare their scores with those of remitted depressed patients without suicidal ideation. Adult depression patients who had completed 12 weeks of follow-up ($N=138$) were divided into three groups: patients with a history of suicide attempts ($N=23$); patients with current suicidal ideation ($N=59$); and patients without current suicidal ideation ($N=56$). After controlling for covariates, no significant differences were found among the three groups on any measure of temperament or character except self-directedness and self-transcendence. The self-transcendence scores of the lifetime suicide-attempt group were significantly higher compared with those of the suicidal-ideation group; *post hoc* analysis revealed that self-directedness was significantly lower in the suicide-attempt group compared with the non-suicidal group. The results from the present study suggest that remitted depression patients with a history of suicide attempts do not differ from non-attempters in temperament, but do differ in certain character traits.

Editor: Jerson Laks, Federal University of Rio de Janeiro, Brazil

Funding: This research was supported by a grant of the Korea Health 21 R&D, Ministry of Health and Welfare, Republic of Korea (HI10C2020). The funder had no role in study design, data collection and analysis, decision to publish, or preparation of the manuscript.

Competing Interests: The authors have declared that no competing interests exist.

* Email: tyjun@catholic.ac.kr

Introduction

Suicide is a major public health problem worldwide, especially in patients with depression. The World Health Organization (WHO) estimates that 873,000 people commit suicide each year worldwide. This represents 1.4% of the total global burden of disease [1]. 60–70% of suicide victims have severe depression prior to committing suicide [2]. Moreover, as many as two-thirds of people with depression experience suicidal ideation, and 10–15% commit suicide [3]. The suicide rate in South Korea is increasing: the average number of daily deaths was 38.8 [4]. Korea also had the highest rate of suicide among the Organization for Economic Cooperation and Development countries in 2011 [5].

Although a variety of risk factors for suicidal behavior have been identified among persons with depression, including prior suicide attempts, hopelessness, co-morbid alcohol/substance abuse, further depressive episodes, and earlier age of onset of a major depressive disorder (MDD) [6–9], risk prediction is known to be imprecise. Indeed, false-positive and -negative findings are common [10,11]. To predict and prevent suicidality, it is important to understand which personality traits that may be linked to suicidal behavior, and whether suicidality develops in the context of a time-limited psychiatric disorder or as part of a situation-dependent process [12]. Certain predisposing and protective factors for suicidal behavior lie in the structure of personality.

In several previous studies, personality, as represented in Cloninger's temperament and character model and measured by the Temperament and Character Inventory (TCI), has been investigated in suicidal patients. TCI is a widely used inventory that evaluates four major dimensions of temperament: harm avoidance (HA), novelty seeking (NS), reward dependence (RD), and persistence (PE), together with three major character dimensions: self-directedness (SD), cooperativeness (CO), and self-transcendence (ST) [13]. Temperament, as understood in this model, has been inferred largely from genetic studies of personality in humans and neurobiological studies with rodents [14]. The dimensions of temperament have been hypothesized to relate to brain neurotransmitter systems (where HA relates to serotonergic function, RD to noradrenergic function, and NS to dopaminergic function) [13].

Two temperament traits have been repeatedly associated with suicidal behavior: higher NS [15–18] and higher HA [19–22]. Other personality traits, including low RD, SD, and CO and high ST [20,22–24], are also associated with suicidal behavior. However, previous studies have primarily compared psychiatric patients with a history of suicide attempts either to patients without a history of suicide attempts or to healthy controls. All of these studies evaluated TCI during the acute phase of the patients' illnesses; hence, TCI scores may have been affected by patients' mood. [19,25], and depressed mood has been shown to be associated with higher HA scores and lower SD and CO scores [26–28].

To date, no study has specifically compared remitted depression patients who have attempted suicide to patients with and without suicidal ideation in the context of Cloninger's temperament and character model as measured by the TCI. The aim of the present study was to compare the personality traits, indexed by TCI scores, of Korean patients with remitted major depressive disorder across three groups: patients with a history of suicide attempts (suicide-attempt group); patients with current suicidal ideation but without a history of suicide attempts (suicidal-ideation group); and patients with neither current suicidal ideation nor a history of suicide attempts (non-suicidal group).

Materials and Methods

The present study used data from the ongoing Clinical Research Center for Depression study (CRESCEND), whose design has been detailed elsewhere [29]. A summary of the study design is presented below.

1. Subjects

Between January 2006 and August 2008, CRESCEND enrolled 1,183 patients with depressive disorders (major depressive disorder, dysthymic disorder, and depressive disorder not otherwise specified) from 18 South Korean hospitals (16 university hospitals and two general hospitals). Enrolment occurred in a naturalistic clinical environment from both outpatient and inpatient settings irrespective of depression subtype or physical co-morbidities. The study was approved by all of the relevant university and/or hospital institutional review boards and was conducted according to the Declaration of Helsinki and good clinical practices. All participants reviewed the consent form, and written informed consent was obtained by research staff prior to their participation.

2. Inclusion and exclusion criteria

All patients with depressive disorders reviewed at the study hospitals were approached regarding participation. The clinicians assessing and diagnosing the patients applied the Diagnostic and Statistical Manual of Mental Disorders, Fourth Edition (DSM-IV) criteria [30]. CRESCEND used broad inclusion and minimal exclusion criteria in an effort to reflect the actual clinical situation in Korea. The inclusion criteria were (i) outpatients and inpatients >7 years of age and (ii) a DSM-IV diagnosis of depressive disorder (MDD with or without psychotic features, dysthymic disorder, or a depressive disorder not otherwise specified). The exclusion criteria were as follows: (i) a current or lifetime DSM-IV diagnosis of co-morbid schizophrenia, other psychotic disorder, bipolar disorder, organic psychosis, or dementia; (ii) a medical or neurologic illness of sufficient severity to interfere with the evaluations and interviews of the study; and (iii) pregnant or breastfeeding women. For analysis purposes, we selected only adult patients (≥20 years of age) who were in remission week 12, when this study was conducted, and excluded patients with other clinically diagnosed Axis I or II co-morbidities. Remission was determined by a Hamilton Depression Rating Scale (HAMD) [31] score of ≤7.

3. Assessments

The CRESCEND research protocol recommended assessments at baseline, 1, 2, 4, 8, 12, 24, and 52 weeks and annually thereafter. The analysis described herein was restricted to data obtained at baseline and week 12 because the TCI was only completed at week 12. Socio-demographic and clinical characteristics were evaluated at baseline. Baseline and week 12 scores were used in this analysis.

4. Determination of suicidality

We categorized patients into three groups: patients without current suicidal ideation and without a history of suicide attempts (non-suicidal group); patients with current suicidal ideation but without a history of suicide attempts (suicidal-ideation group); and patients with a history of suicide attempts with or without current suicidal ideation (suicide-attempt group). To determine suicidality, we investigated patients' suicide attempt histories, and we administered the Beck Scale for Suicide Ideation (SSI-B) [32] to measure current suicidal ideation. The participants and their families were asked whether patients had ever attempted suicide. A suicide attempt was defined as self-destructive behavior with at least some intent to die [33]. The SSI-B, a structured, self-administered scale, was used to identify patients with current suicidal ideation. A rating of "0" for item 4 indicates no active suicidal intent, and for item 5, indicates no avoidance of death if presented with a life-threatening situation. Thus, patients with suicidal ideation are rated as having either active or passive thoughts about killing themselves [34].

5. Statistical Analysis

Descriptive statistics are provided for socio-demographic data and psychometric tests. The chi-square test, Fisher's exact test, and analysis of variance (ANOVA) were conducted to compare the groups across categorical and continuous variables. The three groups' TCI scores were compared via analysis of covariance (ANCOVA), with sociodemographic variables that were significant at baseline and clinical variables significant at week 12 used as covariates. If two or more significant variables exhibited strong correlations ($p<0.1$), we excluded variables with low variance and/or significance. Finally, a *post hoc* analysis was performed to compare the three groups. Statistical significance was set at $p< 0.05$ for all tests. All statistical analyses were conducted using the Statistical Analysis System software package (SAS, version 9.1; SAS Institute, Inc., Cary, NC, USA).

Results

Of 1,183 total participants, 253 (21.4%) patients who had attempted suicide and 407 (34.4%) other patients completed follow-up to the week 12 visit. Information from the TCI was available for 325 patients (79.9%); 138 patients (42.5%) met the inclusion and exclusion criteria for the analysis described herein. The majority of the patients were female ($n = 138$; 85.5%), and 23 patients (16.7%) had a history of suicide attempts. Included patients were more likely to be employed and had lower baseline scores on the CGI-S, HAMD, BDI, and SSI-B and higher scores on the SOFAS and WHOQOL compared with the excluded patients (data not shown).

The baseline socio-demographic and clinical characteristics of the non-suicidal, suicidal-ideation, and suicide-attempt groups are summarized in Table 1. There were no significant differences in socioeconomic status, years of education, employment status, family history of depression or other psychiatric illnesses, current physical co-morbidities, or history of adverse life events among groups. There were significant differences among the three groups with respect to age ($df = 2$, $F = 7.316$, $p = 0.001$), age of onset ($df = 2$, $F = 3.262$, $p = 0.046$), marital status ($df = 2$, $\chi^2 = 10.736$,

$p = 0.005$), and religious status ($df = 2$, $\chi^2 = 7.278$, $p = 0.026$). Among the baseline psychiatric symptom scales, the HAMA ($df = 2$, $F = 5.721$, $p = 0.004$), BDI ($df = 2$, $F = 5.625$, $p = 0.005$), WHOQOL-BREF ($df = 2$, $F = 5.497$, $p = 0.005$), and SSI-B ($df = 2$, $F = 33.161$, $p < 0.001$) differed significantly across the three groups.

Post hoc analysis indicated that the suicide-attempt group was significantly younger compared with the suicidal-ideation ($p = 0.004$) and non-suicidal ($p = 0.001$) groups. Age of onset was higher in the suicidal-ideation group compared with the suicide-attempt group ($p = 0.042$). Patients in the suicide-attempt group were more likely to be unmarried/divorced/widowed ($p = 0.005$) and to have no religious affiliation ($p = 0.026$) compared with the other groups. Compared with the non-suicidal group, the baseline HAMA total score was higher in the suicidal-ideation ($p = 0.015$) and suicide-attempt ($p = 0.019$) groups. Baseline total BDI scores were higher in the suicidal-ideation group compared with the non-suicidal group ($p = 0.004$), and baseline WHOQOL scores were significantly lower in the suicide-attempt group compared with the non-suicidal group ($p = 0.005$).

At week 12, the total HAMD, BDI, CGI-S, WHOQOL-BREF, and SOFAS scores were not significantly different across groups. However, total HAMA scores were higher in the suicide-attempt group compared with the non-suicidal group ($p = 0.009$).

In the second phase of the analysis, ANCOVA was performed to compare group TCI scores at week 12, with age, gender, and week 12 HAMA total scores used as covariates. Age of onset, marital status and religion were excluded because they were correlated with age (data not shown), although they were significantly different across groups at baseline (Table 2). There were no significant group differences in scores for any TCI item. Based on the results of the *post-hoc* analysis, there were no significant differences between the three groups in temperament and character dimensions, with the exception of ST and SD (Table 2). ST scores in the suicidal-ideation group were significantly lower compared with the suicide-attempt group ($p = 0.035$), and the SD scores of the suicide-attempt group were significantly lower compared with the non-suicidal group ($p = 0.033$).

Discussion

The aim of present study was to evaluate patients who were currently in remission from MDD, with or without suicidal ideation and prior suicide attempts, to identify a distinct personality profile for suicide risk based on the TCI. We compared TCI scores in remitted MDD patients with and without suicidal ideation and in patients who had attempted suicide. The suicide-attempt group had higher ST scores compared with the suicidal-ideation group and had lower SD scores compared with the non-suicidal group. Interestingly, there were no significant group differences in HA, NS, RD, CO, and PE scores among groups.

Several previous studies have reported that high HA, NS, and ST and low SD scores were associated with the risk for suicide [19,24,35]. Some researchers have suggested that the association between HA and suicidal behavior is questionable because the association may be dependent on underlying psychopathology and diagnostic status [24,28,36,37]. Studies that have reported high NS and HA in suicidal patients have included patients with various diagnoses; furthermore, a study that only included patients with MDD did not exclude patients with Axis I or II co-morbidities [15,16,20,24]. Moreover, the previous studies evaluated TCI in patients who were symptomatic for depression. Hirano et al. [27] reported that the level of depression was positively correlated with HA score and, further, that scores for HA changed significantly toward normal values in treatment responders, but were stable in treatment non-responders. In a recent meta-analysis, HA scores decreased with effective treatment in patients with MDD [14]. Therefore, high HA scores in the suicidal risk groups of previous studies may have been confounded by the presence of current depressive symptoms. Although the analysis controlled for severity of depression, there was a significant difference in such severity between groups [19]. Moreover, the inclusion criteria applied in the present study, which included only remitters, may have excluded a possible confounder in that high HA scores have previously been associated with increased risk of treatment-resistant depression [14]. With respect to NS, some discrepancies have been found in the direction of the association between NS and suicidality. Many studies have suggested a protective effect of NS [38,39]; however, Brezo et al. [35] found only weak support for the importance of impulsivity and aggression in suicidal ideation, personality traits were mainly measured by the NS and CO dimensions of the TCI [13,36].

In the present study, the suicide-attempt group had higher ST scores compared with the suicidal-ideation group and lower SD scores compared with the non-suicidal group. In a study with schizophrenic patients, high ST was associated with previous suicide attempts [40], and suicidality has been found to be associated with high ST in many other previous studies [15,19,23,41]. This is in line with the results from the present study. SD subsumes personality features such as responsibility, resourcefulness, and self-acceptance [36]. Low SD has been linked to lack of conviction, which is important for problem solving, and to vulnerability to the environment [13]. Previous studies have reported a correlation between low SD and severity of psychiatric symptomatology [42–44]. Moreover, low SD is the principal TCI correlate of Axis II pathology [45–47]. Because we included remitted patients without Axis I or II comorbidity, our results suggest that low SD is related to suicidality and not to the severity of depressive symptoms and personality problems. This result is in accordance with previous studies that reported had lower SD among suicide attempters compared with non-attempters [15,22,44,48]. Moreover, the relatively high ST and low SD scores of suicide attempters in the present study should be viewed in the context of previous studies' reports of an association between high ST and suicidality, as high ST is associated with low SD and is characterized by illogical, immature, and suspicious behavior [15,41].

It is unclear why suicidal ideation was observed so frequently (42.8%, $n = 59$) in remitted depressive patients in the present study. However, the widely accepted relationship between impulsivity and suicidality [49,50] may provide an explanation. In recent studies, Ekinci et al. [51,52] investigated impulsivity, temperament, and character in euthymic patients with major depressive disorder. They reported that impulsivity scores were higher in remitted depressive patients compared with a healthy control group, and also that elevated impulsivity scores were associated with a history of suicide attempts. Accordingly, trait impulsivity may continue to influence suicidal ideation in remitted depressive patients. Moreover, there is evidence of a close relationship between trait anxiety and trait impulsivity [53,54], which could also be an important risk factor for suicide ideation [55]. The higher HAMA score at week 12 in the suicidal-ideation and suicide-attempt groups, compared with the non-suicidal-ideation group, may reflect group differences in impulsivity.

The present study had a number of strengths. First, the study used data from the CRESCEND study, which is the largest-scale depression cohort study ever conducted in Asia and includes a wide range of data pertaining to the socio-demographic and

Table 1. Socio-demographic and clinical characteristics.

	Non suicidal group (N=56)		Suicidal-ideation group (N=59)		Suicide-attempt group (N=23)		
	Mean (*N*)	***SD* (%)**	**Mean (*N*)**	***SD* (%)**	**Mean (*N*)**	***SD* (%)**	***p*-value**
Age (years)	50.7	15.6	49.1	16.5	36.2	14.8	0.001*
Female gender	45	80.4	53	89.8	20	87.0	0.379
Age at onset (years)	38.3	12.1	42.3	19.0	28.3	14.5	0.046*
Education (years)	10.6	4.7	9.9	4.5	11.3	4.0	0.423
Number of previous depressive episodes	6.2	21.9	1.9	2.1	1.5	1.5	0.488
Duration of illness	8.1	8.5	6.7	7.2	9.2	5.7	0.671
Currently married	42	75.0	43	72.9	9	39.1	0.005*
Living alone	52	92.9	51	86.4	19	82.6	0.328
No religious affiliation	13	23.2	15	25.4	12	52.2	0.026*
Annual household income, US$>19,000	31	55.4	31	52.5	12	52.2	0.944
Currently unemployed	11	19.6	8	13.6	4	17.4	0.684
Previous history of depression	20	35.7	23	39.0	13	56.5	0.219
Family history of depression	11	19.6	9	15.3	3	13.0	0.788
Family history of other psychiatric illness	6	10.7	8	13.6	1	4.3	0.583
Adverse life event	11	19.6	12	20.3	8	34.8	0.299
Current physical disorder	13	23.20	18	30.50	7	7	0.648
Baseline assessment scale scores							
CGI-S	4.4	1.1	4.3	1.1	4.6	1.0	0.558
HAMD	16.7	6.0	19.0	5.4	18.8	7.2	0.096
HAMA	13.7	5.8	17.3	7.0	18.3	7.8	0.004*
BDI	21.5	9.5	28.5	11.3	26.7	11.4	0.005*
SSI-B	2.8	3.2	9.9	6.6	15.0	8.3	0.000*
WHOQOL-BREF	69.0	8.8	65.3	9.3	61.7	8.5	0.005*
SOFAS	60.3	10.3	62.1	11.0	56.4	13.2	0.115
Week 12 assessment scale scores							
HAMD	3.8	2.3	3.8	2.0	4.4	2.4	0.487
HAMA	3.5	2.5	4.7	3.0	6.0	5.6	0.009*
CGI-S	1.7	0.9	1.8	0.8	2.1	1.2	0.174
BDI	7.0	6.5	9.2	8.7	8.7	8.4	0.315
SSI-B	1.3	2.6	2.8	5.1	5.3	5.9	0.002*
WHOQOL-BREF	70.6	10.7	68.4	12.1	69.1	12.5	0.591
SOFAS	78.3	10.0	78.1	7.3	76.3	7.8	0.614

CGI-S = Clinical Global Impression Scale; HAMD = Hamilton Depression Rating Scale; HAMA = Hamilton Anxiety Rating Scale; BDI = Beck Depression Inventory, SSI-B = Beck Scale for Suicidal Ideation; SOFAS = Social and Occupational Functioning Assessment Scale; WHOQOL-BREF = World Health Organization Quality of Life assessment instruments.
*$p<0.05$.

Table 2. Temperament and character inventory scores (ANCOVA with covariates of age, gender, and week 12 Hamilton Anxiety Rating Scale total score).

	Group 1 Non-suicidal (N=56)		Group 2 Suicidal ideation (N=59)		Group 3 Suicide attempts (N=23)				Group 1 vs. 2	Group 1 vs. 3	Group 2 vs. 3
	mean	*SD*	mean	*SD*	mean	*SD*	*F*	*P*	*Post hoc* comparison		
Novelty seeking	22.0	4.6	22.8	5.2	23.5	5.1	0.049	0.953	0.805	0.958	0.796
Harm avoidance	13.0	7.4	14.2	5.8	14.0	7.0	0.709	0.494	0.557	0.259	0.43
Reward dependence	10.2	4.2	9.0	3.1	9.2	3.1	0.434	0.649	0.358	0.556	0.675
Persistence	3.6	2.1	3.5	1.7	4.0	1.8	1.976	0.143	0.911	0.156	0.067
Self-directedness	24.1	9.6	19.4	5.8	17.6	6.5	2.281	0.106	0.118	0.035*	0.388
Cooperativeness	16.0	9.3	13.6	6.9	13.1	5.7	0.237	0.789	0.496	0.576	0.892
Self-transcendence	19.0	5.9	17.9	6.3	20.1	5.2	2.451	0.09	0.817	0.189	0.033*

*$p<0.05$.

clinical characteristics of depressed Korean patients. Second, we excluded depressed patients with psychiatric comorbidities to control for the confounding effects of personality disorders or other Axis I disorders, such as anxiety disorders, eating disorders, and substance misuse-related disorders. Third, we included only patients who were in remission from depressive episodes, and assessed TCI at week 12 to control for the possible effects of depressive symptom severity.

The present study also has several limitations. First, we included only Korean patients because cultural issues may lead to variation when assessing dimensions of temperament or character [26]. In a meta-analytic study comparing Cloninger's temperament dimensions across 20 countries [56], differences were particularly apparent between Asian and Western countries. The lowest mean score for RD was observed in the Japanese sample, and the highest mean score in PE was observed in the US sample. Moreover, the Asian sample had lower scores compared with other countries for NS, RD, and PE, and higher scores for HA. Inconsistency in the present results compared with previous studies reporting an association between suicidality and high HA and NS scores may be due to the low scores for HA and NS seen in the Korean sample. This is likely to reduce generalizability. Second, clinical diagnosis was a feature of the present study: this limits the reliability of the diagnosis of depression and other possible comorbid psychiatric disorders. Use of structured diagnostic interview schedules may increase the reliability and validity of diagnoses. Third, given the size of our samples, we could not stratify patients who had attempted suicide by the severity of their suicide attempts. Fourth, the patients included in our analysis had different baseline characteristics compared with excluded patients. Included patients were more likely to be female and employed, and they had lower baseline scores on the CGI-S, HAMD, BDI, and SSI-B and higher scores on the SOFAS and WHOQOL compared with excluded patients. In a previous study investigating TCI in remitted depressive patients [51], socio-demographic variables, including education, age, and gender, did not significantly contribute to TCI scores. However, the inclusion of patients with milder depressive symptoms and a higher degree of functioning, may limit the generalizability of the results of this study. Furthermore, detailed information pertaining to treatment was not included. Multiple, uncontrolled treatments can limit the interpretative validity of results. In a previous study, persistent suicidality was associated with treatment with selective serotonin reuptake inhibitors, a higher baseline SSI-B score and no HAMD- or HAMA-indexed remission episodes [57]. The present results should be interpreted in this context. Finally, certain TCI scores are likely to change over time [36]. We could not investigate changes in TCI scores in an attempt to limit this bias because TCI was only administered at week 12.

In conclusion, we did not observe differences among patients who attempted suicide and those with and without suicidal ideation in any of the dimensions of the TCI, with the exception of ST and SD. Longitudinal studies that include younger age groups are required to disentangle the personality profile of individuals with high suicidality from underlying psychopathology. The findings of the present study may further the delineation of this complex phenotype.

Acknowledgments

We thank the clinicians and research workers who participated in the CRESCEND study.

The English in this document has been checked by at least two professional editors, both native speakers of English. For a certificate, please see: http://www.textcheck.com/certificate/3xx5E8

Author Contributions

Conceived and designed the experiments: YSW TYJ YHJ HRS TSK JBK MSL JMK SJJ. Performed the experiments: YSW TYJ YHJ HRS TSK JBK MSL JMK. Analyzed the data: YSW TYJ HRS. Contributed reagents/materials/analysis tools: YSW TYJ HRS. Wrote the paper: YSW TYJ.

References

1. World Health Organization. Director-General's Office. Communications Office. (2006) World Mental Health Day 2006: Building awareness, reducing risks: suicide and mental illness. Geneva: World Health Organization. 2 pp.
2. Sudak HS (2009) Psychiatric emergencies: Suicide. In: Sadock BJ, Sadock VA, editors. Kaplan and Sadock's Comprehensive Textbook of Psychiatry. Philadelphia: Lippincott Williams & Wilkins. pp. 2723.
3. Sadock BJ, Kaplan HI, Sadock VA (2007) Kaplan & Sadock's synopsis of psychiatry: behavioral sciences/clinical psychiatry. Philadelphia: Wolter Kluwer/Lippincott Williams & Wilkins. xv, 1470 pp.
4. Korea S (2013) Causes of Death Statistics in 2012.
5. OECD Suicide: OECD Publishing.
6. Beck AT, Steer RA, Kovacs M, Garrison B (1985) Hopelessness and eventual suicide: a 10-year prospective study of patients hospitalized with suicidal ideation. Am J Psychiatry 142: 559–563.
7. Claassen CA, Trivedi MH, Rush AJ, Husain MM, Zisook S, et al. (2007) Clinical differences among depressed patients with and without a history of suicide attempts: findings from the STAR*D trial. J Affect Disord 97: 77–84.
8. Malone KM, Haas GL, Sweeney JA, Mann JJ (1995) Major depression and the risk of attempted suicide. J Affect Disord 34: 173–185.
9. Mann JJ, Waternaux C, Haas GL, Malone KM (1999) Toward a clinical model of suicidal behavior in psychiatric patients. Am J Psychiatry 156: 181–189.
10. (2003) Practice guideline for the assessment and treatment of patients with suicidal behaviors. Am J Psychiatry 160: 1–60.
11. Pokorny AD (1983) Prediction of suicide in psychiatric patients. Report of a prospective study. Arch Gen Psychiatry 40: 249–257.
12. Heeringen Kv (2001) Understanding suicidal behaviour: the suicidal process approach to research, treatment, and prevention. Chichester: John Wiley. xiv, 322 pp.
13. Cloninger CR, Svrakic DM, Przybeck TR (1993) A psychobiological model of temperament and character. Arch Gen Psychiatry 50: 975–990.
14. Kampman O, Poutanen O (2011) Can onset and recovery in depression be predicted by temperament? A systematic review and meta-analysis. J Affect Disord 135: 20–27.
15. Becerra B, Paez F, Robles-Garcia R, Vela GE (2005) [Temperament and character profile of persons with suicide attempt]. Actas Esp Psiquiatr 33: 117–122.
16. Grucza RA, Przybeck TR, Spitznagel EL, Cloninger CR (2003) Personality and depressive symptoms: a multi-dimensional analysis. J Affect Disord 74: 123–130.
17. Guillem E, Pelissolo A, Notides C, Lepine JP (2002) Relationship between attempted suicide, serum cholesterol level and novelty seeking in psychiatric in-patients. Psychiatry Res 112: 83–88.
18. van Heeringen K, Audenaert K, Van de Wiele L, Verstraete A (2000) Cortisol in violent suicidal behaviour: association with personality and monoaminergic activity. J Affect Disord 60: 181–189.
19. Conrad R, Walz F, Geiser F, Imbierowicz K, Liedtke R, et al. (2009) Temperament and character personality profile in relation to suicidal ideation and suicide attempts in major depressed patients. Psychiatry Res 170: 212–217.
20. Engstrom C, Brandstrom S, Sigvardsson S, Cloninger CR, Nylander PO (2004) Bipolar disorder. III: Harm avoidance a risk factor for suicide attempts. Bipolar Disord 6: 130–138.
21. Rothenhausler HB, Stepan A, Kapfhammer HP (2006) Soluble interleukin 2 receptor levels, temperament and character in formerly depressed suicide attempters compared with normal controls. Suicide Life Threat Behav 36: 455–466.
22. van Heeringen C, Audenaert K, Van Laere K, Dumont F, Slegers G, et al. (2003) Prefrontal 5-HT2a receptor binding index, hopelessness and personality characteristics in attempted suicide. J Affect Disord 74: 149–158.
23. Anderson CB, Carter FA, McIntosh VV, Joyce PR, Bulik CM (2002) Self-harm and suicide attempts in individuals with bulimia nervosa. Eat Disord 10: 227–243.
24. Calati R, Giegling I, Rujescu D, Hartmann AM, Moller HJ, et al. (2008) Temperament and character of suicide attempters. J Psychiatr Res 42: 938–945.
25. Corruble E, Duret C, Pelissolo A, Falissard B, Guelfi JD (2002) Early and delayed personality changes associated with depression recovery? A one-year follow-up study. Psychiatry Res 109: 17–25.
26. Farmer A, Mahmood A, Redman K, Harris T, Sadler S, et al. (2003) A sib-pair study of the Temperament and Character Inventory scales in major depression. Arch Gen Psychiatry 60: 490–496.
27. Hirano S, Sato T, Narita T, Kusunoki K, Ozaki N, et al. (2002) Evaluating the state dependency of the Temperament and Character Inventory dimensions in patients with major depression: a methodological contribution. J Affect Disord 69: 31–38.
28. Hansenne M, Reggers J, Pinto E, Kjiri K, Ajamier A, et al. (1999) Temperament and character inventory (TCI) and depression. J Psychiatr Res 33: 31–36.
29. Kim JM, Kim SY, Stewart R, Yoo JA, Bae KY, et al. (2011) Improvement within 2 weeks and later treatment outcomes in patients with depressive disorders: the CRESCEND study. J Affect Disord 129: 183–190.
30. American Psychiatric Association., American Psychiatric Association. Task Force on DSM-IV. (1994) Diagnostic and statistical manual of mental disorders: DSM-IV. Washington, DC: American Psychiatric Association. xxv, 886 pp.
31. Hamilton M (1960) A rating scale for depression. J Neurol Neurosurg Psychiatry 23: 56–62.
32. Beck AT, Kovacs M, Weissman A (1979) Assessment of suicidal intention: the Scale for Suicide Ideation. J Consult Clin Psychol 47: 343–352.
33. Oquendo MA, Waternaux C, Brodsky B, Parsons B, Haas GL, et al. (2000) Suicidal behavior in bipolar mood disorder: clinical characteristics of attempters and nonattempters. J Affect Disord 59: 107–117.
34. Steer RA, Beck AT, Brown GK, Beck JS (1993) Classification of suicidal and nonsuicidal outpatients: a cluster-analytic approach. J Clin Psychol 49: 603–614.
35. Brezo J, Paris J, Turecki G (2006) Personality traits as correlates of suicidal ideation, suicide attempts, and suicide completions: a systematic review. Acta Psychiatr Scand 113: 180–206.
36. Cloninger CR (1994) The temperament and character inventory (TCI): a guide to its development and use. St. Louis, MO: Center for Psychobiology of Personality, Washington University. 184 pp.
37. Smith DJ, Duffy L, Stewart ME, Muir WJ, Blackwood DH (2005) High harm avoidance and low self-directedness in euthymic young adults with recurrent, early-onset depression. J Affect Disord 87: 83–89.
38. Allen MH, Chessick CA, Miklowitz DJ, Goldberg JF, Wisniewski SR, et al. (2005) Contributors to suicidal ideation among bipolar patients with and without a history of suicide attempts. Suicide Life Threat Behav 35: 671–680.
39. Csorba J, Dinya E, Ferencz E, Steiner P, Bertalan G, et al. (2010) Novelty seeking: difference between suicidal and non-suicidal Hungarian adolescent outpatients suffering from depression. J Affect Disord 120: 217–220.
40. Aukst Margetic B, Jakovljevic M, Ivanec D, Tosic G, Margetic B (2011) Novelty seeking and medication adherence in patients with schizophrenia. Psychiatry Res 186: 141–143.
41. Bulik CM, Sullivan PF, Joyce PR (1999) Temperament, character and suicide attempts in anorexia nervosa, bulimia nervosa and major depression. Acta Psychiatr Scand 100: 27–32.
42. Abbate-Daga G, Piero A, Gramaglia C, Fassino S (2005) Factors related to severity of vomiting behaviors in bulimia nervosa. Psychiatry Res 134: 75–84.
43. Abbate-Daga G, Piero A, Gramaglia C, Gandione M, Fassino S (2007) An attempt to understand the paradox of anorexia nervosa without drive for thinness. Psychiatry Res 149: 215–221.
44. Evren C, Evren B (2006) The relationship of suicide attempt history with childhood abuse and neglect, alexithymia and temperament and character dimensions of personality in substance dependence. Nord J Psychiatry 60: 263–269.
45. Casey JE, Joyce PR (1999) Personality disorder and the Temperament and Character Inventory in the elderly. Acta Psychiatr Scand 100: 302–308.
46. Svrakic DM, Whitehead C, Przybeck TR, Cloninger CR (1993) Differential diagnosis of personality disorders by the seven-factor model of temperament and character. Arch Gen Psychiatry 50: 991–999.
47. de la Rie SM, Duijsens IJ, Cloninger CR (1998) Temperament, character, and personality disorders. J Pers Disord 12: 362–372.
48. Grucza RA, Przybeck TR, Cloninger CR (2005) Personality as a mediator of demographic risk factors for suicide attempts in a community sample. Compr Psychiatry 46: 214–222.
49. Horesh N, Rolnick T, Iancu I, Dannon P, Lepkifker E, et al. (1997) Anger, impulsivity and suicide risk. Psychother Psychosom 66: 92–96.
50. Oquendo MA, Mann JJ (2000) The biology of impulsivity and suicidality. Psychiatr Clin North Am 23: 11–25.
51. Ekinci O, Albayrak Y, Ekinci AE (2012) Temperament and character in euthymic major depressive disorder patients: the effect of previous suicide attempts and psychotic mood episodes. Psychiatry Investig 9: 119–126.
52. Ekinci O, Albayrak Y, Caykoylu A (2011) Impulsivity in euthymic patients with major depressive disorder: the relation to sociodemographic and clinical properties. J Nerv Ment Dis 199: 454–458.
53. Farmer RF (1998) Depressive symptoms as a function of trait anxiety and impulsivity. J Clin Psychol 54: 129–135.
54. Apter A, Plutchik R, van Praag HM (1993) Anxiety, impulsivity and depressed mood in relation to suicidal and violent behavior. Acta Psychiatr Scand 87: 1–5.
55. Schaefer KE, Esposito-Smythers C, Riskind JH (2012) The role of impulsivity in the relationship between anxiety and suicidal ideation. J Affect Disord 143: 95–101.
56. Miettunen J, Kantojarvi L, Veijola J, Jarveline MR, Joukamaa M (2006) International comparison of Cloninger's temperament dimensions. Personality and Individual Differences 41: 1515–1526.

Prevalence of Depression, Suicidal Ideation, Alcohol Intake and Nicotine Consumption in Rural Central India. The Central India Eye and Medical Study

Jost B. Jonas[1,2,¶]*, **Vinay Nangia**[1,¶]*, **Marcella Rietschel**[3,¶], **Torsten Paul**[3], **Prakash Behere**[1,4], **Songhomitra Panda-Jonas**[1,2]

1 Suraj Eye Institute, Nagpur, Maharashtra, India, **2** Department of Ophthalmology, Medical Faculty Mannheim of the Ruprecht-Karls-University Heidelberg, Mannheim, Germany, **3** Department of Genetic Epidemiology in Psychiatry, Central Institute of Mental Health, Medical Faculty Mannheim of the Ruprecht-Karls-University Heidelberg, Mannheim, Germany, **4** Department of Psychiatry, Datta Meghe Institute of Medical Sciences, Wardha, Maharashtra, India

Abstract

Background: To investigate the prevalence of depression, suicidal ideations, alcohol and nicotine consumption in adults in an agrarian society mostly unchanged by the effects of urbanization.

Methods: The Central India Eye and Medical Study is a population-based study in rural Central India close to the tribal belt and included 4711 subjects (aged 30+ years). Depression was assessed by the Center for Epidemiologic Studies Depression Scale (CESD), suicidal ideation by six standardized questions, nicotine use by the Fagerstroem Nicotine Tolerance Questionnaire (FTNQ), and alcohol consumption by the Alcohol Use Disorders Identification Test (AUDIT).

Results: Mild to moderate depression (CESD sum score: 15–21) was detected in 1862 (39.6%) individuals (33.5% of men, 44.8 of women), and major depression (CESD sum score >21) in 613 (13.0%) individuals (8.1 of men, 17.3% of women). Suicide attempt was reported by 199 (4.2%) participants and suicidal thoughts during the last 6 months by 238 (5.1%) individuals. There were 887 (18.9%) smokers and smokeless tobacco was consumed by 1968 (41.8%) subjects. Alcohol consumption was reported by 1081 (23.0%) participants; 283 (6.0%) subjects had an AUDIT score ≥8 (hazardous drinking), and 108 (4.63%) subjects a score ≥13 (women) or ≥15 (men) (alcohol dependence).

Conclusions: In rural Central India, prevalence of major depression was comparable to figures reported from other developing countries. Prevalence of smoking and hazardous alcohol consumption was higher than as reported from urban regions. Measures should be taken to address the relatively high prevalence of suicide attempts and thoughts on suicide in rural Central India.

Editor: Osama Ali Abulseoud, Mayo Clinic, United States of America

Funding: Support was provided by an unrestricted grant from Om Drishti Trust Nagpur; Heidelberg Engineering Co. Heidelberg, Germany; Rotary Sight Saver Netherlands; Orbis India; and Carl Zeiss Meditec Co., Jena, Germany. The funders had no role in study design, data collection and analysis, decision to publish, or preparation of the manuscript.

Competing Interests: The authors advise of the following: The authors received unrestricted grants from Heidelberg Engineering Co. Heidelberg, Germany and Carl Zeiss Meditec Co., Jena, Germany. Co-author Jost B. Jonas is an Editor of PLOS ONE. This does not alter the authors' adherence to PLOS ONE policies on sharing data and materials.

* Email: nagpursuraj@gmail.com (VN); jost.jonas@medma.uni-heidelberg.de (JBJ)

These authors contributed equally to this work.

¶ These authors share first authorship on this work.

Introduction

Depression with a lifetime prevalence of 2% to 15% is one of the most important risk factors for substantial disability and is one of the major leading causes of disease burden in 2010 [1–5]. Smoking has become the leading cause of preventable death with yearly about 5 million premature deaths worldwide [1,2,6–8]. Alcohol consumption, among other risk factors such as dietary risks, tobacco smoking, high blood pressure, high fasting plasma glucose and physical inactivity, belongs to the leading risk factors related to DALYs [1,2,9–13]. Results from the Global Burden of Disease study showed that especially mental health disorders constitute an enormous and growing problem in developed and developing regions [14]. Despite the worldwide importance of depression, suicide, smoking and alcohol consumption, and although India is the second largest nation by the number of inhabitants, relatively little has been known about the prevalence of depression, suicide ideation, alcohol and nicotine consumption in India. It holds true in particular for the rural population in the under-developed regions of the Indian subcontinent. The present study was therefore conducted to assess the prevalence of depression, nicotine and alcohol abuse and possibly associated health issues in adults living in rural Central India in villages bordering the so-called tribal belt. Since the living conditions in these communities have not markedly changed within the last 100 years, the study additionally offered the possibility of assessing the prevalence of depression, smoking and alcohol consumption in an environment which has remained mostly untouched by factors associated with a developed technical and medical infrastructure.

Methods

The Central India Eye and Medical Study (CIEMS) is a population-based cross-sectional study in Central India [15]. The Medical Ethics Committee of the Medical Faculty Mannheim of the Ruprecht-Karls-University Heidelberg and the ethical committee of Suraj Eye Institute/Nagpur approved the study and all participants gave informed written consent, according to the Declaration of Helsinki. The study was carried out in 8 villages in the rural region of Central Maharashtra at a distance of about 40 km from Nagpur. The villages were at the border of tribal regions. All villagers aged 30+ were invited to participate in the study which included a bus ride to the hospital, a one-day long examination, meals, and a return bus ride to the village in the evening all free of charge. All examinations were carried out on site in the hospital. Trained social workers interviewed the participants with the help of a standardized questionnaire including 200 questions on the socioeconomic background, living conditions, daily food, smoking or other types of tobacco consumption, alcohol consumption, amount and type of daily physical activity, known diagnosis of major diseases, and intake of medication. Addressing the questionnaire usually took about 30 to 40 minutes with the help of an experienced interviewer. If the study participants appeared to be fatigued, a break was made to make the study participant refresh.

The psychiatric status was assessed by the use of several questionnaires. Current depressive mood disorders were recorded by the Center for Epidemiologic Studies Depression Scale (CES-D) with a 20-item self-report depression scale [16]. A clinical episode of major depression was defined as a score of >21 in the CES-D. Six standardized questions concerning suicidal thoughts, suicidal behavior and suicidal attempts during the last 6 months and lifetime were asked. Individuals identified with suicidal thoughts were visited during the repeated visits to the villages as well as after the end of the study since the Suray Eye Institute continued serving visually handicapped villagers with cataract surgery. We used the Fagerstrom Test for Nicotine Dependence (FTND) to assess the smoking behavior [17]. In addition to the FTND, the history of former nicotine consumption (age of onset of tobacco consumption, cessation age, estimated pack years) and consumption of different tobacco products like hookah, bidis and smokeless tobacco products like snuff, chewing tobacco and bethel was recorded by 9 additional standardized questions. To determine alcohol consumption, the Alcohol Use Disorders Identification Test (AUDIT) was utilized [18]. The Audit is a 10-item self-report questionnaire with a sum score of 8 or more being associated with harmful or hazardous drinking, and a score of 13 or more in women and 15 or more in men, being likely to indicate alcohol dependence. In addition to the AUDIT, the history of former alcohol consumption (starting age of alcohol consumption, cessation age) and the current drinking behavior (e. g. type of drink) was assessed by a further 4 standardized questions.

Statistical analysis was performed using a commercially available statistical software package (SPSS for Windows, version 21.0, SPSS, Chicago, IL). We examined the mean values (presented as mean ± standard error for frequency parameters; presented as mean ± standard deviation for other parameters). All P-values were 2-sided and were considered statistically significant when the values were less than 0.05.

Results

Out of total population of 13,606 villagers, 5885 subjects fulfilled the inclusion criterion of an age of 30+ years. Out of these 5885 subjects, 4711 people participated, resulting in a response rate of 80.1% (Table 1). The representativeness of the study population compared to the total population of India had been examined in previous investigations with no major difference detected between the population structure of the study and the general Indian population (Table 1) [15].

There were 2520 (53.5%) women. Mean age of the study participants was 49.5±13.4 years (Table 2). Among the 1174 non-participants were 685 (58.3%) men; mean age was 48.6±14.1 years (median: 45 years; range: 30–95 years). The group of study participants and the group of non-participants did not differ significantly in age ($P = 0.06$), while the proportion of men was significantly ($P<0.001$) higher in the group of non-participants. Further details about the sub items of the non-psychiatric questionnaire, the socioeconomic background and the medical records were presented previously [15].

The mean body mass index was 19.7±3.4 kg/m^2. Mean duration of daily work was 7.4±2.2 hours. The subjects went to work by foot or by bike in 6.6±1.2 days per week. 2394 (50.8%) subjects were purely vegetarians, 35 (0.7%) subjects reported to eat fish and eggs in addition to vegetables, but no meat, and 2275 (48.3%) subjects had a mixed diet. Mean reported monthly income was 1584±1233 Rupee (1 US$ was roughly the equivalent of 50 Rupee). The reported monthly family income was less than 1500 Rupee for 2377 subjects (50.4%). Hinduism was the predominant religion (97.2% of the study population). Out of the total 4711 subjects, 1623 (34.5%) subjects reported to be illiterate, 1310 (27.8%) subjects to have visited school up the 5th standard, 533 (11.3%) subjects to have visited school between the 6th to 8th standard, 1070 (22.7%) subjects to have attended school between the 9th and 12th standard, and 165 (3.5%) subjects reported to have received a higher level of education such as graduation. Out of the 4711 subjects, 139 (3.0%) participants had a mobile. The majority of the study population lived in houses made out of mud without bricks and mortar ("kacha"; 1109 (23.5%) subjects) or made partially out of mud ("semi pucca2330 (49.5%) subjects). Out of the total 4711 subjects, 2206 (46.9%) subjects indicated that they did not have a toilet facility in their houses. Water source was a public tap, hand pump or well for 1719 (36.5%) subjects.

Depression

Data on depression were available on 4698 (99.7%) subjects with a mean age of 49.5±13.4 years. The group of subjects with data on depression and the group of subjects without assessment of depression (mean age: 55.2±13.9 years) did not differ significantly in age ($P = 0.67$).

The mean of the valid CESD sum scores was 14.1±7.5 points (median: 15; range: 0–58) (Fig. 1, 2). Men had a mean CESD sum score of 12.3±6.9 points (median: 13; range: 0–51), while female participants had a mean CESD sum score of 15.7±7.6 points (median: 16; range: 0–58). 1862 individuals (39.57%) showed a CESD sum score between 15 and 21 points indicating a mild to moderate depression within the last week, while 613 individuals (13.03%) scored >21 points in the CESD, indicating the possibility of a major depression. With respect to gender 734

Table 1. Demographic data of the Central India Eye and Medical Study (Part I) and the whole of India according to the National Census - India (2001).

	Central India Eye and Medical Study			India (Total; in Millions)			India (Rural; in Millions)		
Age	**Total**	**Males**	**Females**	**Total**	**Males**	**Females**	**Total**	**Males**	**Females**
30–34 Years	405 (17%)	173 (16%)	232 (18%)	74.3 (19%)	37.4 (19%)	36.9 (19%)	51.8 (19%)	25.7 (18%)	26.1 (19%)
35–39 Years	381 (16%)	154 (14%)	227 (18%)	70.6 (18%)	36.0 (18%)	34.5 (18%)	49.0 (18%)	24.9 (18%)	24.1 (18%)
40–44 Years	336 (14%)	161 (15%)	175 (14%)	55.7 (14%)	29.9 (15%)	25.9 (14%)	38.6 (14%)	20.4 (15%)	18.1 (13%)
45–49 Years	256 (11%)	118 (11%)	138 (11%)	47.4 (12%)	24.9 (12%)	22.5 (12%)	33.0 (12%)	17.0 (12%)	15.9 (12%)
50–54 Years	248 (10%)	123 (11%)	125 (10%)	36.6 (9%)	19.9 (10%)	16.7 (9%)	25.8 (9%)	13.8 (10%)	12.0 (9%)
55–59 Years	141 (6%)	66 (6%)	75 (6%)	27.7 (7%)	13.6 (7%)	14.1 (7%)	20.0 (7%)	9.6 (7%)	10.3 (8%)
60–64 Years	214 (9%)	91 (8%)	123 (10%)	27.5 (7%)	13.6 (7%)	13.9 (7%)	20.7 (7%)	10.1 (7%)	10.5 (8%)
65–69 Years	172 (7%)	66 (6%)	106 (8%)	19.8 (5%)	9.5 (5%)	10.3 (5%)	14.8 (5%)	7.1 (5%)	7.7 (6%)
70–74 Years	176 (7%)	95 (9%)	81 (6%)	14.7 (4%)	7.5 (4%)	7.2 (4%)	11.1 (4%)	5.7 (4%)	5.4 (4%)
75–79 Years	48 (2%)	40 (4%)	8 (1%)	6.6 (2%)	3.3 (2%)	3.3 (2%)	4.8 (2%)	2.4 (2%)	2.4 (2%)
80+ Years	37 (2%)	27 (2%)	10 (1%)	8.0 (2%)	3.9 (2%)	4.1 (2%)	6.0 (2%)	3.0 (2%)	3.0 (2%)
Total	2414 (100%)	1114 (100%)	1300 (100%	388.9 (100%)	199.4 (100%)	189.5 (100%)	275.5 (100%)	139.8 (100%)	135.7 (100%)

men (33.52%) and 1128 (44.83) women scored between 15 and 21 points, while 178 men (8.13%) and 435 females (17.29%) scored more than 21 points in the CESD.

For 4702 (99.8%) of the 4711 participants three standardized questions concerning suicidal behavior and suicidal attempts during their lifetime could be assessed. 199 participants (4.2%) admitted to have made an attempt at suicide. Out of these, 79 (39.7%) were men. For 3890 of the 4711 participants, three standardized questions concerning suicidal thoughts during the last 6 months or earlier were recorded. Out of these, 238 (5.1% total; 83 men (34.9%)) reported to have thought of committing suicide in the last 6 months. The most often reported reason for attempts at suicide were family related (68.4%), financial problems (22.4%) and long illness (7.9%) for men, and family related (91.7%), financial problems (5.8%) and long illness (0.8%) for women. Reasons for thoughts of committing suicide were similar: family related (79.0%), financial problems (8.6%) and long illness (9.9%) for men, and family related (93.5%), financial problems (2.6%) and long illness (3.9%) for men.

Smoking

With respect to smoking, 887 (18.84%) subjects reported to be or to have been smokers, with 184 (20.74%) being former smokers, and with 398 (44.87%) subjects who had tried to quit smoking previously without success. The mean package year number was 26.6±20.6 (median: 20.0). The mean starting age for smoking was 22.4±9.2. Stratified by gender, 883 men (40.3%) and 4 (0.02%) women reported current or former smoking. Of the 883 male smokers, 701 (79.3%) were current smokers, while of the 4 female smokers 3 still smoked on the examination date. Smokeless tobacco was consumed by 1968 (41.8%) subjects, with 1792 (91.1%) subjects being current users and 176 (8.9%) subjects being former users. Out of the 1968 users of smokeless tobacco, 275 (14.0%) subjects additionally smoked cigarettes/bidis. Gender distribution of the smokeless tobacco users was 1066 men (48.7%) and 902 women (35.8%). A complete Fagerstrom Test for Nicotine Dependence (FTND) could be calculated for 855 smokers (96.4%). The mean of the 855 valid FTND sum scores was 3.87±2.5 points (median: 4). A FTND sum score between 0 and 3 points (low level of addiction) was reported by 424 smokers (49.59%), a score between 4 and 6 points (moderate level of nicotine addiction) was reported by 281 smokers (32.87%), and 150 smokers (17.5%) scored between 7 and 10 FTND points (high level of addiction). Concerning smokeless tobacco no valid sum score was available. For 1957 smokeless tobacco users (99.44%), the mean number of daily consumptions was 4.23±2.2 times (median: 4).

Alcohol consumption

3628 (77.0%) participants reported to have never drunken alcohol; 287 (6.1%) participants reported on a consumption of alcohol once per month or less often, 264 (5.6%) participants an alcohol consumption of 2–4 times/month, 310 (6.6%) subjects an alcohol consumption of 2–3 times/week; 166 (3.5%) subjects an alcohol consumption of 4 times/week; and 54 (1.1%) subjects declared a daily alcohol consumption. Mean AUDIT sum scores was 1.4±3.8 points (median: 0). For the 1081 individuals reporting to drink alcohol the AUDIT sum score was 6.0±5.8 points (median: 4). An AUDIT sum score of 8 or more (harmful or hazardous drinking) was scored by 283 subjects (6.0% of the study population/26.2% of the individuals consuming alcohol). An AUDIT sum score of ≥13 in women or ≥15 or more in men (alcohol dependence) was achieved by 108 subjects (4.6% of the

Table 2. Demographic Parameters and Data on Daily Activities, Smoking and Alcohol Consumption, and Depression in the Central India Eye and Medical Study.

Parameter	Mean ± Standard Deviation	Median	Range
Age (Years)	49.5±13.4	47.0	30, 100
Body Mass Index (kg/m^2)	19.7±3.4	19.1	11.0, 46.3
Duration of Daily Work (Hours)	7.4±2.2	8	0.8, 18
Walking or Biking to Work (Days per Week)	6.6±1.2	7	1, 7
Diet	Purely vegetarians: 2394 (50.8%) subjects; Eating fish and eggs in addition to vegetables, but no meat: 35 (0.7%) subjects, Mixed diet: 2275 (48.3%) subjects		
Reported Monthly Income (Rupee)	1584±1233	1350	200, 15000
Family Income	<1500 Rupee: 2372 (50.5%); 1500–5000 Rupee: 2153 (45.8%); >5000 Rupee: 166 (3.5%)		
Family Type	Joint: 1968 (41.8%); Nuclear: 2607 (55.4%); Single: 133 (2.8%)		
Religion	Hindu: 4562 (96.9%); Muslim: 121 (2.6%); Others: 6 (0.6%)		
Level of Education	Illiterate: 1623 (34.5%); School up 5th standard: 1310 (27.8%); School between 6th to 8th standard: 533 (11.3%); School between 9th and 12th standard: 1070 (22.7%); Higher level of education: 165 (3.5%)		
Possession of Mobile Telephone	139 (3.0%) participants		
Housing	Houses made out of mud ("kacha"): 1109 (23.5%); Houses made partially out of mud ("semi pucca"): 2330 (49.5%)		
House Ownership	Own house: 4486 (95.6%); Rented house: 194 (4.1%); Mortgaged: 13 (0.1%)		
Light Source	Electricity: 4315 (92.0%); Kerosene, gas or oil: 333 (3.5%);		
Room for Cooking in the House	Yes: 4209 (89.7%); No: 485 (10.3%)		
Toilet Facility	No toilet facility in the houses: 2206 (46.9%) subjects		
Water Source	Public tap, hand pump or well: 1719 (36.5%); Pipe, Hand pump or well in the residency/compound: 2904 (62.6%); Other: 18 (0.4%)		
Agricultural Land Ownership	No land; 2062 (44.0%); <2 acres: 482 (10.3%); 2.0–4.9 acres: 833 (17.8%); 5+ acres: 1313 (28.0%)		
Durable Goods Ownership	Mattress, pressure cooker, chair cot/bed, table or clock: 569 (14.3%); Bicycle, electric fan, radio/Transistor, sewing machine: 2941 (63.8%); Moped/scooter, motorcycle, fixed telephone or mobile telephone: 965 (20.9%); Car, tractor: 41 (0.9%); None: 92 (2.0%)		
Livestock Ownership	Yes: 1920 (41.0%); No: 2762 (59.0%)		
Irrigated Land Ownership	No: 2049 (58.8%); Owns at least some irrigated land: 1433 (41.2%);		
Depression Score CESD	14.1±7.5	15	0, 58
Smoking	Current and/or former smokers: 887 (18.9%) (883 men; 4 women); Former smokers: 184 (20.7%); Current smokers with unsuccessful try to quit: 398 (44.9%)		
Package Years	26.6±20.6	20.0	
Fagerstrom Test for Nicotine Dependence	3.87±2.5 points	4	
Fagerstrom Test for Nicotine Dependence	0–3: 424 smokers (49.6%); 4–6: 281 smokers (32.9%); 7–10: 150 smokers (17.5%)		
Smokeless Tobacco	1957 (mean daily consumptions: 4.23±2.2 times (median: 4)		
Alcohol Consumption			
No Alcohol	3628 (77.0%) participants		
consumption of alcohol once per month or less often,	287 (6.1%) participants		
alcohol consumption of 2–4 times/month,	264 (5.6%) participants		
alcohol consumption of 2–3 times/week	310 (6.6%) subjects.		
alcohol consumption of 4 times/week	166 (3.5%) subjects		
daily alcohol consumption	54 (1.1%) subjects		
AUDIT sum score (1081 individuals)	6.0±5.8 points (median: 4)		
AUDIT sum score of 8 or more (harmful or hazardous drinking)	283 subjects (6.0% of the study population/26.2% of the individuals consuming alcohol).		
AUDIT sum score of ≥13 in women or ≥15 or more in men (alcohol dependence)	108 subjects (4.6% of the study population; 51 women (8.9% of women consuming alcohol), 57 men (11.2% of men consuming alcohol).		

study population; 51 women (8.9% of women consuming alcohol), 57 men (11.2% of men consuming alcohol).

Discussion

In our rural Central Indian study, 13.0% of the participants fulfilled the criteria for a major depression and an additional 39.6% of the study population showed mild to moderate depression. Suicide attempt was reported by 199 (4.2%) participants and suicidal thoughts during the last 6 months by 238 (5.1%) participants. Alcohol consumption was reported by 1081 (23.0%) participants; 283 (6.0%) subjects had an AUDIT sum score of ≥8 (harmful or hazardous drinking), and 108 (4.63%) subjects scored an AUDIT sum of ≥13 in women and ≥15 in men indicating alcohol dependence.

The figure of 13.0% for the prevalence of major depression is in agreement with results reported for developing countries by the WHO and the GBD [1,2]. Previous studies from India estimated the prevalence of depression in Indian community samples [19–24]. The most recent and largest population-based study reported by Poongothai and colleagues in 2009 screened more than 24,000 subjects in the city of Chennai (South India) and reported an overall prevalence of depression of 15.1% [19]. Earlier studies which mostly used screening instruments with poorer sensitivity, reported lower frequencies: Nandi and colleagues who performed their studies in the same region in 1972 reported prevalence rates for depression of 5.0% which by 1992 had increased to 7.4% [20]. A review by Math and Chandrashekar in 2006 suggested that the data reported on prevalence rates for psychiatric disorders from epidemiological studies was inconclusive with a high discrepancy in the prevalence rates, ranging from 9.5 to 370/1000 populations in India [23]. They concluded that the prevalence of mental disorders reported in epidemiological surveys could be considered lower estimates rather than accurate reflections of the true prevalence in the population.

The WHO estimated that 170 000 people die of suicide in India out of nearly 900 000 people worldwide, with about another 200 000 subjects in China and 140 000 in high-income countries [25]. In a recent survey on suicide mortality in India, Patel and colleagues found that about 3% of surveyed deaths in individuals aged 15 years or older were due to suicide [26]. A 15-year-old subject in India had a cumulative risk of about 1.3% of dying before the age of 80 years by suicide, with men having a higher risk (1.7%) than had women (1.0%). According to the recent global Burden of Disease Study GBD 2010, suicide was the most common cause of death among Indian women aged between 15 and 49 years, followed by maternal disorders, fire, tuberculosis, and diarrhea [27,28]. Beside these and other studies on the death rate by suicide in India [29–31], none of the major investigations have addressed the prevalence of suicide thoughts and unsuccessful suicide attempts in the Indian population, in particular not in the rural population. A WHO publication based on data collected by India's National Crime Records Bureau, Ministry of Home Affairs showed a rising suicide rate from 1980–2009 [32]. In 1980, there was a total rate of 6.3 suicides per 100.000 people, in 2009 the total rate was 10.5 per 100.000. In this publication the suicide

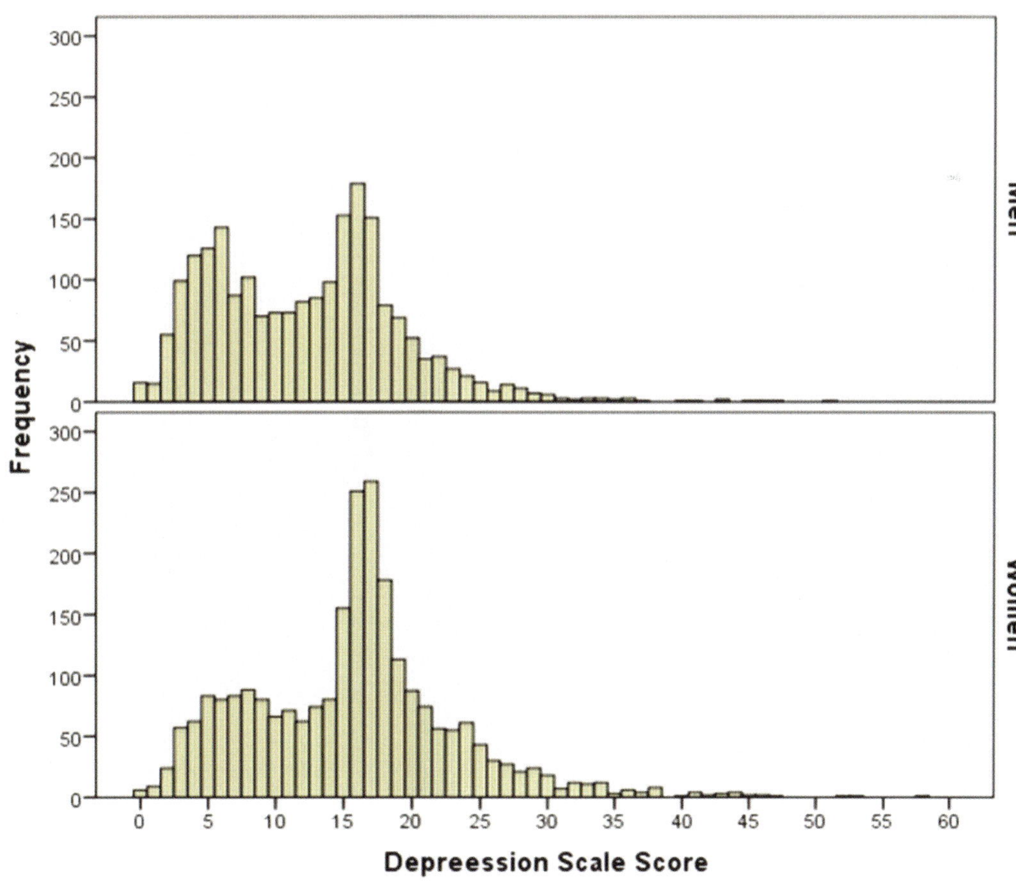

Figure 1. Histograms Showing the Distribution of the Depression Scale Score Stratified by Gender in the Central India Eye and Medical Study.

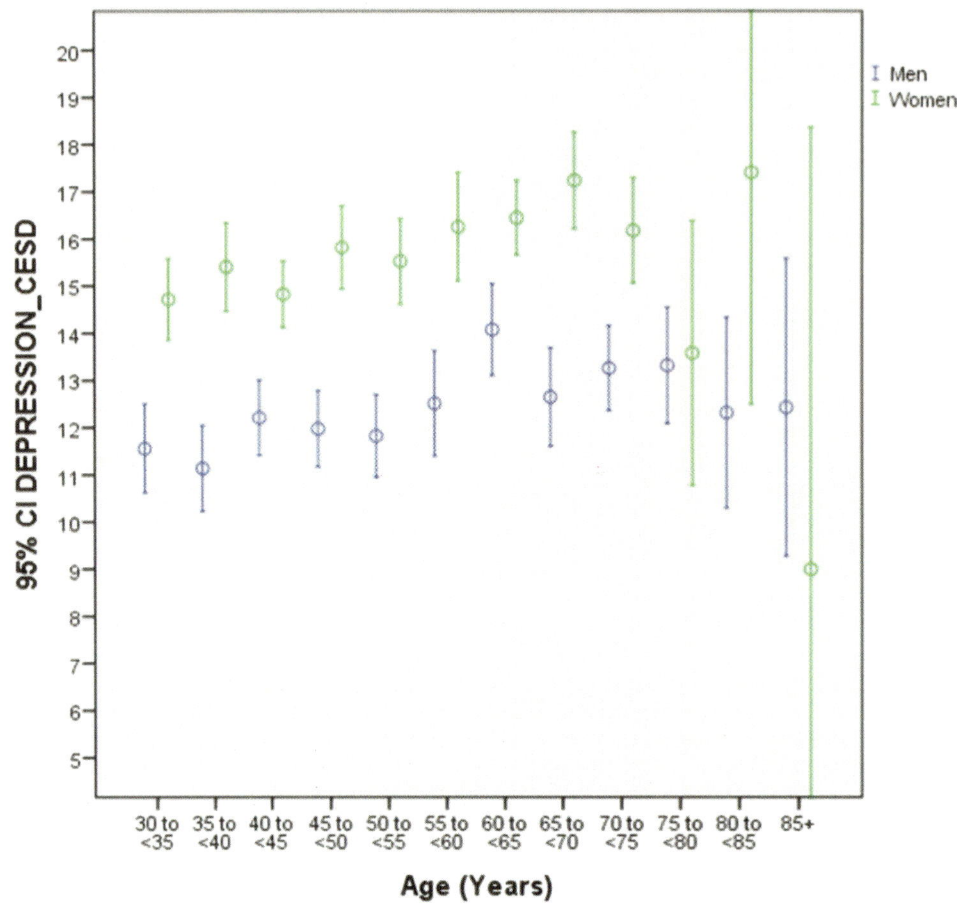

Figure 2. Graph Showing the Distribution of the Depression Score Stratified by Age and Gender in the Central India Eye and Medical Study.

rate for women only showed a slight increase from 1980 to 2009 with a peak in the year 2000, while the rate of suicides among the male population nearly doubled (7.3 in 1980 to 13.0 in 2009).

In the study population, 19% of the individuals reported to be or to have been smokers, with the majority of smokers being men (40.3% of men versus 0.02% of women). Smokeless tobacco was consumed by 1968 (41.8%) subjects. These figures were higher than those reported in the Indian National Family Health Survey-2 from 1998–99 [33]. That survey on 315,598 individuals 15 years or older revealed that 30% of the population (47% men and 14% of women) either smoked or chewed tobacco. It also showed that individuals with no education were 2.7 times more likely to smoke and chew tobacco than those with postgraduate education, and that scheduled tribes had a 23% higher probability to consume tobacco than other social groups [34]. Compared with the figures from a survey focused on 14 low-income and middle-income countries including India, 48.6% of men and 11.3% of women were tobacco users [35]. Again these figures were lower than those for our rural study population. It indicates that our study population had a relatively high prevalence of using tobacco corresponding to the association between lower socio-economic background or lower educational level and tobacco use [34,36].

Out of our study population, 77.0% of the participants reported to have never drunken alcohol, while an AUDIT sum score of 8 or more (harmful or hazardous drinking) was scored by 6.0% of the study population or 26.2% of the individuals consuming alcohol. In the Indian National Sample Survey as a representative survey of 471,143 people over the age of 10 years in 1995–96 revealed a national prevalence of regular use of smoking tobacco is estimated to be 16.2%, chewing tobacco 14.0%, and alcohol 4.5%. Men were 9.7 times more likely to regularly use alcohol [36]. Respondents belonging to scheduled castes and tribes (recognized disadvantaged groups), people from rural areas and those without formal education were significantly more likely to report regular use of alcohol [37,38].

Potential limitations of our study should be discussed. First, a major concern in any prevalence study is nonparticipation. The Central India Eye and Medical Study had a reasonable response rate of 80.1%, however, differences between participants and non-participants can lead to a selection artifact. Second, our study included only those who resided in a purely rural region, a region that can be considered to be markedly rural based on responses to the questionnaire regarding socioeconomic background and lifestyle. The study did not include subjects from an urban region, so we can provide no information on any differences between rural and urban regions with respect to the examined parameters. Third, our study as cross-section investigation does not allow firm statements on a longitudinal association, i.e. temporal causation cannot be established with the current cross-sectional design. Fourth, our study only included participants over the age of 30 years and therefore the frequency we report only refer to this age-group. This is important as cohort effects exist for major depression and generally age at onset is declining. Fifth, epidemiological studies using questionnaires such as the CES-D, usually assessed "depressive symptoms" rather than "depression", so the findings of our study can give information only about depressive symptoms. To make a definitive diagnosis of depression would need additional tests. Sixth, due to the study design, our investigation could not assess relationships between outcome parameters, such as a potential association between smoking and prevalence of depression, or an association between alcohol consumption and depression.

In conclusion, the rural Central Indian population living in a purely agrarian society showed a prevalence of major depression of 13.0% (8.1 of men, 17.3% of women). About 4% of the study population reported about suicide attempt, and 5% indicated to have had suicidal thoughts during the last 6 months. Approximately 20% of the population was present or former smokers. Harmful or hazardous drinking or alcohol dependence was reported by 12% and 5% of the study population, respectively. As in other population and societies, depression was a very common psychiatric disorder. Measures should be taken to address the relatively high prevalence of suicide attempts and thoughts on suicide. Future research focused on the general population, longitudinal (prospective), multi-center, co-morbid studies, assessment of disability, functioning, family burden and quality of life studies involving a clinical service providing approach, is required.

Author Contributions

Conceived and designed the experiments: JBJ VN MR PB SPJ. Performed the experiments: JBJ VN MR PB SPJ. Analyzed the data: JBJ MR TP. Contributed reagents/materials/analysis tools: JBJ VN. Wrote the paper: JBJ VN MR TP PB SPJ.

References

1. Murray CJ, Vos T, Lozano R, Naghavi M, Flaxman AD, et al. (2012) Disability-adjusted life years (DALYs) for 291 diseases and injuries in 21 regions, 1990–2010: a systematic analysis for the Global Burden of Disease Study 2010. Lancet 380: 2197–2223.
2. Lim SS, Vos T, Flaxman AD, Danaei G, Shibuya K, et al. (2012) A comparative risk assessment of burden of disease and injury attributable to 67 risk factors and risk factor clusters in 21 regions, 1990–2010: a systematic analysis for the Global Burden of Disease Study 2010. Lancet 380: 2224–2260.
3. Lieb K, Zanarini MC, Schmahl C, Linehan MM, Bohus M (2004) Borderline personality disorder. Lancet 364: 453–461.
4. Moussavi S, Chatterji S, Verdes E, Tandon A, Patel V, et al. (2007) Depression, chronic diseases, and decrements in health: results from the World Health Surveys. Lancet 370: 851–858.
5. Patton GC, Coffey C, Romaniuk H, Mackinnon A, Carlin JB, et al. (2014) The prognosis of common mental disorders in adolescents: a 14-year prospective cohort study. Lancet 383: 1404–1411.
6. Peto R, Lopez AD, Boreham J, Thun M, Heath C Jr (1992) Mortality from tobacco in developed countries: indirect estimation from national vital statistics. Lancet 339: 1268–1278.
7. Glassman AH, Covey LS, Stetner F, Rivelli S (2001) Smoking cessation and the course of major depression: a follow-up study. Lancet 357: 1929–1932.
8. Williamson DF, Madans J, Anda RF, Kleinman JC, Giovino GA, et al. (1991) Smoking cessation and severity of weight gain in a national cohort. N Engl J Med 324: 739–745.
9. Renaud S, de Lorgeril M (1992) Wine, alcohol, platelets, and the French paradox for coronary heart disease. Lancet 339: 1523–1526.
10. Biederman J, Faraone SV (2005) Attention-deficit hyperactivity disorder. Lancet 366: 237–248.
11. Room R, Babor T, Rehm J (2005) Alcohol and public health. Lancet 365: 519–530.
12. Hawton K, van Heeringen K (2009) Suicide. Lancet 373: 1372–1381.
13. Moran P, Coffey C, Romaniuk H, Olsson C, Borschmann R, et al. (2012) The natural history of self-harm from adolescence to young adulthood: a population-based cohort study. Lancet 379: 236–243.
14. Lim SS, Vos T, Flaxman AD, Danaei G, Shibuya K, et al. (2012) A comparative risk assessment of burden of disease and injury attributable to 67 risk factors and risk factor clusters in 21 regions, 1990–2010: a systematic analysis for the Global Burden of Disease Study 2010. Lancet 380: 2224–2260.
15. Jonas JB, Nangia V, Joshi PP, Matin A, Panda-Jonas S (2010) Diabetes mellitus in rural India. Epidemiology 21: 754–755.
16. Radloff LS (1977) 'The CES-D scale: A self report depression scale for research in the general population'. Applied Psychological Measurement 1: 385–401.
17. Heatherton TF, Kozlowski LT, Frecker RC, Fagerstrom KO (1991) The Fagerstrom Test for Nicotine Dependence: A revision of the Fagerstrom Tolerance Questionnaire. Br J Addict 86: 1119–1127.
18. Saunders JB, Aasland OG, Babor TF, de la Fuente JR, Grant M (1993) Development of the alcohol use disorders identification test (AUDIT): WHO collaborative project on early detection of persons with harmful alcohol consumption—II. Addiction 88: 791–803.
19. Poongothai S, Pradeepa R, Ganesan A, Mohan V (2009) Prevalence of depression in a large urban South Indian population - The Chennai Urban Rural Epidemiology Study (CURES-70). PloS One 4: E7185.
20. Nandi DN, Banerjee G, Mukherjee SP, Ghosh A, Nandi PS, et al. (2000) Psychiatric morbidity of a rural Indian community changes over a 20 year interval. Br J Psych 176: 351–356.
21. Nandi PS, Banerjee G, Mukherjee SP, Nandi S, Nandi DN (1997) A study of psychiatric morbidity of the elderly population of a rural community in West Bengal. Indian J Psych 39: 122–129.
22. Tiwari SC (2000) Geriatric Psychiatric morbidity in rural Northern India: Implications for the future. Int Psychogeriatrics 12: 35–48.
23. Math SB, Chandrashekar CR, Bhugra D (2007) Psychiatric epidemiology in India. Indian J Med Res 126: 183–192.
24. Ganguli HC (2000) Epidemiological findings on prevalence of mental disorders in India. Indian J Psychiatry 42: 14–20.
25. WHO (2008) The global burden of disease: 2004 update. Geneva: World Health Organization, 2008.
26. Patel V, Ramasundarahettige C, Vijayakumar L, Thakur JS, Gajalakshmi V, et al. (2012) Suicide mortality in India: a nationally representative survey. Lancet 379: 2343–2351.
27. Salomon JA, Wang H, Freeman MK, Vos T, Flaxman AD, et al. (2010) Healthy life expectancy for 187 countries, 1990–2010: a systematic analysis for the Global Burden Disease Study 2010. Lancet 380: 2144–2162.
28. Lozano R, Naghavi M, Foreman K, Lim S, Shibuya K, et al. (2012) Global and regional mortality from 235 causes of death for 20 age groups in 1990 and 2010: a systematic analysis for the Global Burden of Disease Study 2010. Lancet 380: 2095–2128.
29. Lester D, Natarajan M, Agarwal K (1999) Suicide in India. Arch Suicide Res 5: 91–96.
30. Aaron R, Joseph A, Abraham S, Muliyil J, George K, et al. (2004) Suicides in young people in rural southern India. Lancet 363: 111–118.
31. Borges G, Nock MK, Haro Abad JM, Hwang I, Sampson NA, et al. (2010) Twelve-month prevalence of and risk factors for suicide attempts in the world health organization world mental health surveys. J Clin Psychiatry 71: 1617–1628.
32. World Health Organization website. Available: http://www.who.int/entity/mental_health/media/indi.pdf. Accessed 2014 Mar 3.
33. Rani M, Bonu S, Jha P, Nguyen SN, Jamjoum L (2003) Tobacco use in India: prevalence and predictors of smoking and chewing in a national cross sectional household survey. Tob Control 12:e4.
34. Subramanian SV, Nandy S, Kelly M, Gordon D, Davey Smith G (2004) Patterns and distribution of tobacco consumption in India: cross sectional multilevel evidence from the 1998–9 national family health survey. BMJ 328: 801–806.
35. Giovino GA, Mirza SA, Samet JM, Gupta PC, Jarvis MJ, et al. (2012) Tobacco use in 3 billion individuals from 16 countries: an analysis of nationally representative cross-sectional household surveys. Lancet 380: 668–679.
36. Neufeld KJ, Peters DH, Rani M, Bonu S, Brooner RK (2005) Regular use of alcohol and tobacco in India and its association with age, gender, and poverty. Drug Alcohol Depend 77: 283–291.
37. Ghosh S, Samanta A, Mukherjee S (2012) Patterns of alcohol consumption among male adults at a slum in Kolkata, India. J Health Popul Nutr 30: 73–81.
38. Srinath Reddy K, Perry CL, Stigler MH, Arora M (2006) Differences in tobacco use among young people in urban India by sex, socioeconomic status, age, and school grade: Assessment of baseline survey data. Lancet 367: 589–594.

'Two Pains Together': Patient Perspectives on Psychological Aspects of Chronic Pain while Living with HIV

Jessica S. Merlin[1,2]*, Melonie Walcott[1], Christine Ritchie[3,4], Ivan Herbey[1], Stefan G. Kertesz[5,6], Eric Chamot[7], Michael Saag[1], Janet M. Turan[7]

1 Division of Infectious Diseases, Department of Medicine, University of Alabama at Birmingham, Birmingham, Alabama, United States of America, **2** Division of Gerontology, Geriatrics, and Palliative Care, University of Alabama at Birmingham, Birmingham, Alabama, United States of America, **3** Division of Geriatrics, Department of Medicine, University of California at San Francisco, San Francisco, California, United States of America, **4** Jewish Home of San Francisco Center for Research on Aging, San Francisco, California, United States of America, **5** Birmingham VA Medical Center, Birmingham, Alabama, United States of America, **6** Division of Preventive Medicine, Department of Medicine, University of Alabama at Birmingham, Birmingham, Alabama, United States of America, **7** School of Public Health, University of Alabama at Birmingham, Birmingham, Alabama, United States of America

Abstract

Objective: Chronic pain is common in HIV-infected individuals. Understanding HIV-infected patients' chronic pain experience not just from a biological, but also from a psychological perspective, is a critical first step toward improving care for this population. Our objective was to explore HIV-infected patients' perspectives on psychological aspects of chronic pain using in-depth qualitative interviews.

Methods: Investigators engaged in an iterative process of independent and group coding until theme saturation was reached.

Results: Of the 25 patients with chronic pain interviewed, 20 were male, 15 were younger than age 50, and 15 were African-American. Key themes that emerged included the close relationship between mood and pain; mood and pain in the context of living with HIV; use of alcohol/drugs to self-medicate for pain; and the challenge of receiving prescription pain medications while dealing with substance use disorders.

Conclusions: The results suggest that psychological approaches to chronic pain treatment may be well received by HIV-infected patients.

Editor: Shao-Jun Tang, University of Texas Medical Branch, United States of America

Funding: This research was supported by the University of Alabama at Birmingham (UAB) Center for AIDS Research (CFAR), an National Institutes of Health funded program (P30 A1027767) that was made possible by the following institutes: National Institute of Allergy and Infectious Diseases, National Cancer Institute, National Institute of Child Health and Human Development, National Heart, Lung, and Blood Institute, National Institute on Drug Abuse, National Institute of Mental Health, National Institute on Aging, and the NIH Office of AIDS Research. JSM is supported by 1K12HS02169401 (Agency for Healthcare Research and Quality). CSR is supported by 7K07AG031779 (National Institute on Aging). Funding was also provided by the Mary Fisher CARE Fund at UAB. The funders had no role in study design, data collection and analysis, decision to publish, or preparation of the manuscript.

Competing Interests: The authors have declared that no competing interests exist.

* Email: jmerlin@uab.edu

Introduction

Chronic pain is defined as pain of at least 3 months' duration, not associated with ongoing tissue injury. [1] Chronic pain in HIV-infected patients is a common, disabling condition. It occurs in between 39–85% of HIV-infected patients,[2–4] and HIV-infected patients with chronic pain have up to 10 times greater odds of functional impairment. [5] Chronic pain often occurs in the context of medical, psychiatric, and addiction comorbidities, which add an additional layer of complexity for both the patient and provider.[6–8].

The clinical approach to chronic pain has historically drawn from a biomedical model. [9] For example, despite limited evidence of efficacy, chronic opioid therapy is commonly prescribed in both the general population and in HIV-infected patients. [10] [11] Psychological approaches such as cognitive behavioral therapy [12] and pain self-management [13,14] have been used in the general population with promising results in randomized controlled trials. [15] However, such interventions have not seen widespread implementation and dissemination and are often inadequately reimbursed. Furthermore, psychological interventions have not been adapted to HIV-infected patients who are likely to have a unique chronic pain experience, due to unique

HIV-related biological factors, complex social challenges, and high degrees of medical, psychiatric, and addiction comorbidity. [16].

The Biopsychosocial (BPS) Framework is an explanatory conceptual framework based on systems theory that has been applied to medical and psychiatric illnesses, [17] including chronic pain. [18] Understanding HIV-infected patients' chronic pain experience not just from a biological, but also from a psychological and social perspective, is a critical first step toward improving their care. Therefore, we recently adapted and tailored this framework to HIV-infected patients with chronic pain by identifying factors common to both conditions. [16] Our goal in the current manuscript is to explore patients' perspectives on the psychological aspects of pain, using the psychological portion of the BPS framework as a guide.

Methods

Study Design

We conducted qualitative interviews, and used individual interviews as the topics covered were of a sensitive nature, and we sought to obtain in-depth information regarding patient perspectives on the chronic pain experience. Our study methods have been described in detail previously. [19].

Research Context

This study took place at a comprehensive HIV clinic, which includes HIV primary care and psychiatric and addiction services, in an urban center in the Southern US. Most clinic patients participate in the Center for AIDS Research Network of Integrated Clinical Systems (CNICS) study, which involves completion of Patient Reported Outcome (PRO) measures every 6 months on touch-screen computers.

Inclusion criteria and sampling

Inclusion criteria were a) age ≥19 (Alabama's legal age of majority), b) participation in CNICS, and c) at least mild chronic pain based on a Brief Chronic Pain Screening tool (BCPS). [19] Participant selection was also designed to ensure representation of "patients who are likely to be the target of future chronic pain interventions, and who are vulnerable to worse pain-related outcomes."[19–21] Therefore, we used PROs to purposively sample individuals with *and* without various symptoms of a major mood disorder, defined as depressive symptoms (PHQ-9≥10) or anxiety symptoms/panic (PHQ-Anxiety module), [22] and illicit substance use (ASSIST, excluding marijuana) (23). Participants provided informed consent and were reimbursed $20.

Interview Design and Data Collection/Analysis

The qualitative interview guide was based on the BPS Framework for Chronic Pain in HIV (Table 1) and modified emergently during the study. Hour-long interviews were conducted by an experienced qualitative interviewer (MW), audio-recorded, transcribed verbatim, and coded using NVivo 10.0 while interviews were still ongoing. Transcripts were initially coded by IH, who developed the codebook while remaining blinded to the interview guide. Subsequently, three investigators (JSM, MW, IH) engaged in an iterative process of independent and group coding. Interviews were conducted until theme saturation was reached. Results presented are limited to psychological themes, and to participants who reported at least mild chronic pain as defined above.

Ethics Statement

This protocol was approved by the University of Alabama at Birmingham's Institutional Review Board, which specifically approved this study. All participants provided written informed consent.

Results

Of the 25 participants, 5 were female, 10 were age 50 or greater, 15 were African-American, the median CD4+ T-cell count was 571 cells/mm3, and 20 had an undetectable viral load (Table 2). The majority (16) had a mood disorder, and nearly half (12) reported actively using illicit substances. Six reported mild pain, 4 reported moderate pain, and 14 reported severe pain (1 did not report pain severity).

Major psychological themes that emerged were mood and relationships between alcohol/illicit substance use and pain.

MOOD (Depression and Anxiety)

Themes that emerged in this category were: a) the close relationship between mood and pain, and b) mood and pain in the context of living with HIV.

a) Close relationship between mood and pain. Many participants described a strong connection between mood – mostly depression, but also anxiety – and pain. One participant's comment clearly articulates the challenging nature of the coexistence of mood disturbance and pain:

> *I mean because I'm already feeling down, and then my pain makes me ache. And then I'm down and I'm aching. That's two pains together. That's not good.* 49-year-old African American male

The three main sub-themes that emerged regarding the close relationship between mood and pain were: 1) bidrectionality, 2) the relationship between physical and emotional pain, 3) coping with mood disturbance and pain.

1. Bidirectionality. The connection between mood and pain was often explained as bidirectional. Specifically, participants explained that having pain can exacerbate pre-existing mood disorders, and that difficulties with mood can also make pain worse. For example:

> *I really have to work on my depression, and the depression gets worse when the pain gets worse. … I know that for a fact. There's no two ways about it. The pain gets worse, so does the depression…. And it's hard to handle both of 'em at one time. …. I've been suffering with [depression] about as long as I have the pain…. And it – as the day goes on, the pain gets worse. The depression gets worse. …. I tell you living in pain everyday, it'll – it depressed the hell out of ya.* 56-year-old white male

2. Relationship between physical and emotional pain. Participants readily described the concept of not only physical, but also emotional pain. Their comments indicate that physical and emotional pain are two very closely related constructs. Some participants described that at times, physical and emotional pain are indistinguishable:

> *Interviewer: What is the relationship between your depression and your pain? …*

Table 1. In-Depth Interview Guide Psychological Probes.

Psychological distress	Tell me more about your mood. Does pain affect your mood? (Probe: do you think that the people close to you think that pain affects your mood, or detect changes in your mood related to pain?)
Substance use	How do you think using drugs or alcohol is related to pain? What effect do you think drug or alcohol use has on your pain?
Environmental stressors	Is pain affected by other things that cause stress in your life? (Probe: your job, your family, money, housing situation, access to food, etc? If so, how?)
Anger	In our everyday lives, there are things that make us angry. Do these things affect your pain? (Probe: if so, how?)
Fear/Traumatic life events	Have you ever been in any situation that was extremely frightening or horrifying, or one in which you felt extremely helpless? (Probe: If yes, what was it? Your chronic pain started X years ago-was that before or after this event?)

Participant: Both of them are the same to me. … I be depressed all the time, every day. The pain is the same way. I be in pain every day, all day. 46-year-old African-American female

Participant: When you consider peoples' pain, a lot of it is emotional…. If you're happy your bones are happy…. If you're sad your bones are sad. 49-year-old African-American male

Still others explained that emotional distress actually creates a painful sensation:

Participant: Uhm, and it's just you know, with depression comes just, it's like almost a weight, uhm, uhm, or pressure that can translate to, to physical pain at times…when it gets bad … I don't know if it, if it's something that I would necessarily always refer to as, as a physical pain more than an emotional pain. But at times, sometimes that, that line between the two becomes a little blurred. … And it, uhm, it's kind of hard to tell what exactly hurts. 31-year-old white male

However, a few participants drew a sharp distinction between physical and emotional pain:

Participant: The depression really is painful. Does that make sense to you? … You know, there is a different kind of pain than your leg hurting, you know? 37-year-old white male

3. Mechanisms for relationship between mood and pain. Participants offered some potential mechanisms to explain the relationship between pain and mood. These related to effects on physical and social functioning. In describing this relationship some participants noted that worse mood contributes to reluctance to participate in physical or social activities, leading to impaired physical and social function. Others noted that depression independently leads to impaired function, and decreased function further worsens pain.

Another participant explained the relationship between his anxiety and pain, and the mediating role of depression:

Anxiety affects my pain by keeping me from doing things like driving and things like that, that I really shouldn't be afraid of doing…. That makes me depressed, so that makes me want to just sit and muddle in my pain. 50-year-old white male

On the flip side, a few participants acknowledged that being in a good mood helped them to cope with their pain better:

If I'm in a good mood uh I can kinda deal with [pain] more…. If I'm in a bad mood it's just like nothing else really

Table 2. Characteristics of Participants with Chronic Pain, as identified by the Brief Chronic Pain Screening Tool (BCPS) Results (N = 25).

	Mild-moderate-very severe pain for at least 3 months (N = 25)*
Female	5
African-American	15
Age ≥50	10
CD4+ T-cell count (median, IQR)	587 (421–792) cells/mL
VL <200 copies/mL	14
Pain**	25
Mood disorder†	16
Substance use††	12

*BCPS results typically dichotomized as mild-moderate-severe pain for at least 3 months (= chronic pain), and none or any pain less than three months (= not chronic pain).
**Based on the EuroQOL pain measure indicating mild, moderate or severe pain within the 6 months prior to enrollment.
†Based on a PHQ-9≥10 or a PHQ-Anxiety module consistent with anxiety symptoms/panic within the 6 months prior to enrollment.
††Based on an ASSIST reporting use of opiates, heroin, cocaine, or amphetamines within the 6 months prior to enrollment.

matters other than, you know, tryin' to get comfort. 48-year-old African-American male

b) Mood and Pain in the Context of Living with HIV. The majority of participants appeared to conceptualize their HIV and their chronic pain as two distinct health conditions and did not attribute their pain to their HIV, and did not think that their HIV caused pain. However, some participants reported that having HIV is depressing, having pain is depressing, and the combined effect of having both at the same time can be difficult to manage:

I am hurting all the time and hurting all the time when you have HIV and stuff like that you want to live a normal life but you know you cannot live a normal life. And sometimes you are out there and you forget about it and then reality kicks in and you have to say whoa, pull yourself back. 47-year-old African-American male

Well, just I've got enough problems dealing with HIV, and trying to get myself clean, and then you throw in the pain on top of that, well, that's just something I don't need, right now. And it just I mean, you can only take so many hard licks from one day, before you just gotta give up. And, if you got that damn pain sitting there, just gnawing, it's like somebody's gnawing on a bone, and you got that sitting there. 56-year-old white male

Relationships between Alcohol/Illicit Substance Use and Pain

Another category that emerged initially and was then specifically probed was the relationship between alcohol/illicit substance abuse and pain. In this category, themes that emerged were: a) the use of alcohol/drugs to self-medicate for pain, and b) the challenge of receiving prescription pain medications while dealing with current or past history of substance use disorders.

a) Use of alcohol/drugs to self-medicate for pain

A minority of participants reported that pain actually led them to use alcohol or drugs, in an attempt to alleviate their suffering. One participant described how in his case alcohol worked to help him manage his pain:

I would just drink [alcohol] it until my mind – it takes your mind differently. After you've had a few you get a good buzz going on and you don't think about the pain no more. 34-year-old African-American male

Another participant explained how pain actually fueled the development of his addiction to illicit drugs:

Well, [pain and drug use] go hand in hand. Because when I hurt I wanna stop hurting so… and I know that… I know what will help me stop hurting…But and that's the problem now is I use it when I'm not hurting…. It did go hand in hand for me but now it just became a, a problem or addiction." 45-year-old African-American male

Most participants who discussed the role of illicit substances felt that self-medication in this way is only a temporary fix. After the drug has worn off, the person is left with their original pain:

You know, you know, drugs doesn't help because uh if you try to alleviate the pain with – with drinkin' alcohol 'cause you gonna just – it's gonna be a hurtin' drunk. 52-year-old African-American male with severe chronic pain

For the few minutes that I'm using drugs, I don't hurt…. And I might, uh, it might last, the pain might be gone for thirty minutes, hour…. But that's only because cocaine done numb the feeling, I guess…But it, it always comes back which caused me to keep going get more cocaine 45-year-old African-American male

One participant felt that after getting off drugs his pain was even worse:

Uh actually … when I was doin' the drugs [crack cocaine] I – I didn't notice the pain. But now that I'm not I do feel – feel it a little more intensely. 48-year-old African American male

b) Prescription pain medication and substance use. Participants reported that clinicians are reluctant to prescribe opioids for individuals with substance use, often discovered on a urine drug screen. In some cases, this caused frustration, as the patient felt they really needed medications to deal with the pain.

Several participants reported their own fear of receiving prescription pain medications due to a personal history of substance use. They feared that the pain medications would start them back on the road to addiction.

Those pills, that methadone, that's a substance to me. To me that's a substance. I don't want that…. When they gave me that first, I told that Dr. X, because he put me on that first to see how I would do. I told him "No, I don't want that." I don't want it. 49-year-old African-American male

I don't wanna get back on drugs again…. I don't want 'em treatin' me with narcotics…. Because I been on 'em before and I don't want back on 'em….

Interviewer: You think the doctors would treat you with narcotics again?

Participant: If I wanted 'em to probably. … I'm not gonna do it…Back when I was gettin' my teeth pulled down here he was givin' me Lortabs for pain. I didn't take 'em. I didn't take 'em. I just took aspirins 'cause I didn't wanna get strung out again…I cut my hand not long ago and had to go get stitches in it out in the yard. And she gave me a bunch a Lortabs for pain, that doctor did. I didn't – I didn't take 'em. I don't even remember if I filled the script. I mighta filled the script once or twice but a lot of 'em I didn't fill just in case it got to hurtin' real bad. But I didn't take 'em. 51-year-old white male

On the flip side, one participant understood the clinicians' logic, but nevertheless wished they would prescribe:

They won't put me on narcotics, 'cause I'm – I was addicted to crack cocaine for a while…So, they an – they're not real enthusiastic about giving me the dem – uh the uh, hydrocodone…So, just have to suffer. …Well, [SIGH] I – you know, I can see the reason, because I am an addict, and I always will be. But I was an addict to crack cocaine…. I just don't really see why they can't give me the narcotics now, because that's what gets me out of the pain, and I wouldn't want but one a day, because I can – I can take it up to twelve to one o'clock, but after twelve to one o'clock, I could take that, and I would be pain free the rest of the night. But because I'm an addict, you know, and I can see where they're coming from, you know, because but uh, and I've got several cousins, and uh, they've all been addicted to pain killers, and I wouldn't wanna get in their shape. Their livers are bad. Their uh, they're always chasing the dope, and I know how that comes in to being, cause I chase crack before, but uh, it's either stay in pain, or take the narcotics. 56-year-old white male

Another participant also drew a direct link between the use of opioids for pain and the development of addiction to illicit substances:

Lortabs gets you started…Then once you can't get them anymore you go out there and find that heroin or that Dilaudid… Because uh the more drugs they give ya to treat your pain the worse off you get…It's just a spiral down…-Before long it's all you want, that's all you want. That's all you gotta have. Don't care about nothin' else. Don't wanna do nothin' else…You just want that next shot. 51-year-old white male

Discussion

This is the first study to focus on psychological aspects of chronic pain among HIV-infected individuals. Our results highlight the importance of the relationship between chronic pain, mood, and substance use in a sample of HIV-infected individuals enriched with individuals with mood disorders and substance use.

This study is consistent with previously published evidence that mood disorders, particularly depression, are common and complex chronic diseases in individuals with HIV. [23] The high level of comorbidity between depression and chronic pain in the general population has also been well-established. [24] Additionally, there are studies that suggest that patients with severe depression and chronic musculoskeletal pain, [25] fibromyalgia, [20] and low back pain [26] have worse functional outcomes, and that depression severity mediates the role of post-traumatic stress disorder on pain interference. [27] The close, often bidirectional relationship between mood and pain that patients described has also been observed quantitatively. [14] Furthermore, our patients expressed a nuanced understanding and candidness about this relationship, and about the concepts of both physical and emotional pain.

Historically, providers have addressed pain mainly from a biomedical perspective, [9] focusing on the importance of gathering objective evidence of biological causal factors. [28] In our experience, providers assume that patients are equally wedded to this biomedical model, and are not as open to acknowledging psychosocial influences. Patients' interest in operating within the biomedical model may relate to how providers use diagnostic testing in patients with chronic pain. Patients often observe providers who use positive diagnostic test results to confirm the existence of the pain, and the lack of a positive diagnostic test to cast doubt on the pain's existence. [29] Prior studies have suggested that while providers focus on convincing patients with negative test results that there is no biological basis for their pain, patients insist that there is a biological basis in order to gain credibility. [30].

Patients in our study also clearly articulated the relationship between pain and substance use. They acknowledged the practice of self-medicating using alcohol and illicit substances, the ineffectiveness of this approach, and the risk of addiction. Patients' willingness to address these issues was recently echoed in another study of physician-patient communication regarding chronic opioid therapy. [31] Despite patients' ability to discuss topics related to pain and addiction, HIV primary care providers often feel unprepared to address opioid misuse and addiction in patients with chronic pain. [32].

Our study suggests that patients make a direct connection between mood, alcohol/substance use, and pain, and seem to understand the way in which these factors work together to impact their health. Providers may feel that such conversations may be interpreted as telling patients that their pain is "all in their head" [33]. While statements such as that should certainly be avoided, an open-ended, non-judgmental approach to discussing the psychosocial aspects of pain, similar to that used in this study, could facilitate provider-patient communication about this difficult topic. Further research into effective communication strategies about chronic pain between patients and providers is needed. [34].

Despite the importance of psychological aspects of pain, the most readily available pain treatments are biomedical, and do not address mood or substance use. For example, the most commonly prescribed medications for pain in the US are opioids, which have increased in use dramatically over the past 10 years. [10] Opioids are more commonly prescribed for HIV-infected patients with chronic pain than HIV-uninfected patients, [11] and HIV-infected individuals are more likely to receive high dose opioids. [35] Despite their frequency and intensity of use, a recent Cochrane review concluded that among participants who continued the opioid, results were insufficient to draw conclusions regarding function, and there was only weak evidence to substantiate improvement in pain. [36] Likewise, HIV-infected individuals with chronic pain on chronic opioid therapy have worse pain than those not on chronic opioid therapy. [37] In addition to these major efficacy concerns, opioids carry serious risks, including misuse and overdose.[38–42] This is especially concerning in patients with a history of substance use – a common comorbidity in HIV-infected patients. [43].

Our study suggests that HIV-infected patients understand the limited efficacy of both licit and illicit substances in the management of pain, and would welcome a behavioral approach addressing the psychological aspects of pain highlighted here. Evidence-based behavioral interventions are among the most effective non-pharmacologic chronic pain treatments investigated in the general population. [24] While most participants in our study did not perceive their pain to be caused by their HIV, they did underscore the importance of chronic pain in the context of living with HIV. Other studies have shown that the prevalence and complexity of depression is higher among HIV-infected patients than in the general population. [23,44] Based on our findings, depression may actually play a key role in the relationship between HIV and chronic pain. This supports existing knowledge and practice and affirms that treating depression and incorporating psychological approaches to pain management is critical in HIV-infected patients. Therefore, given the importance of the context of HIV, chronic pain behavioral interventions specifically tailored to HIV-infected patients, particularly ones that incorporate treatment of depression and substance abuse, should be developed.

Author Contributions

Conceived and designed the experiments: JSM MW CR IH SGK EC MS JMT. Performed the experiments: JSM MW CR IH SGK EC MS JMT. Analyzed the data: JSM MW CR IH SGK EC MS JMT. Contributed reagents/materials/analysis tools: JSM MW CR IH SGK EC MS JMT. Contributed to the writing of the manuscript: JSM MW CR IH SGK EC MS JMT.

References

1. Vervest AC, Schimmel GH (1988) Taxonomy of pain of the IASP. Pain 34: 318–321.
2. Merlin JS, Cen L, Praestgaard A, Turner M, Obando A, et al. (2012) Pain and physical and psychological symptoms in ambulatory HIV patients in the current treatment era. J Pain Symptom Manage 43: 638–645.
3. Miaskowski C, Penko JM, Guzman D, Mattson JE, Bangsberg DR, et al. (2011) Occurrence and characteristics of chronic pain in a community-based cohort of indigent adults living with HIV infection. J Pain 12: 1004–1016.
4. Merlin JS, Westfall AO, Raper JL, Zinski A, Norton WE, et al. (2012) Pain, Mood, and Substance Abuse in HIV: Implications for Clinic Visit Utilization, ART Adherence, and Virologic Failure. J Acquir Immune Defic Syndr 61: 164–170.
5. Merlin JS, Westfall AO, Chamot E, Overton ET, Willig JH, et al. (2013) Pain is Independently Associated with Impaired Physical Function in HIV-Infected Patients. Pain Med.
6. Bair MJ, Robinson RL, Katon W, Kroenke K (2003) Depression and pain comorbidity: a literature review. Arch Intern Med 163: 2433–2445.
7. Manchikanti L, Cash KA, Damron KS, Manchukonda R, Pampati V, et al. (2006) Controlled substance abuse and illicit drug use in chronic pain patients: An evaluation of multiple variables. Pain Physician 9: 215–225.
8. Dominick CH, Blyth FM, Nicholas MK (2012) Unpacking the burden: understanding the relationships between chronic pain and comorbidity in the general population. Pain 153: 293–304.
9. Vivian CT (2007) Talk of psychological factors: Tell the whole story. BMJ 335: 900.
10. Kuehn BM (2007) Opioid prescriptions soar: increase in legitimate use as well as abuse. JAMA 297: 249–251.
11. Silverberg MJ, Ray GT, Saunders K, Rutter CM, Campbell CI, et al. (2012) Prescription long-term opioid use in HIV-infected patients. Clin J Pain 28: 39–46.
12. Eccleston C, Williams AC, Morley S (2009) Psychological therapies for the management of chronic pain (excluding headache) in adults. Cochrane Database Syst Rev: CD007407.
13. Kroenke K, Bair M, Damush T, Hoke S, Nicholas G, et al. (2007) Stepped Care for Affective Disorders and Musculoskeletal Pain (SCAMP) study: design and practical implications of an intervention for comorbid pain and depression. Gen Hosp Psychiatry 29: 506–517.
14. Kroenke K, Wu J, Bair MJ, Krebs EE, Damush TM, et al. (2011) Reciprocal relationship between pain and depression: a 12-month longitudinal analysis in primary care. J Pain 12: 964–973.
15. Kroenke K, Bair MJ, Damush TM, Wu J, Hoke S, et al. (2009) Optimized antidepressant therapy and pain self-management in primary care patients with depression and musculoskeletal pain: a randomized controlled trial. JAMA 301: 2099–2110.
16. Merlin JS, Zinski A, Norton WE, Ritchie CS, Saag MS, et al. (2013) A Conceptual Framework for Understanding Chronic Pain in Patients with HIV. Pain Pract.
17. Adler RH (2009) Engel's biopsychosocial model is still relevant today. J Psychosom Res 67: 607–611.
18. Gatchel RJ, Peng YB, Peters ML, Fuchs PN, Turk DC (2007) The biopsychosocial approach to chronic pain: scientific advances and future directions. Psychol Bull 133: 581–624.
19. Merlin JS, Walcott MM, Herbey I, Chamot E, Ritchie C, et al. (2014) Qualitative Investigation of a Brief Chronic Pain Screening Tool in HIV-Infected Patients. AIDS Patient Care STDS.
20. Alok R, Das SK, Agarwal GG, Salwahan L, Srivastava R (2011) Relationship of severity of depression, anxiety and stress with severity of fibromyalgia. Clin Exp Rheumatol 29: S70–72.
21. Morasco BJ, Corson K, Turk DC, Dobscha SK (2011) Association between substance use disorder status and pain-related function following 12 months of treatment in primary care patients with musculoskeletal pain. J Pain 12: 352–359.
22. Martin A, Rief W, Klaiberg A, Braehler E (2006) Validity of the Brief Patient Health Questionnaire Mood Scale (PHQ-9) in the general population. Gen Hosp Psychiatry 28: 71–77.
23. Gaynes BN, O'Donnell J, Nelson E, McGuinness T, Edwards M, et al. (2013) Psychiatric Comorbidity in Depressed HIV Individuals: Common and Clinically Consequential. 8th International Conference on HIV Prevention and Treatment Adherence. Miami, FL.
24. Turk DC, Wilson HD, Cahana A (2011) Treatment of chronic non-cancer pain. Lancet 377: 2226–2235.
25. Stubbs D, Krebs E, Bair M, Damush T, Wu J, et al. (2010) Sex Differences in Pain and Pain-Related Disability among Primary Care Patients with Chronic Musculoskeletal Pain. Pain Med 11: 232–239.
26. Verra ML, Angst F, Staal JB, Brioschi R, Lehmann S, et al. (2011) Differences in pain, function and coping in Multidimensional Pain Inventory subgroups of chronic back pain: a one-group pretest-posttest study. BMC Musculoskelet Disord 12: 145.
27. Morasco BJ, Lovejoy TI, Lu M, Turk DC, Lewis L, et al. (2013) The relationship between PTSD and chronic pain: mediating role of coping strategies and depression. Pain 154: 609–616.
28. Bergman AA, Matthias MS, Coffing JM, Krebs EE (2013) Contrasting Tensions Between Patients and PCPs in Chronic Pain Management: A Qualitative Study. Pain Med.
29. Rhodes LA, McPhillips-Tangum CA, Markham C, Klenk R (1999) The power of the visible: the meaning of diagnostic tests in chronic back pain. Soc Sci Med 48: 1189–1203.
30. Kenny DT (2004) Constructions of chronic pain in doctor-patient relationships: bridging the communication chasm. Patient Educ Couns 52: 297–305.
31. Matthias MS, Krebs EE, Collins LA, Bergman AA, Coffing J, et al. (2013) "I'm not abusing or anything": patient-physician communication about opioid treatment in chronic pain. Patient Educ Couns 93: 197–202.
32. Lum PJ, Little S, Botsko M, Hersh D, Thawley RE, et al. (2011) Opioid-prescribing practices and provider confidence recognizing opioid analgesic abuse in HIV primary care settings. J Acquir Immune Defic Syndr 56 Suppl 1: S91–97.
33. Servan-Schreiber D, Tabas G, Kolb R (2000) Somatizing patients: part II. Practical management. Am Fam Physician 61: 1423–1428, 1431–1422.
34. Frantsve LM, Kerns RD (2007) Patient-provider interactions in the management of chronic pain: current findings within the context of shared medical decision making. Pain Med 8: 25–35.
35. Edelman EJ, Gordon K, Becker WC, Goulet JL, Skanderson M, et al. (2012) Receipt of Opioid Analgesics by HIV-Infected and Uninfected Patients. J Gen Intern Med 28: 82–90.
36. Noble M, Treadwell JR, Tregear SJ, Coates VH, Wiffen PJ, et al. (2010) Long-term opioid management for chronic noncancer pain. Cochrane Database Syst Rev: CD006605.
37. Koeppe J, Armon C, Lyda K, Nielsen C, Johnson S (2010) Ongoing pain despite aggressive opioid pain management among persons with HIV. Clin J Pain 26: 190–198.
38. Li L, Setoguchi S, Cabral H, Jick S (2013) Opioid use for noncancer pain and risk of myocardial infarction amongst adults. J Intern Med 273: 511–526.
39. Li L, Setoguchi S, Cabral H, Jick S (2013) Opioid Use for Noncancer Pain and Risk of Fracture in Adults: A Nested Case-Control Study Using the General Practice Research Database. Am J Epidemiol 178: 559–569.
40. Reddy RG, Aung T, Karavitaki N, Wass JA (2010) Opioid induced hypogonadism. BMJ 341: c4462.
41. Dunn KM, Saunders KW, Rutter CM, Banta-Green CJ, Merrill JO, et al. (2010) Opioid prescriptions for chronic pain and overdose: a cohort study. Ann Intern Med 152: 85–92.
42. Gudin J (2012) Opioid therapies and cytochrome p450 interactions. J Pain Symptom Manage 44: S4–14.
43. Galvan FH, Burnam MA, Bing EG (2003) Co-occurring psychiatric symptoms and drug dependence or heavy drinking among HIV-positive people. J Psychoactive Drugs 35 Suppl 1: 153–160.
44. Gaynes BN, Pence BW, Eron JJ, Miller WC (2008) Prevalence and comorbidity of psychiatric diagnoses based on reference standard in an HIV+ patient population. Psychosom Med 70: 505–511.

17

Evaluation of the Validity of Job Exposure Matrix for Psychosocial Factors at Work

Svetlana Solovieva[1,2]*, Tiina Pensola[1], Johanna Kausto[1,2], Rahman Shiri[1,2], Markku Heliövaara[3], Alex Burdorf[4], Kirsti Husgafvel-Pursiainen[1,2], Eira Viikari-Juntura[2]

1 Centre of Expertise for Health and Work Ability, Finnish Institute of Occupational Health, Helsinki, Finland, **2** Disability Prevention Centre, Finnish Institute of Occupational Health, Helsinki, Finland, **3** National Institute for Health and Welfare, Helsinki, Finland, **4** Erasmus MC, University Medical Center Rotterdam, Rotterdam, The Netherlands

Abstract

Objective: To study the performance of a developed job exposure matrix (JEM) for the assessment of psychosocial factors at work in terms of accuracy, possible misclassification bias and predictive ability to detect known associations with depression and low back pain (LBP).

Materials and Methods: We utilized two large population surveys (the Health 2000 Study and the Finnish Work and Health Surveys), one to construct the JEM and another to test matrix performance. In the first study, information on job demands, job control, monotonous work and social support at work was collected via face-to-face interviews. Job strain was operationalized based on job demands and job control using quadrant approach. In the second study, the sensitivity and specificity were estimated applying a Bayesian approach. The magnitude of misclassification error was examined by calculating the biased odds ratios as a function of the sensitivity and specificity of the JEM and fixed true prevalence and odds ratios. Finally, we adjusted for misclassification error the observed associations between JEM measures and selected health outcomes.

Results: The matrix showed a good accuracy for job control and job strain, while its performance for other exposures was relatively low. Without correction for exposure misclassification, the JEM was able to detect the association between job strain and depression in men and between monotonous work and LBP in both genders.

Conclusions: Our results suggest that JEM more accurately identifies occupations with low control and high strain than those with high demands or low social support. Overall, the present JEM is a useful source of job-level psychosocial exposures in epidemiological studies lacking individual-level exposure information. Furthermore, we showed the applicability of a Bayesian approach in the evaluation of the performance of the JEM in a situation where, in practice, no gold standard of exposure assessment exists.

Editor: James Coyne, University of Pennsylvania, United States of America

Funding: The study was financially supported by the Finnish Work Environment Fund (project no 109364). The funders had no role in study design, data collection and analysis, decision to publish, or preparation of the manuscript.

Competing Interests: The authors have declared that no competing interests exist.

* Email: svetlana.solovieva@ttl.fi

Introduction

During the past three decades, the effects of psychosocial factors at work on health have received considerable attention in research. Psychosocial factors at work are numerous, with psychological job demands, job control (decision latitude), efforts and rewards [1,2] comprising the key dimensions. Another factor of importance is social support at work [3].

The job strain model, introduced by Karasek in 1979 [4], is one of the most studied occupational stress models. According to the model, workers with a combination of high psychosocial job demands and low control over a job (high job strain) have a higher risk of developing an illness as compared to workers with low psychosocial job demands and high job control (low job strain) [1]. The job strain model has been successfully used to predict the risk of cardiovascular disease [5,6], major mental disorders [7], type II diabetes [8] and musculoskeletal diseases [9]. The effects of the individual components of the job strain model on health have also been evaluated, although the results have often been inconsistent across the studies and health outcomes [7,9].

The interpretation of the observed associations between psychosocial factors at work and health mainly depends on the validity of the assessment methods of the risk factors. Self-reported questionnaires are widely used to measure psychosocial factors at work [10]. Self-reports provide subjective information representing a worker's perception of occupational stress and are therefore susceptible to reporting bias. The subjective assessment of psychosocial factors at work has been the largest concern in the debate on the interpretation of associations and on the possible causal role of these factors for illness. It has been suggested that common source bias due to subjective measures of psychosocial factors at work increases the likelihood of false positive findings, particularly in cross-sectional studies with the self-reported health outcomes [11–13]. Workers having health problems are more likely to report certain psychosocial exposures than healthy workers. Such tendency might lead to differential misclassification, which results either in an overestimation or underestimation of the true effect [14], particularly, when exposures and outcome are measured simultaneously.

The assessment of psychosocial factors at work with a job exposure matrix (JEM), where exposure level is assigned based on the job-specific average of exposure, is not prone to information bias and may therefore guarantee some degree of objectivity. The major advantage of the JEM in epidemiological studies is that it can be applied to the populations with lacking exposure information. However, such method of exposure assessment induces Berkson type error, which may not cause notable bias on the effect estimates but weakens the precision of the estimates [15]. A JEM neglects both within worker (over time variation) and between worker (variation in tasks, activities and work processes) variation in a job [16] and therefore may result in false positive and negative exposure assignments for a considerable proportion of the subjects. A non-differential misclassification bias induced by JEM will attenuate the observed associations towards null [15,17,18]. Knowing the magnitude of measurement error (e.g. sensitivity and specificity) and exposure prevalence, the extent of non-differential bias can be estimated [15,19].

Several psychosocial job exposure matrices have been developed and used in epidemiological studies [20–26]. Even though the JEM measures are more objective than self-reported ones, they cannot be seen as a gold standard in the context of psychosocial factors at work [13]. Therefore, the question of the reliability of the associations between JEM-based exposures and health outcomes is always warranted. The validity of psychosocial JEM measures in the absence of a gold standard method is challenging to evaluate and, as a result, has rarely been examined and reported [24–28]. Furthermore, the magnitude of misclassification bias of psychosocial JEM measures on effect estimates has not been examined so far.

The aims of the study were 1) to examine the accuracy of a developed gender-specific job exposure matrix in the assessment of psychosocial factors at work applying the Bayesian approach, 2) to evaluate the theoretical impact of exposure misclassification on exposure-outcome associations and 3) to examine the ability of the matrix to detect known associations between psychosocial factors at work and health outcomes.

Materials and Methods

Study population

We utilized two large Finnish population samples. The Health 2000 (H2000) Study was used to construct the JEM and to examine the inter-method agreement, and the national Finnish Work and Health (FWH) Surveys were used to test the performance of the matrix. The study populations consisted of 18–64 year-old individuals, who had been working during the preceding 12 months.

The Health 2000 Study is a large Finnish population-based study carried out in 2000–01. The main objective of the study was to obtain representative information on the current health status of the whole non-institutional adult population in Finland. The survey consisted of several questionnaires, a home interview, and a health examination. A nationally representative sample of the population was obtained using a two-stage stratified cluster sampling design. The original samples consisted of 8028 subjects aged 30 years or over and 1894 subjects aged 18–29. The participation rates were 87% and 90%, respectively. A detailed comprehensive description of the methods and processes has been published elsewhere [29,30]. The sample of this study comprised 4619 persons aged 18–64 who were working during the preceding 12 months and for whom information on occupational titles and exposures were available. The age and gender distribution of the study population matched those of the employed persons in Finland in the year 2000.

The national Finnish National Work and Health Surveys have been conducted every third year since 1997 to collect information on perceived working conditions and the health of the working-age population, For the 1997–2003 Surveys, random samples of subjects aged 25–64 years independent of their working status (e.g., working, unemployed, retired or student) were drawn from the Finnish population register. For the 2009 Survey a random sample of subjects aged 20–64 years was drawn from Finnish employment statistics. The sample size has varied between 2031 and 2355 persons from year to year with a response rate of 58–72% [31]. At each survey, a phone number was not found for about 10–16% of subjects. The proportion of non-participants in each survey was slightly higher among men than women and among subjects aged 24–34 years than among the older subjects. Age, gender, education, socioeconomic status and occupational sector of the respondents were compared with the Census data. No major differences were found. Thus, the respondents to the FWH Surveys represent rather well the targeted population. The data from all five surveys were combined. Hence, the total number of the interviewed persons with information on occupation during 1997–2009 was 11326.

The H2000 Study and the FWH Surveys have all obtained ethical approval from the appropriate ethics committees.

Classification of occupations

Occupations in both surveys were classified on the 4-digit level (including few occupations coded with 5 digits) according to the Classification of Occupations 2001 by Statistics Finland, which is based on the International Standard Classification of Occupations (ISCO-88). The classification is based on ten categories of professional skills. In total, the classification includes 444 job titles.

Psychosocial exposures

Psychosocial exposures in the H2000 Study were measured with a Finnish version of the Job Content Questionnaire (JCQ) [32]. The JCQ has been shown to be a valid and reliable instrument to assess job stress and social support in many occupational settings worldwide [10,13]. Responses were given on a five point Likert-scale from 1 (fully agree) to 5 (fully disagree).

Psychological *job demands* scale is the sum of the following five items: "work fast", "work hard", "excessive work", "not enough time", and "hectic job". In the current study, Cronbach's alpha for the scale was 0.76 for men and 0.81 for women. *Job control* scale is the sum of two subscales. Decision authority was measured with three items: "allows own decisions", "decision freedom", and "a lot of say on the job"), and skill discretion was measured with five items: "learn new things", "requires creativity", "high skill level", "variety", and "develop own abilities". Cronbach's alpha for the scale was 0.85 for men and 0.86 for women. Since *monotonous (repetitive) work* was weakly correlated with the other five items of the skill discretion scale we treated it as a separate exposure. Job demands, job control and monotonous work were dichotomized using gender-specific median cut-off points.

Job strain was operationalized using the quadrant approach proposed by Karasek and Theorell [1]. It defines workers who are above the median on job demands and below the median on job control as having a high strain job. Other categories are: low strain (low demands and high control), passive (low demands and low control) and active (high demands and high control). Low strain job was used as the reference category in the analyses.

Social *support* at work was measured with four items: "support from supervisor", "supervisor appreciates", "support from co-workers", "discussion on work". Cronbach's alpha for the scale was 0.80 for men and 0.82 for women. Social support was dichotomized at a gender-specific median in order to define low and high support.

Development of the job exposure matrix (JEM)

We constructed a gender-specific matrix with exposure estimates at each intersection between rows (occupational groups) and columns (psychosocial exposures). The exposure axis of the matrix included the above mentioned five psychosocial risk factors at work. The occupation axis of the matrix was based on the original job titles or occupational groups.

Previous studies showed that ten individuals with the same job title will be sufficient for a reliable estimation of exposures [33,34]. The exposure estimates for job demands, job control, monotonous work and social support at work were calculated as a median score of exposures in each occupation which included at least 10 subjects in order to obtain reasonably precise estimates. The exposure estimates for job strain were calculated as the proportion of exposed to passive, active and high strain work. The job titles with a small number (<10) of respondents were grouped based on the similarities of these job titles with regard to work tasks (including supervising), work environment, and required educational level. The gender differences in the exposures were also considered. If there was no reasonable way to merge the occupation with other occupations within the gender (such as female frontier guards), the exposure estimates of both genders in that occupation/occupational group were combined.

The sample size of the H2000 Study was large enough to enable us to develop a gender-specific job exposure matrix and to keep several job titles unmerged. Out of 444 possible job titles, altogether 363 (300 among men and 267 among women) were available in the Health 2000 Study. There were 61 job titles among men and 58 among women with at least 10 subjects. These job titles covered 69% of the study sample. After merging the smaller groups the number of job titles or occupational groups reduced to 110 among men and 101 among women.

The exposure estimates for job demands, job control, monotonous work and social support at work were dichotomized using gender-specific median as a cut-off point. The categories of job strain were obtained based on the dichotomized JEM-based job demands and job control.

Health outcomes

Based on the current evidence we chose two health outcomes that are known to be associated with psychosocial factors at work. Both cross-sectional and longitudinal studies have shown that high level of psychological demands and job strain are associated with major mental disorders [7,35–37]. Suggestive evidence for a relationship of job demands, job control and monotonous work with low back pain has also been reported [9,38,39].

Depressive symptoms. In both studies, depressive symptoms were assessed with the following question: "Have you had melancholy or depression during the last month (30 days)?". The response categories ranged from 1 = not at all to 5 = very often. The occurrence of depressive symptoms was dichotomized as no (categories 1 and 2) or yes (categories from 3 to 5).

Low back pain. In the H2000 Study information on low back pain was inquired with the following question: "Have you had pain in your back during the past month (30 days)?" (yes/no). In the FWH Surveys, data on low back pain were collected with an interview using the question: "Have you during the past month (30 days) had long-lasting or recurrent pain in the lumbar spine?" (yes/no).

Data analyses

In the H2000 Study, the inter-method agreement between self-reported and JEM measures was examined using intra-class correlation (ICC). Two-way mixed total ICC agreements were computed. In the FWH Surveys, the performance of the matrix was evaluated by examining the accuracy of the matrix in the identification of exposed/non-exposed individuals, estimating exposure misclassification error, and looking at the ability of the matrix to detect associations of psychosocial factors at work with one-month prevalence of depression or low back pain (predictive validity) [40]. The accuracy of the JEM was evaluated using five indicators: sensitivity (Se), specificity (Sp), Youden's J index, likelihood ratio positive (LR+) and likelihood ratio negative (LR−).

Sensitivity (ability of the test to identify positive results) and specificity (ability of the test to identify negative results) are usually determined against a reference standard test (gold standard). Errors in measuring the sensitivity and specificity of a test will arise if the reference test itself does not have 100% sensitivity and 100% specificity. Since there is no gold standard measure for psychosocial factors at work, we estimated sensitivity and specificity using a Bayesian approach, proposed by Joseph et al. [41]. As the first step, the posterior distribution of sensitivity and specificity of the JEM measures was calculated using self-reported and JEM measures of exposures from H2000 Study. For these analyses, the prior distribution of the parameters was derived based on the assumption that the self-reported measures have almost perfect sensitivity and specificity and no prior information on sensitivity and specificity of JEM measures is available. As the second step, the posterior distribution of sensitivity and specificity of the JEM measures was calculated using data from FWH Surveys. For these analyses the prior distributions of the parameters were derived based on the posterior distributions obtained in the first step. At each step, the posterior medians and their 95% Bayesian credible intervals were estimated using Gibbs sampler algorithm with WinBUGS software version 1.4.3.

The estimated sensitivity and specificity were used to calculate Youden's J index as well as LR+ and LR−. The Youden's J index ($J = Se + Sp - 1$) has been used as a measure of the effectiveness of the JEM to discriminate between exposed and non-exposed individuals. The possible range of the Youden's J index value is between 0 (totally useless) and 1 (perfect). Likelihood ratio positive is the probability of an exposed person to be classified as exposed divided by the probability of a non-exposed person to be classified as exposed. Likelihood ratio negative is the probability of an exposed person to be classified as non-exposed divided by the probability of a non-exposed person to be classified as non-exposed. A likelihood ratio equal to 1 will indicate that the JEM measure is unable to distinguish between exposed and non-exposed. A $LR > 1$ will indicate that the JEM is likely to identify exposed and $LR < 1$ will indicate that the JEM is likely to identify non-exposed. The higher LR+ value and lower the LR− value, the better is the JEM performance.

To estimate the theoretical magnitude of exposure misclassification, biased odds ratios (OR′) were calculated based on the obtained estimates of sensitivity (Se) and specificity (Sp) and assumed "true prevalence" (Pr) and "true odds ratios" (OR) using

Table 1. Prevalence of self-reported and JEM-based psychosocial exposures.

Exposures	Men			Women		
	H2000 Study		FWH Surveys	H2000 Study		FWH Surveys
	Self-reported	JEM	JEM	Self-reported	JEM	JEM
	Prev. (95% CI)	Prev. (95% CI)	Prev. (95% CI)	Prev. (95% CI)	Prev. (95% CI)	Prev. (95% CI)
High job demands	43.1 (41.1, 45.0)	33.1 (29.4, 33.3)	32.2 (31.0, 33.4)	44.2 (42.2, 46.3)	35.3 (33.4, 37.3)	36.0 (34.7, 37.3)
Low job control	52.6 (50.5, 54.7)	49.8 (47.8, 51.9)	49.8 (48.5, 51.1)	56.1 (54.1, 58.1)	56.5 (54.5, 58.5)	55.4 (54.1, 56.7)
Job strain						
Low strain job	26.2 (24.4, 28.1)	36.3 (34.3, 38.3)	36.3 (34.1, 36.6)	23.8 (22.1, 25.6)	24.6 (22.9, 26.4)	25.6 (24.4, 26.3)
Passive job	30.7 (28.8, 32.7)	32.4 (30.5, 34.4)	32.5 (31.3, 33.8)	32.0 (30.1, 33.9)	40.0 (38.1, 42.1)	38.4 (37.2, 39.7)
Active job	21.2 (19.5, 22.9)	13.9 (12.5, 15.4)	14.9 (14.0, 15.8)	20.0 (18.4, 21.7)	18.9 (17.3, 20.5)	19.0 (18.0, 20.1)
High strain job	21.9 (20.2, 23.6)	17.4 (15.9, 19.1)	17.3 (16.3, 18.3)	24.2 (22.5, 26.0)	16.4 (15.0, 18.0)	16.9 (16.0, 18.0)
Low social support	47.3 (45.3, 49.4)	48.5 (46.4, 50.1)	48.4 (47.1, 49.7)	44.2 (42.2, 46.2)	37.1 (35.2, 39.1)	37.5 (36.2, 38.7)
Monotonous work	28.5 (26.6, 30.4)	17.2 (15.7, 18.8)	17.1 (16.1, 18.1)	31.8 (29.9, 33.7)	24.0 (22.3, 25.8)	22.1 (21.0, 23.2)

H2000 Study- the Health 2000 Study; FWH Surveys- the Finnish Work and Health Surveys.

the following formula [19]:

$$OR' = \frac{((Se*OR*Pr+(1\text{-}Sp)*(1\text{-}Pr))*((1\text{-}Se)*Pr+Sp*(1\text{-}Pr))}{((Se*Pr+(1\text{-}Sp)*(1\text{-}Pr))*((1\text{-}Se)*OR*Pr+Sp*(1\text{-}Pr))}$$

The true prevalence was fixed at 0.50 for high job demands, low job control and low social support, at 0.33 for monotonous work and at 0.25 for high strain job. The true odds ratios were fixed at three values OR = 1.5, OR = 2 and OR = 3. The relative difference between biased and true estimates was calculated ((OR′-OR)/OR) and used as quantitative measure for the magnitude of exposure misclassification.

Logistic regression analyses with age, education and year of survey (the FWH Surveys) adjusted odds ratios (OR) and 95% confidence intervals (CIs) were carried out to study the associations between the JEM measures and one-month prevalence of depression or low back pain. These analyses were performed using SAS version 9.1. The effect estimates were adjusted for misclassification error using WINPEPI COMPARE2 program, version 3.08 [42].

All analyses were performed separately for men and women.

Results

In both genders, the prevalence of high job demands, high job strain and monotonous work measured by job exposure matrix was statistically significantly lower than that assessed by self-reports (Table 1). In women, the prevalence of low social support was lower for JEM measures than for self-reported measures. There were no differences in the distribution of exposures assessed by JEM between the two study populations, reflecting a similar job distribution in both surveys. In general, total agreement between self-reported and JEM measures assessed by ICC was slightly better among women than men, with the largest ICC values observed for job control followed by monotonous work (Table 2).

Bayesian estimates of sensitivity and specificity and magnitude of exposure misclassification error

The Bayesian estimates of sensitivity and specificity were calculated based on the data from the Health 2000 Study and The Finnish Work and Health Surveys and are shown in the form of posterior medians and 95% Bayesian intervals (Table 3). The posterior estimates were very similar in both study populations. The specificity of JEM measures was higher than sensitivity for all exposures except job control among women. Specificity ranged from 0.62 to 0.90 in men, and from 0.68 to 0.86 in women. Sensitivity was the lowest for high strain job (0.46) in men and for low social support (0.52) in women. The best matrix performance assessed by Youden's J index and likelihood ratios was found for high strain job, particularly in women. The JEM was least effective in identification of men exposed to high demands (J = 0.17) and women exposed to low social support (J = 0.15).

The theoretical effect of exposure misclassification error on estimated ORs is shown in Table 4. In both genders, the smallest misclassification error was observed for high job strain, followed by that for low job control. The largest misclassification error was found for low social support (both genders) and high job demands (men). In general, when the true OR is equal to 1.5, the effect of misclassification error on point estimates is relatively small, though there is a high likelihood of false negative findings. A statistically significant association can be detected only for low job control and high job strain in women. With the increase of true OR, there is a larger reduction in the biased odds ratios, but at the same time the likelihood of false negative findings is lowered.

Table 2. Intra-class correlation (ICC) between individual-based and group-based measures of psychosocial exposures for men and women in the H2000 Study.

	Men	Women
Job demands	0.31	0.40
Job control	0.53	0.60
Monotonous work	0.45	0.51
Social support	0.36	0.33
Job strain	0.21	0.29

H2000 Study- the Health 2000 Study.

Table 3. Posterior medians and lower and upper limits of the posterior equally tailed 95% credible intervals (Bayesian confidence interval).

		H2000 Study		FWH Surveys				
		Sensitivity	Specificity	Sensitivity	Specificity	J[1]	LR+[2]	LR−[3]
High demands	Men	0.41 (0.38–0.44)	0.76 (0.74–0.78)	0.41 (0.39–0.44)	0.76 (0.74–0.78)	0.17	1.71 (1.53–1.91)	0.78 (0.73–0.82)
	Women	0.49 (0.46–0.52)	0.75 (0.73–0.78)	0.49 (0.46–0.52)	0.75 (0.73–0.78)	0.24	2.00 (1.77–2.25)	0.68 (0.63–0.72)
Low control	Men	0.67 (0.64–0.70)	0.69 (0.67–0.72)	0.67 (0.64–0.69)	0.70 (0.67–0.72)	0.37	2.20 (2.01–2.42)	0.48 (0.43–0.52)
	Women	0.75 (0.73–0.78)	0.68 (0.65–0.71)	0.76 (0.73–0.78)	0.68 (0.65–0.71)	0.44	2.35 (2.14–2.59)	0.36 (0.32–0.40)
High strain job	Men	0.58 (0.52–0.64)	0.87 (0.84–0.91)	0.60 (0.55–0.65)	0.82 (0.77–0.86)	0.42	3.34 (2.52–4.45)	0.49 (0.42–0.57)
	Women	0.77 (0.71–0.82)	0.88 (0.84–0.92)	0.78 (0.73–0.83)	0.86 (0.81–0.90)	0.64	5.75 (4.13–8.03)	0.25 (0.19–0.31)
Low social support	Men	0.60 (0.57–0.63)	0.62 (0.59–0.65)	0.60 (0.57–0.63)	0.62 (0.59–0.65)	0.22	1.59 (1.45–1.74)	0.65 (0.59–0.71)
	Women	0.48 (0.45–0.51)	0.72 (0.70–0.74)	0.44 (0.42–0.46)	0.71 (0.69–0.73)	0.15	1.52 (1.40–1.65)	0.79 (0.75–0.83)
Monotonous work	Men	0.35 (0.32–0.39)	0.90 (0.88–0.91)	0.36 (0.32–0.39)	0.90 (0.88–0.91)	0.26	3.39 (2.84–4.01)	0.72 (0.68–0.76)
	Women	0.46 (0.42–0.50)	0.86 (0.84–0.88)	0.46 (0.42–0.50)	0.86 (0.84–0.88)	0.32	3.31 (2.79–3.91)	0.63 (0.58–0.68)

The sensitivity and specificity of JEM-based measures for men and women in the H2000 Study and the FWH Surveys.
H2000 Study- the Health 2000 Study; FWH Surveys- the Finnish Work and Health Surveys;
[1]J - Youden's index = sensitivity+specificity − 1.
[2]LR+ likelihood ratio positive.
[3]LR− likelihood ratio negative.

Table 4. Biased odds (OR′) ratios according to sensitivity and specificity of the job exposure matrix when the true odds ratios (OR) were assumed to equal 1.5, 2 or 3.

	OR = 1.5		OR = 2.0		OR = 3.0	
	Men	Women	Men	Women	Men	Women
High job demands[1]	1.08	1.11	1.13	1.18*	1.21*	1.28*
Low job control[1]	1.16	1.20*	1.28*	1.35*	1.45*	1.58*
Monotonous work[2]	1.17	1.17	1.30*	1.31*	1.50*	1.52*
Low social support[1]	1.09	1.07	1.16	1.11	1.25*	1.17*
High job strain[3]	1.18	1.27*	1.34*	1.53*	1.60*	1.99*

[1]Prevalence of exposure is assumed to equal 0.50.
[2]Prevalence of exposure is assumed to equal 0.33.
[3]Prevalence of exposure is assumed to equal 0.25.
*Statistical significance at the 5% level (two-sided test) of the biased odds ratios is calculated for a study population of 5000 men and 5000 women.

Predictive validity of the JEM measures

The one-month prevalence of depression was statistically significantly higher in the H2000 Study as compared with the FWH Surveys, while the prevalence of low back pain during the preceding 30 days was similar (Table 5). In both study populations, women tended to report depression and LBP more frequently than men.

In the H2000 Study, associations between all self-reported psychosocial factors at work and depression were statistically significant in both genders (Table 5). In the FWH Surveys, the point estimates of associations between the JEM-based exposures and depression were reduced by 22–65% as compared with those for self-reported exposures in the H2000 Study, particularly in women. The smallest drop was found for low job control (men) and monotonous work (women), while the largest reduction in estimates was observed for low social support in women. After correction for exposure misclassification, the odds ratios obtained with JEM regained their statistical significance for low job control (both genders), monotonous work (women), and high job demands, low social support and high strain job (men). However, women with high job demands or low social support assessed by JEM had reduced odds of depression. Similarly, monotonous work seemed to be associated with lower risk of depression in men.

All self-reported psychosocial factors at work, except monotonous work, were statistically significantly associated with LBP in women (Table 5). In men, high job demands, low job control and low social support tended to increase the odds of LBP, although the association was statistically significant for high job strain only. The estimated odds for JEM-based exposures were reduced by 6–21% in men and by 12–32% in women as compared with those for self-reported exposures. Unexpectedly, for monotonous work, the odds ratios obtained with JEM were increased by 21% as compared to odds ratios obtained with self-reports. After correction for exposure misclassification error, all JEM-based exposures in men and all except high job demands in women were statistically significantly associated with LBP. Women with low social support had a low prevalence of LBP.

Discussion

We comprehensively validated a gender-specific job exposure matrix that we constructed for the assessment of psychosocial factors at work. The matrix showed a good accuracy in identification of individuals exposed to low job control and high job strain, while its performance for job demands and social support was relatively low. The largest misclassification error was found for low social support (women) and high job demands (men). The difference between the odds ratios based on self-reports and JEM was larger for depression than for low back pain, especially in women. Without correction for exposure misclassification, the JEM was able to detect the association between job strain and depression in men and that between monotonous work and low back pain in both genders. The predictive ability of the matrix substantially improved after correction for possible misclassification bias.

Although several psychosocial JEMs exist, their validity is poorly explored. Most of the previous studies on the validation of JEMs examined their ability to detect known associations between JEM measures and health outcomes (predictive validity) [24–28]. Few studies evaluated inter-method agreement between JEM and self-reported measures [24,43]. There are several parameters that can be used to evaluate the performance of an exposure assessment method, of which sensitivity, specificity, Youden's J index and likelihood ratios are the most commonly applied. Considering all performance indicators, the performance of our JEM was good for job control and job strain and was rather low for job demands and social support. These findings are in line with the results of the previous studies that reported higher validity of the JEM measures for job control and job strain than for job demands and social support [13,43,44]. The relatively low validity of job demands may suggest that variation of this factor between occupations is smaller than that within occupation [20,21]. However, the poor performance for social support may alternatively reflect that some psychosocial factors are highly individually oriented in that a particular job may be perceived as very strenuous for some whereas not for others.

Among performance indicators, sensitivity and specificity are the key ones, because all others are calculated based on them. Theoretically, sensitivity and specificity should be determined against a reference test (gold standard). In practice, the sensitivity and specificity of the JEMs are usually evaluated against self-reports, even if it is well known that the self-reported exposures may be subject to information bias. In the current study, we used the Bayesian approach to estimate sensitivity and specificity of JEM measures. The similarity of estimates obtained in both of our study samples suggests their robustness. The sensitivity of the JEM-based estimates for job control and high strain job was acceptable, while it was reduced for job demands, monotonous work and social support. The specificity of all our JEM-based estimates varied from good to very good and was substantially higher,

Table 5. The association of psychosocial exposures measured at individual (ind) level and at group level (job exposure matrix (JEM)) with one-month prevalence of depression and low back pain among men and women.

		High demands		Low control		Monotonous work		Low social support		High strain job	
	Prevalence (95% CI)	**OR**	**95% CI**	**OR**	**95% CI**	**OR**	**95% CI**	**OR**	**95% CI**	**OR**	**95% CI**
Men											
Depressive symptoms											
H2000 (ind)[1]	13.9 (12.3–15.5)	1.98	1.51–2.59	1.52	1.16–2.01	1.45	1.07–1.95	2.07	1.59–2.74	3.07	2.05–4.62
FWH (JEM)[2]	10.6 (9.8–11.5)	1.15	0.96–1.37	1.19	0.98–1.43	0.95	0.75–1.21	1.11	0.93–1.31	1.34	1.04–1.72
FWH (JEM)[3]		2.08	1.74–2.48	1.33	1.12–1.59	0.81	0.67–0.99	1.54	1.30–1.72	1.70	1.34–2.15
Low back pain											
H2000 (ind)[1]	26.8 (25.0–28.7)	1.19	0.99–1.44	1.13	0.93–1.37	1.01	0.81–1.26	1.16	0.96–1.41	1.37	1.04–1.80
FWH (JEM)[2]	29.8 (28.6–31.0)	1.04	0.92–1.18	1.06	0.94–1.21	1.22	1.05–1.42	1.06	0.94–1.19	1.10	0.92–1.30
FWH (JEM)[3]		1.20	1.07–1.34	1.73	1.54–1.95	2.38	2.10–2.69	1.50	1.33–1.68	1.77	1.51–2.09
Women											
Depressive symptoms											
H2000 (ind)[1]	18.7 (17.0–20.5)	1.55	1.22–1.95	1.49	1.17–1.90	1.29	1.00–1.67	2.75	2.16–3.50	2.38	1.68–3.37
FWH (JEM)[2]	15.9 (14.9–16.9)	0.99	0.85–1.15	1.07	0.91–1.28	1.01	0.84–1.22	0.97	0.83–1.13	1.09	0.87–1.37
FWH (JEM)[3]		0.88	0.76–1.01	1.33	1.15–1.54	1.24	1.05–1.45	0.79	0.69–0.92	1.20	0.96–1.50
Low back pain											
H2000 (ind)[1]	29.7 (27.8–31.6)	1.29	1.08–1.55	1.27	1.05–1.54	1.16	0.95–1.43	1.28	1.07–1.54	1.68	1.28–2.20
FWH (JEM)[2]	31.4 (30.2–32.)	1.00	0.89–1.13	1.12	0.99–1.27	1.19	1.03–1.38	1.00	0.89–1.12	1.14	0.95–1.38
FWH (JEM)[3]		0.92	0.82–1.03	1.76	1.56–1.97	2.38	2.10–2.71	0.83	0.74–0.94	1.52	1.27–1.81

Odds ratios (OR) and their 95% confidence intervals (95% CI).
H2000 – the Health 2000 Study; FWH- the Finnish Work and Health Surveys;
[1]ORs calculated based on self-reports and adjusted for age and education.
[2]ORs calculated based on JEM and adjusted for age, education and year of survey.
[3]ORs calculated based on JEM adjusted for exposure misclassification bias.

especially in women, as compared to those found in a French study [24].

The studies that examined the predictive validity of the psychosocial JEM measures have consistently reported weaker associations between JEM measures and health outcomes than what has been found for the corresponding self-reported factors [24–28]. In general, the associations of JEM measures for job strain and job control with health outcomes were better reproducible than the associations for job demands. However, even unexpected results of a protective effect of high job demands assessed by JEM on anxiety disorders [25] and self-rated health [24] have been reported.

When JEM is used to study the association between an exposure and a health outcome, there is always some loss of information because the individual values are replaced with the group-based (job title) ones. Both self-reported exposures and JEM are prone to classification errors whose consequences on effect estimates need to be considered when interpreting the association between the exposure and the outcome. The measurement error in exposures assessed by JEM is always of a Berkson type, while the error of self-reported measures is of a classical type. The group-specific average of exposures used in our JEM was obtained based on nationally representative self-reported exposure data; therefore, the measurement error of our JEM has both classical and Berkson component, with the latter being dominant. The classical and Berkson errors bias the effect estimates differently [15]. The Berkson error has almost no effect on the point estimate, while it severely affects the estimate's precision. In case of classical error, the direction and magnitude of bias are more difficult to assess. We observed a larger difference between the self-reported and JEM-based exposures in the ORs for depressive symptoms than for LBP. This may suggest the presence of a higher common source bias in self-reported exposure measures among those reporting depressive symptoms than among those reporting LBP. As a result, for depressive symptoms, the risk estimates based on JEM measures may be closer to the true risk than the risk estimates based on self-reports. These benefits support the use of the JEM in epidemiological studies.

The ability of the JEM to detect known associations between risk factors and health outcomes primarily depends on the magnitude of misclassification error. Even though studies have examined the predictive validity of psychosocial JEM measures, none of them examined the effect of exposure misclassification on observed associations. Our results suggest that, due to misclassification error, we were not able to observe associations between job demands, job control and social support assessed by JEM with either depression or low back pain. However, after correction for misclassification bias, the ability of the matrix to detect the expected associations improved substantially. Furthermore, the bias-adjusted effect estimates for low job control and high job strain in our study were about the same as those reported in previous meta-analyses [7,9].

Conclusions

Our results suggest that JEM more accurately identifies occupations with low control and high strain than those with high demands or low social support. Although the JEM is a rather crude exposure assessment method, it can be a useful source of job-level psychosocial exposures in epidemiological studies lacking individual-level exposure. Furthermore, we showed the applicability of a Bayesian approach in the evaluation of the performance of the JEM in a situation where, in practice, no gold standard of exposure assessment exists.

Acknowledgments

We would like to thank Dr. Timo Kauppinen for his expertise in the development of the job exposure matrix.

Author Contributions

Conceived and designed the experiments: SS TP JK RS AB KH-P EV-J. Performed the experiments: SS TP JK RS AB KH-P EV-J. Analyzed the data: SS. Contributed reagents/materials/analysis tools: MH EV-J. Wrote the paper: SS TP EV-J KH-P. Contributed substantially to the interpretation of the findings and critically revised the manuscript: SS TP JK RS MH AB KH-P EV-J.

References

1. Karasek RA, Theorell T (1990) Healthy Work: Stress, Productivity, and the Reconstruction of Working Life. New York: Basic Books.
2. Siegrist J (1996) Adverse health effects of high-effort/low-reward conditions. J Occup Health Psychol 1:27–41.
3. Johnson JV, Hall EM (1988) Job strain, work place social support, and cardiovascular disease: a cross-sectional study of a random sample of the Swedish working population. Am J Public Health 78: 1336–42.
4. Karasek RA (1979) Job demands, job decision latitude, and mental strain: Implications for job redesign. Adm Sci Q 24:285–308.
5. Diène E, Fouquet A, Esquirol Y (2012) Cardiovascular diseases and psychosocial factors at work. Arch Cardiovasc Dis 105:33–9.
6. Kivimäki M, Nyberg ST, Batty GD, Fransson EI, Heikkilä K, et al. (2012) Job strain as a risk factor for coronary heart disease: a collaborative meta-analysis of individual participant data. Lancet 380(9852):1491–7.
7. Stansfeld S, Candy B (2006) Psychosocial work environment and mental health—a meta-analytic review. Scand J Work Environ Health 32:443–62.
8. Cosgrove MP, Sargeant LA, Caleyachetty R, Griffin SJ (2012) Work-related stress and Type 2 diabetes: systematic review and meta-analysis. Occup Med (Lond) 62:167–73.
9. Lang J, Ochsmann E, Kraus T, Lang JW (2012) Psychosocial work stressors as antecedents of musculoskeletal problems: a systematic review and meta-analysis of stability-adjusted longitudinal studies. Soc Sci Med 75:1163–74.
10. Tabanelli MC, Depolo M, Cooke RM, Sarchielli G, Bonfiglioli R, et al. (2008) Available instruments for measurement of psychosocial factors in the work environment. Int Arch Occup Environ Health 82:1–12.
11. Landsbergis P, Theorell T, Schwartz J, Greiner BA, Krause N (2000) Measurement of psychosocial workplace exposure variables. Occup Med 15:163–88.
12. Macleod J, Davey Smith G (2003) Psychosocial factors and public health: a suitable case for treatment? J Epidemiol Community Health 57:565–70.
13. Theorell T, Hasselhorn HM (2005) On cross-sectional questionnaire studies of relationships between psychosocial conditions at work and health–are they reliable? Int Arch Occup Environ Health 78:517–22.
14. Blair A, Stewart P, Lubin JH, Forastiere F (2007) Methodological issues regarding confounding and exposure misclassification in epidemiological studies of occupational exposures. Am J Ind Med 50:199–207.
15. Armstrong BG (1998) Effect of measurement error on epidemiological studies of environmental and occupational exposures. Occup Environ Med 55:651–6.
16. Tielemans E, Heederik D, Burdorf A, Vermeulen R, Veulemans H, et al. (1999) Assessment of occupational exposures in a general population: comparison of different methods. Occup Environ Med 56:145–151.
17. Siemiatycki J, Dewar R, Richardson L (1989) Costs and statistical power associated with five methods of collecting occupation exposure information for population-based case-control studies. Am J Epidemiol 130:1236–46.
18. Bouyer J, Dardenne J, Hémon D (1995) Performance of odds ratios obtained with a job-exposure matrix and individual exposure assessment with special reference to misclassification errors. Scand J Work Environ Health 21:265–71.
19. Flegal KM, Brownie C, Haas JD (1986) The effects of exposure misclassification on estimates of relative risk. Am J Epidemiol 123:736–51.
20. Schwartz JE, Pieper CF, Karasek RA (1988) A procedure for linking psychosocial job characteristics data to health surveys. Am J Public Health 78:904–9.
21. Johnson JV, Stewart WF (1993) Measuring work organization exposure over the life course with a job-exposure matrix. Scand J Work Environ Health 19:21–8.
22. Mariani M (1999) Replace with a database: O*NET replaces the Dictionary of Occupational Titles. Occup Outlook Quarterly 43:3–9.
23. Kauppinen T, Toikkanen J, Pukkala E (1998) From cross-tabulations to multipurpose exposure information systems: a new job-exposure matrix. Am J Ind Med 33:409–17.
24. Niedhammer I, Chastang JF, Levy D, David S, Degioanni S, et al. (2008) Study of the validity of a job-exposure matrix for psychosocial work factors: results

from the national French SUMER survey. Int Arch Occup Environ Health 82:87–97.

25. Wieclaw J, Agerbo E, Mortensen PB, Burr H, Tuchsen F, et al. (2008) Psychosocial working conditions and the risk of depression and anxiety disorders in the Danish workforce. BMC Public Health 8:280.
26. Rijs KJ, van der Pas S, Geuskens GA, Cozijnsen R, Koppes LL, et al. (2013) Development and Validation of a Physical and Psychosocial Job-Exposure Matrix in Older and Retired Workers. Ann Occup Hyg 2013 Dec 11. [Epub ahead of print], doi:10.1093/annhyg/met052.
27. Theorell T, Tsutsumi A, Hallquist J, Reuterwall C, Hogstedt C, et al. (1998) Decision latitude, job strain, and myocardial infarction: a study of working men in Stockholm. The SHEEP Study Group. Stockholm Heart epidemiology Program. Am J Public Health 88:382–8.
28. Cohidon C, Santin G, Chastang JF, Imbernon E, Niedhammer I (2012) Psychosocial exposures at work and mental health: potential utility of a job-exposure matrix. Occup Environ Med 54:184–91.
29. Aromaa A, Koskinen S (2004) Population and methods. Health and functional capacity in Finland. In: Aromaa A. and Koskinen S, editors. Baseline result of the Health 2000 Helath Examination Survey. Helsinki: The National Public Health Institute pp. 11–23.
30. Laiho J, Djerf K, Lehtonen R (2006) Sampling design. In: Heistaro S, editor. Methodology report Health 2000 Survey. Helsinki: the National Public Health Institute B26: 13–5.
31. Perkiö-Mäkelä M, Hirvonen M, Elo A-L, Kauppinen K, Kauppinen T, et al. (2010) Työ ja terveys -haastattelututkimus. 2009; Helsinki: Työterveyslaitos (in Finnish).
32. Karasek R, Brisson C, Kawakami N, Houtman I, Bongers P, et al. (1998) The Job Content Questionnaire (JCQ): an instrument for internationally comparative assessments of psychosocial job characteristics. J Occup Health Psychol 3:322–55.
33. Le Moual N, Bakke P, Orlowski E, Heederik D, Kromhout H, et al. (2000) Performance of population specific job exposure matrices (JEMs): European collaborative analyses on occupational risk factors for chronic obstructive pulmonary disease with job exposure matrices (ECOJEM). Occup Environ Med 57:126–32.
34. Solovieva S, Pehkonen I, Kausto J, Miranda H, Shiri R, et al. (2012) Development and validation of a job exposure matrix for physical risk factors in low back pain. PLoS One 7(11):e48680.
35. Bonde JP (2008) Psychosocial factors at work and risk of depression: a systematic review of the epidemiological evidence. Occup Environ Medicine 65:438–45.
36. Netterstrom B, Conrad N, Bech P, Fink P, Olsen O, et al. (2008) The relation between work-related psychosocial factors and the development of depression. Epidemiologic reviews 30:118–32.
37. Niedhammer I, Sultan-Taïeb H, Chastang JF, Vermeylen G, Parent-Thirion A (2013). Fractions of cardiovascular diseases and mental disorders attributable to psychosocial work factors in 31 countries in Europe. Int Arch Occup Environ Health 2013 Apr 27. [Epub ahead of print], doi 10.1007/s00420-013-0879-4
38. Hartvigsen J, Lings S, Leboeuf-Yde C, Bakketeig L (2004). Psychosocial factors at work in relation to low back pain and consequences of low back pain; a systematic, critical review of prospective cohort studies. Occup Environ Med 61:e2.
39. Macfarlane GJ, Pallewatte N, Paudyal P, Blyth FM, Coggon D, et al. (2009) Evaluation of work-related psychosocial factors and regional musculoskeletal pain: results from a EULAR Task Force. Ann Rheum Dis 68:885–91.
40. Bouyer J, Hémon D (1993) Studying the performance of a job exposure matrix. Int J Epidemiol 22 (Suppl 2):S65–71.
41. Joseph L, Gyorkos TW, Coupal L (1995) Bayesian estimation of disease prevalence and the parameters of diagnostic tests in the absence of a gold standard. Am J Epidemiol 141:263–72.
42. Abramson JH (2011) WINPEPI updated: computer programs for epidemiologists, and their teaching potential. Epidemiol Perspect Innov 8:1.
43. Cifuentes M, Boyer J, Gore R, d'Errico A, Tessler J, et al. (2007) Inter-method agreement between O*NET and survey measures of psychosocial exposure among healthcare industry employees. Am J Ind Med 50:545–53.
44. Ostry AS, Marion SA, Demers PA, Hershler R, Kelly S, et al. (2001) Measuring psychosocial job strain with the job content questionnaire using experienced job evaluators. Am J Ind Med 39:397–401.

18

Relative Deprivation, Poverty, and Subjective Health

Masashige Saito[1]*, Katsunori Kondo[2], Naoki Kondo[3], Aya Abe[4], Toshiyuki Ojima[5], Kayo Suzuki[6] and the JAGES group[¶]

1 Department of Social Welfare, Nihon Fukushi University, Aichi, Japan, **2** Center for Preventive Medical Science, Chiba University, Chiba, Japan, **3** Department of Health Economics and Epidemiology Research, The University of Tokyo, Tokyo, Japan, **4** Department of Empirical Social Security Research, National Institute of Population and Social Security Research, Tokyo, Japan, **5** Department of Community Health and Preventive Medicine, Hamamatsu University School of Medicine, Shizuoka, Japan, **6** Department of Social Studies, Aichi Gakuin University, Aichi, Japan

Abstract

To evaluate the association between relative deprivation (lacking daily necessities) and subjective health in older Japanese adults, we performed a cross-sectional analysis using data from the Japan Gerontological Evaluation Study (JAGES). The data were obtained from functionally independent residents aged ≥65 years from 24 municipalities in Japan (n = 24,742). Thirteen items in three dimensions were used to evaluate relative deprivation of material conditions. Approximately 28% of older Japanese people indicated that they lacked some daily necessities (non-monetary poverty). A two-level Poisson regression analysis revealed that relative deprivation was associated with poor self-rated health (PR = 1.3–1.5) and depressive symptoms (PR = 1.5–1.8) in both men and women, and these relationships were stronger than those observed in people living in relative poverty (monetary poverty). The interaction effect between relative deprivation and relative poverty was not associated with poor health. As a dimension of the social determinants of health, poverty should be evaluated from a multidimensional approach, capturing not only monetary conditions but also material-based, non-monetary conditions.

Editor: Takeru Abe, Waseda University, Japan

Funding: This study was supported in part by Grant-in-Aid for Scientific Research (KAKENHI 26285138 and 23243070) from the Japan Society for the Promotion of Science, and Health Labour Sciences Research Grant, Comprehensive Research on Aging and Health (H25-Choju-ippan-003) from the Japanese Ministry of Health, Labour and Welfare. This survey data was supported by MEXT Supported Program for the Strategic Research Foundation at Private Universities 2009–2013, Health Labour Sciences Research Grant, Comprehensive Research on Aging and Health (H22-Choju-shitei-008), JSPS KA-KENHI Grant Number 22330172, 22119506, 22390400, 22592327, 22700694, 23590786, 23700819 & 23243070, and Japan Foundation for Aging and Health. The funders had no role in study design, data collection and analysis, decision to publish, or preparation of the manuscript.

Competing Interests: The authors have declared that no competing interests exist.

* Email: masa-s@n-fukushi.ac.jp

¶ Membership of the JAGES project is provided in the Acknowledgments.

Introduction

The association between poverty and health has been established. A number of studies have revealed that relative income poverty is significantly related to poor health [1–3]. However, this approach has limitations when attempting to capture the diverse and complex aspects of poverty. In reality, older people tend to have comparatively high-quality living conditions due to savings and property ownership, even if their income is low [4]. To overcome this limitation, poverty research has proposed the concept of relative deprivation in material conditions to reflect the multidimensional non-monetary aspects of poverty [5–15]. Townsend [5] developed 60 relative deprivation indices within 12 dimensions composed of items such as "Household does not have a refrigerator" and "Has not had a week's holiday away from home in the last 12 months," and found that poverty in the United Kingdom was more extensive than generally believed or officially reported. The Europe 2020 strategy has adopted the concept of relative deprivation as a material dimension of social exclusion and has set the elimination of severe material deprivation as a goal for the next decade [16].

In investigating relationships between poverty and health, some studies have applied a social indicator approach, such as the Carstairs deprivation score or Townsend deprivation index, to include unemployment rate or proportion of non-car ownership. These previous studies found that relatively deprived areas were associated with standardized mortality rates [17–20], cancer mortality rates [21], suicide rates [22], coronary heart disease [23], dental caries [24], number of sound teeth remaining [25], and depression symptoms [26]. However, there have been few studies analyzing the relationship between an individual's relative deprivation and his or her health. Some studies have shown an association between deprivation in living conditions and poor health [14], low levels of satisfaction with life [27], and poor social support [28]. Furthermore, no studies investigating the different associations between relative deprivation, relative poverty, and health have been conducted, although it has been suggested that people who live in relative deprivation have different character-

Table 1. Distribution of control variable.

Variable	Category	Total	Men	Women
Individual (n = 24,742)				
Sex	men	45.9	-	-
	women	54.1	-	-
Age	65–69	25.4	26.9	24.0
	70–74	29.1	29.5	28.7
	75–79	23.3	23.2	23.4
	80–84	14.1	13.5	14.7
	85 -	8.1	6.8	9.2
Education	>9	47.6	51.8	44.1
	=<9	49.9	46.5	52.9
	unknown	2.4	1.7	3.0
Marital status	married	69.0	84.0	56.0
	divorced	22.6	8.6	34.5
	separated	3.2	2.6	3.8
	never married	2.1	1.9	2.3
	unknown	3.1	2.9	3.4
Disease and/or impairment	no	22.4	24.1	20.8
	yes	68.5	67.6	69.3
	unknown	9.1	8.3	9.9
Self recognition of forgetfulness	no	79.3	79.5	79.1
	yes	16.8	16.5	17.1
	unknown	3.9	4.1	3.8
Social supports	present	85.6	84.4	86.7
	absent	8.1	9.9	6.5
	unknown	6.3	5.7	6.8
Municipality (n = 24)				
Proportion of older people	mean (SD)	24.4 (5.2)	-	-
Population density [1000 p/km^2]	mean (SD)	1.70 (1.36)	-	-
Proportion of person receiving public assistance[‰]	mean (SD)	8.5 (10.7)	-	-

istics than those living in relative poverty [9,13,15]. In order to clarify the relationships between poverty and health, it is important to identify the aspects of poverty that are the strongest predictors of health.

In addition, there have been few studies focusing on relative deprivation among older adults [8,15]. Previous studies comparing younger and older people found that both the prevalence and depth of deprivation were more severe in younger people or single parents of working age [4,13,29]. However, from a life course perspective, the impact of relative deprivation on health should be evidenced in older people because the influence of poverty on health may accumulate over time. Finally, with the exception of a study that analyzed 131,335 people in 11 countries [10], most of the previous related research has been conducted on a relatively small scale. Analysis of relative deprivation should be performed with a large sample in order to derive robust findings, as few cases fall into each of the deprivation indices.

The present study posed three research questions: (1) is relative deprivation associated with poor health, even after monetary poverty is controlled for; (2) is the interaction effect between relative deprivation and relative poverty significantly associated with poor health, and (3) do older people with social support have good health, even if they are relatively deprived? In social psychology and sociology, the concept of relative deprivation has also been used to measure psychosomatic stress related to complaints or dissatisfaction based on comparisons with their reference groups [30–38]. However, our focus on relative deprivation is based on Townsend's definition used in the poverty and social policy research described above.

Methods

Study samples

We used data from the Japan Gerontological Evaluation Study (JAGES), which was cross-sectional in design. JAGES was a postal survey of 112,123 people aged ≥65 who were randomly selected from the older residents of 31 municipalities in Japan. Data were collected from August 2010 to January 2012, with a response rate of 66.3%. For our study, we included 24,742 respondents from 24 municipalities who answered a relative deprivation questionnaire. The average age of the respondents was 74.6 years [standard

Table 2. Distribution of relative deprivation index.

Dimension	Item	Category	n	%	Crude odds ratio (95% CI) self-rated health (1 = fair/poor)	depressive symptom (1 = present)
Lack of daily necessities due to economic reasons	no television	no	23,594	97.6	1.00	1.00
		yes (+)	592	2.4	1.47 (1.22–1.77)	2.25 (1.87–2.72)
	no refrigerator	no	23,781	98.3	1.00	1.00
		yes (+)	405	1.7	1.32 (1.05–1.66)	1.67 (1.32–2.11)
	no air conditioner	no	22,823	94.4	1.00	1.00
		yes (+)	1,363	5.6	1.62 (1.44–1.83)	2.23 (1.97–2.52)
	no microwave oven	no	23,315	96.4	1.00	1.00
		yes (+)	871	3.6	1.62 (1.40–1.88)	1.88 (1.61–2.19)
	no water heater	no	23,213	96.0	1.00	1.00
		yes (+)	973	4.0	1.63 (1.41–1.87)	2.14 (1.85–2.48)
Lack in living environment	private WC	yes	22,606	93.5	1.00	1.00
		no (+)	1,580	6.5	1.40 (1.24–1.57)	1.78 (1.58–2.01)
	private kitchen	yes	22,260	92.0	1.00	1.00
		no (+)	1,926	8.0	1.43 (1.29–1.59)	1.79 (1.60–2.00)
	private bathroom	yes	22,153	91.6	1.00	1.00
		no (+)	2,033	8.4	1.40 (1.27–1.56)	1.83 (1.64–2.04)
	dining room separated from bedroom	yes	20,585	85.1	1.00	1.00
		no (+)	3,601	14.9	1.48 (1.37–1.61)	1.81 (1.67–1.97)
Lack of social life due to economic reasons	no telephone	no	23,229	96.0	1.00	1.00
		yes (+)	957	4.0	1.52 (1.32–1.76)	2.25 (1.94–2.60)
	no ceremonial dress	no	23,644	97.8	1.00	1.00
		yes (+)	542	2.2	1.53 (1.27–1.85)	1.92 (1.58–2.34)
	absence from relative's ceremonial occasions	no	21,952	93.4	1.00	1.00
		yes (+)	1,549	6.6	2.47 (2.22–2.76)	3.27 (2.91–3.67)
	cut-off of essential services in the past year	no	23,509	98.4	1.00	1.00
		yes (+)	388	1.6	2.09 (1.70–2.59)	4.10 (3.27–5.14)
Number of relative deprivation index		none	16,812	72.0	1.00	1.00
		1	3349	14.3	1.61 (1.48–1.75)	1.93 (1.77–2.10)
		2	916	3.9	2.01 (1.74–2.32)	2.68 (2.31–3.12)
		3	480	2.1	2.04 (1.67–2.48)	2.89 (2.36–3.52)
		4	1109	4.8	1.61 (1.40–1.85)	2.04 (1.77–2.36)
		5	271	1.2	2.30 (1.77–2.98)	3.49 (2.66–4.58)
		>=6	401	1.7	1.75 (1.40–2.19)	2.92 (2.33–3.67)
		>=2	3177	13.6	1.86 (1.70–2.02)	2.57 (2.35–2.81)

(+) is related to relative deprivation.

deviation (SD) = 6.4] and 54.1% were women. Our study protocol and questionnaire procedures were approved by the Ethics Committee in Research of Human Subjects at Nihon Fukushi University. Written informed consent was assumed with voluntary return of the questionnaire.

Dependent variables

We used self-rated health and depressive symptoms as indicators of subjective health. Self-rated health and depressive symptoms have been found to be highly valid predictors of mortality, regardless of other medical, behavioral, or psychosocial factors [39,40]. Self-rated health was measured using the question "How do you feel about your current health status: excellent, good, fair, or poor?" Responses were recoded into dichotomous response variables (excellent/good or fair/poor). Depressive symptoms were assessed using the short version of the Geriatric Depression Scale (GDS-15), which was developed for self-administration in the community using a simple yes/no format [41,42]. The validity and

Table 3. Combination of relative deprivation and poverty.

		Self-rated health		Depressive symptom	
	n (%)	fair/poor %	Crude OR (95%CI)	present %	Crude OR (95%CI)
No deprivation or poverty	10,241 (53.7)	16.9	1.00	21.0	1.00
Poverty only	3,987 (20.9)	23.3	1.50 (1.37–1.64)	29.0	1.54 (1.41–1.68)
Deprivation only (= 1)	1,334 (7.0)	23.1	1.48 (1.29–1.70)	32.1	1.78 (1.56–2.03)
Deprivation only (>= 2)	893 (4.7)	25.4	1.68 (1.43–1.97)	36.4	2.16 (1.85–2.52)
Poverty and deprivation (= 1)	1,305 (6.8)	31.4	2.26 (1.98–2.57)	43.2	2.86 (2.51–3.26)
Poverty and deprivation (>= 2)	1,300 (6.8)	33.8	2.51 (2.21–2.86)	48.4	3.53 (3.10–4.02)

reliability of this scale have also been confirmed for Japanese older people, and it is often used in Japanese surveys [43,44]. According to Sheikh et al. [42], scores of ≥5 on the GDS-15 indicated the presence of depressive symptoms of mild to severe depression. Our data showed approximately 30% of respondents had depressive symptoms. It is consistent with preceding Japanese studies [43,44].

Independent variables: relative deprivation and relative poverty

The indicators of relative deprivation used in preceding studies differ, because the standard living condition or decent life varies by culture and times. In reference to preceding research including Japanese studies [5–8,10–12,14], we evaluated thirteen indices that equated "lack of daily necessities," "lack of living environment," and "lack of social life due to economic reasons" with a low standard of living. Although lack of access to medical and health care services is another important element of standard of living, this was excluded from our deprivation indices because we assumed it to be directly reflected in poor health. On the other hand, we included experience of cutoff of essential services as a typical condition of lacking decent life, which is also used as a measure of social exclusion in a Japanese study [45].

Indicators of "lack of daily necessities" included having no television, refrigerator, air conditioner, microwave oven, or water heater. "Lack of living environment" indicators included having no private toilet, kitchen, or bathroom in the house and having a dining room that was not separate from the bedroom. "Lack of social life due to economic reasons" indicators included having no telephone or formal dress, being absent from family celebrations and events during the previous year due to economic reasons, and having essential services such as water, electricity or gas, cut off in the previous year (except in cases of forgetting to make a payment).

Relative poverty was defined as an income of less than half of the median annual equivalent income in the National Survey of Family Income and Expenditure in Japan [46]; the threshold was 1.49 million Japanese yen. This is the definition of relative poverty accepted by the Organisation for Economic Co-operation and Development and is conceptually based on the relative approach of the Luxembourg Income Study [47]. We used annual pre-tax household income. For each response, we calculated the equivalent household income by dividing income by the square root of the number of household members. Responses were categorized into three groups: poverty (28.2%), non-poverty (51.7%), and unknown (20.1%).

Covariates

We used several control variables at the individual level: sex, age, educational attainment (to represent ascribed and achieved statuses), medical treatment (to represent recent physical condition), self-recognition of forgetfulness (to represent prodrome of dementia), and social support (to represent a buffer between poverty and health). Medical treatment was determined by asking "Are you currently receiving any medical treatment?" Self-recognition of forgetfulness was measured by asking "Do people around you notice your forgetfulness, for example, by telling you that you often ask the same thing?" Social support was measured using two questions representing emotional and institutional support: "Do you have someone who listens to your concerns and complaints?" and "Do you have someone who looks after you when you are sick and have to stay in bed for a few days?" Responses of "no" or "nobody" to both questions indicated an absence of social support.

In our data set, individuals were nested within each municipality. Previous studies reported significant associations between individual health and regional characteristics such as social capital and income inequality [48,49]. We used the proportion of older people residing in the area (%), population density in inhabitable areas (1,000 person/km2), and the proportion of persons receiving public assistance (‰) for characteristics at the municipal level. These variables were based on 2010 census and government data for Japan. The distribution of these variables is shown is Table 1.

Statistical analysis

First, we confirmed the distribution of the relative deprivation index and calculated crude odds ratios for subjective health. Second, we applied two-level Poisson regression analysis of random-intercept and fixed-slope models to assess the relationship between relative deprivation and self-rated health and depressive symptoms, adjusting for individual factors and municipal-level covariates (level 1: 24,742 individuals, level 2: 24 municipalities). We adopted multilevel modeling in order to control for intraclass (municipal level) cluster correlation. We also examined the interaction effect of relative deprivation and relative poverty. Individual and municipality fixed parameters were converted to prevalence ratios (PR) with a 95% confidence interval (95%CI).

Table 4. Association of subjective health and relative deprivation by two-level Poisson regression analysis[a)].

	Self-rated health (fair/poor)				Depressive symptom (present)			
	Men		**Women**		**Men**		**Women**	
	PR	**(95%CI)**	*PR*	**(95%CI)**	*PR*	**(95%CI)**	*PR*	**(95%CI)**
FIXED EFFECTS								
Individual level								
Age (ref.: 65–69)								
70–74	1.06	(0.94–1.19)	1.09	(0.97–1.23)	0.92	(0.83–1.02)	1.00	(0.90–1.11)
75–79	1.24***	(1.11–1.40)	1.29***	(1.15–1.46)	1.03	(0.93–1.15)	0.98	(0.88–1.10)
80–84	1.31***	(1.15–1.49)	1.49***	(1.31–1.70)	0.95	(0.84–1.08)	1.02	(0.90–1.15)
85 -	1.23*	(1.05–1.45)	1.54***	(1.33–1.79)	0.95	(0.81–1.13)	1.15*	(1.00–1.33)
Education (ref.: >9 years)								
=<9 years	1.07	(0.98–1.16)	1.19***	(1.09–1.29)	1.16***	(1.07–1.25)	1.09*	(1.01–1.18)
Marital status (ref.: married)								
divorced	0.99	(0.86–1.13)	0.83***	(0.76–0.90)	1.23**	(1.09–1.39)	1.03	(0.95–1.12)
separated	1.22	(0.99–1.51)	0.91	(0.75–1.10)	1.37**	(1.14–1.65)	1.10	(0.92–1.31)
never married	1.17	(0.90–1.53)	0.92	(0.72–1.19)	1.29*	(1.03–1.62)	0.98	(0.77–1.26)
Disease and/or impairment (ref.: no)								
yes	4.76***	(4.05–5.60)	3.90***	(3.34–4.56)	1.33***	(1.21–1.46)	1.28***	(1.16–1.41)
Self recognition of forgetfulness (ref.: no)								
yes	1.47***	(1.34–1.61)	1.65***	(1.52–1.79)	1.71***	(1.57–1.86)	1.83***	(1.69–1.98)
Social supports (ref.: present)								
absent	1.37***	(1.21–1.54)	1.58***	(1.39–1.79)	1.57***	(1.41–1.75)	1.84***	(1.64–2.07)
Relative poverty (ref.: non-poverty)								
poverty (< ¥ 1.49 million)	1.25***	(1.11–1.40)	1.13*	(1.01–1.26)	1.34***	(1.20–1.50)	1.24***	(1.11–1.37)
Relative deprivation score (ref.: none)								
1	1.19*	(1.03–1.37)	1.31***	(1.15–1.50)	1.45***	(1.27–1.65)	1.36***	(1.19–1.55)
>=2	1.34***	(1.16–1.54)	1.27**	(1.10–1.46)	1.62***	(1.42–1.85)	1.43***	(1.25–1.64)
Interaction Effect								
poverty×deprivation (1)	1.08	(0.87–1.34)	0.95	(0.78–1.17)	1.03	(0.84–1.26)	1.00	(0.82–1.22)
poverty×deprivation (>=2)	1.01	(0.82–1.25)	1.06	(0.86–1.31)	0.94	(0.77–1.14)	1.01	(0.82–1.23)
Municipal level								
Proportion of older people [1%]	1.00	(0.99–1.01)	0.99	(0.98–1.00)	1.01*	(1.00–1.02)	1.02**	(1.01–1.03)
Population density [1000 p/km^2]	0.96**	(0.94–0.99)	0.94***	(0.92–0.97)	1.03*	(1.00–1.06)	1.01	(0.99–1.04)
Prop. of receiving public assistance [5‰]	1.03*	(1.00–1.06)	1.04**	(1.01–1.07)	0.96**	(0.93–0.99)	0.95**	(0.93–0.98)

Table 4. Cont.

	Self-rated health (fair/poor)				Depressive symptom (present)			
	Men		Women		Men		Women	
	PR	(95%CI)	*PR*	(95%CI)	*PR*	(95%CI)	*PR*	(95%CI)
RANDOM EFFECTS[b]								
Municipality level variance (standard error)	.039 (.050)		.046 (.042)		.045 (.031)		.035 (.031)	

***$p<.001$ **$p<.01$ *$p<.05$ PR: Prevalence ratio.
[a]Each estimated coefficient of "unknown" category was omitted in above table.
[b]Random effect in null model:
SRH(men) = .147(SE = .034), SRH(women) = .197(SE = .037), GDS(men) = .093(SE = .027), GDS(women) = .101(SE = .026).

Finally, we calculated the proportion of poor health among deprived people with social support. We used the computer software, STATA 12.1 for all analyses.

Results

Table 2 showed that 1.6% to 8.4% of respondents lived in deprived conditions, as defined by the study parameters. A higher percentage of respondents did not have a dining room separate from the bedroom (14.9%). Univariate analysis showed that ORs for respondents living in deprived conditions, according to each relative deprivation index, were approximately 1.3–2.5 times higher for fair/poor self-rated health and 1.7–4.1 times higher for depressive symptoms than respondents who did not live in relative deprivation. In particular, the crude ORs for having essential services cut off and absence from family celebrations and events were relatively high. Relative deprivation scores also showed that respondents who were deprived of one item (14.3%) and two or more items (13.6%) were more likely to report fair/poor self-rated health [OR = 1.61 (95%CI: 1.48–1.75) and OR = 1.86 (95%CI: 1.70–2.02), respectively] and depressive symptoms [OR = 1.93 (95%CI: 1.77–2.10) and OR = 2.57 (95%CI: 2.35–2.81), respectively].

Table 3 shows the associations between subjective health and a combination of relative deprivation and relative poverty. The proportion of respondents with poor health was high with respect to "poverty and deprivation," "deprivation only," "poverty only," and "no deprivation or poverty." Odds ratios for respondents living in poverty and deprivation (two or more deprivation items) were 2.51 (95%CI: 2.21–2.86) and 3.53 (95%CI: 3.10–4.02) times higher for fair/poor self-rated health and depressive symptoms, respectively, than ORs for respondents with no deprivation or poverty.

Table 4 shows the results of a two-level Poisson regression analysis. Random effects showed that municipal-level variance in each model was smaller than that in the null model. This means that part of the municipal-level variance was explained by the individual- and municipal-level variables in the model. Fixed effects showed similar associations for both genders. Respondents with low educational attainment, no social support, under medical treatment, and prodrome of dementia tended to have poor subjective health, although relationships between age and municipal level variables were not consistent.

Relative deprivation was significantly associated with poor health, regardless of the status of relative poverty and other individual- and municipal-level characteristics. In male respondents with two or more deprivation items, rates of fair/poor self-rated health were 1.34 times (95%CI: 1.16–1.54) higher and rates of depressive symptoms were 1.62 times (95%CI: 1.42–1.85) higher than those observed in non-deprived individuals. Similarly, relative deprivation was associated with fair/poor self-rated health [PR = 1.27 (95%CI: 1.10–1.46)] and depressive symptoms [PR = 1.43 (95%CI: 1.25–1.64)] in women. Relative poverty was also related to self-rated health [men: PR = 1.25 (95%CI: 1.11–1.40); women: PR = 1.13 (95%CI: 1.01–1.26)] and depressive symptoms [men: PR = 1.34 (95%CI: 1.20–1.50); women: PR = 1.24 (95%CI: 1.11–1.37)]. The PRs for relative deprivation were comparatively higher than those for relative poverty. The interaction effect between relative poverty and relative deprivation for subjective health was not statistically significant.

Figure 1 shows different associations between subjective health and relative deprivation according to social support. The proportion of respondents with poor health was remarkably lower in those with social support relative to those without. However,

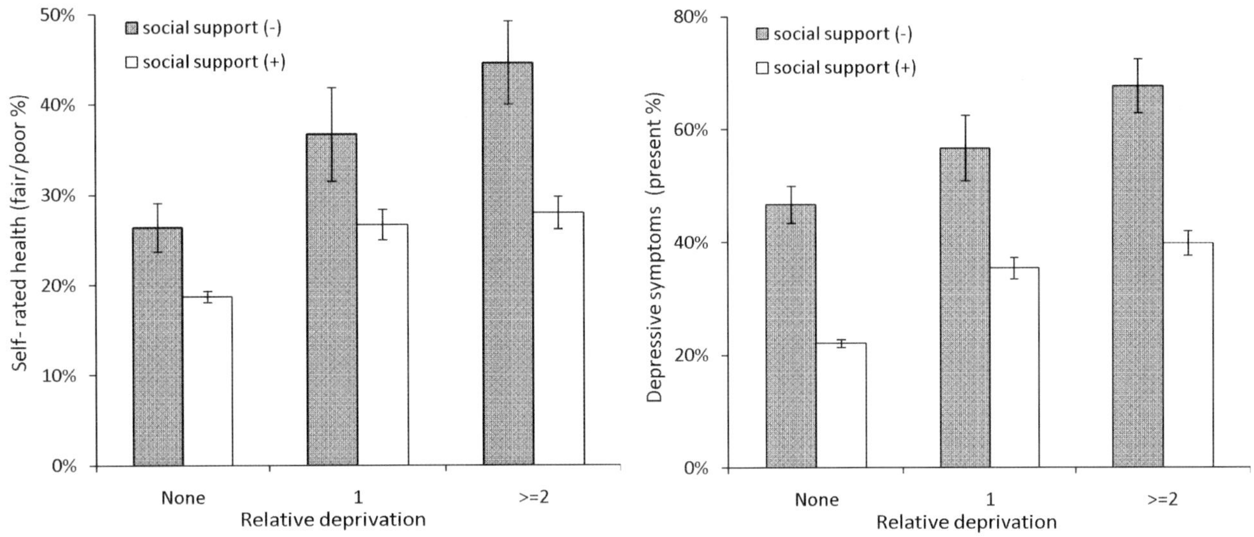

Figure 1. Proportion (95% Confidence Interval) of poor health in relation to relative deprivation and social support. Both figures show a low proportion of poor health in the presence of social support. Meanwhile, the proportion of those with poor health increases as the relative deprivation index score increases even with social support, indicating that social support does not fully cancel out the negative impacts of relative deprivation on health.

relative to non-deprived respondents with any level of social support, the proportions of respondents with poor/fair subjective health were remarkably higher in the relative deprivation groups (1 and $\leq$2, respectively).

Discussion

It was previously thought that all Japanese people were middle class. However, recent surveys have shown that intergenerational inequality exists in Japan [50], and the number of older people on public assistance is increasing [51]. The World Health Organization stated that poverty and relative deprivation have a major impact on health and premature death [52]. On the other hand, most poverty research has been based solely on the concept of relative poverty (monetary poverty) since data on material and environmental poverty was severely limited in Japan.

The present study addressed the concepts of both relative poverty and relative deprivation through a large survey of older Japanese and analyzed the association between health and relative poverty and deprivation. Our results showed that relative deprivation and relative poverty were related to poor health, even after other variables were controlled for. Our results were consistent with preceding findings; Abe [14] found that relative deprivation is closely associated with poor self-rated health and the presence of depressive symptoms using national Japanese representative cross-sectional data of participants aged $\geq$20 years. In particular, our results suggest that the concept of relative deprivation could address a different aspect of poverty that is related to health but is not addressed by the concept of relative poverty. People who have overlapping multidimensional disadvantages are more likely to be socially excluded [9] and to experience premature death [53]. Our results also showed that the negative effects of relative poverty and deprivation on health are additive; people with both relative deprivation and poverty were more disadvantaged with respect to health, but the relationship was not multiplicative.

Our study adds new evidence regarding which elements of poverty have strong impacts on the health of older adults. An important finding is that relative deprivation has a stronger association with subjective health than relative poverty for both sexes. Some studies have revealed that people living in relatively deprived conditions experienced long-term, severe poverty throughout their life course [10,11]. For example, Whelan et al. [10] reported that approximately 40% of persistent income poverty overlapped with lifestyle deprivation in a broadly uniform manner. Consequently, the concept of relative deprivation could capture severe and absolute poverty better than relative poverty, which is based on the distribution of income in society. This could mean that relatively deprived older people might tend to be more disadvantaged, even in good health.

Finally, similar to a preceding study using cross-sectional data from 5,624 women aged 2059 [28], our data confirmed that relative deprivation was associated with the absence of social support [15]. Moreover, our results showed that having social support of any form could mitigate some of the negative impacts of relative deprivation on health. However, it is important to note that even with social support, relatively deprived people have more disadvantages with respect to health than non-deprived people. Therefore, the effects of material and environmental deprivation on poor health cannot be explained only by the absence of social support. As shown in preceding study [30–38], relative deprivation might increase social stresses and anxieties while lowering self-efficacy by depriving a living standard most people in the society enjoy. Furthermore, unlike monetary poverty, poor standard of living such as relative deprivation might closely be related to unhealthy lifestyles including poor eating habit and nutrition and lack of access to healthcare and welfare services.

Compared to relative poverty, which is based on a simple indicator and is often used in international comparative studies, relative deprivation is composed of complex indicators and has limitations for use in comparative studies. In fact, most preceding studies have applied a consensual approach based on public opinion in creating and selecting daily necessities and basic needs indices [4,6,7,10,12–14]. As a result, each relative deprivation indicator was different among preceding studies, although they often reflected the characteristics of that nation and culture.

However, relative deprivation could more accurately represent the phenomenon of poverty due to multidimensional living conditions than it does relative poverty. Although measurements of relative deprivation have been made in order to establish the poverty line, our results suggest that relative deprivation is also important for public health policy as it represents a dimension of the social determinants of health.

Study limitations

The present study has some limitations. First, our relative deprivation indicators did not cover the full range of daily resources among older people in Japan. Although we included indicators used in preceding studies, the indicators should be more sophisticated. Second, while the overall response rate for our data was relatively high, the response rates among the lower income categories were comparatively lower [54]. Therefore, our findings may be underestimated because people living in serious poverty and deprivation may have been less likely to participate in our survey. Third, there is a possibility of selection bias at the municipal level since our data are not representative of the whole country. On the other hand, our subjects were randomly selected in each municipality, and it is important to note that we did perform a large-scale survey concerning non-monetary poverty among older people in more than one municipality. Further research should include longitudinal surveys to reveal whether a causal relationship between relative deprivation and health exits.

Conclusion

Relative deprivation (non-monetary poverty) is an important element in poverty. To the best of our knowledge, this is the first study to investigate the association between health conditions and relative deprivation and poverty among older Asian adults. The results showed that relative deprivation has stronger associations with self-rated health and depressive symptoms than with relative poverty. There was an independent and additive association between relative deprivation and poverty with respect to subjective health, and the presence of social support may not fully mitigate the negative association between relative deprivation and health. Our results suggest that relative deprivation is one social determinant of health that the concept of relative poverty cannot address.

Acknowledgments

The JAGES project (2014) comprises a coordinating group and collaborating investigators in each of the following field centers: Prof. K. Kondo (lead investigator; BZH12275@nifty.ne.jp), Dr H. Hikichi, Mr Y. Miyaguni, Dr Y. Sasaki, Dr Y Nagamine, Dr M. Hanazato, Chiba University; Dr N. Kondo, Dr T. Ashida, Dr D. Takagi, Dr Y. Tani, Tokyo University; Prof. T. Ojima, Dr E. Okada, Hamamatsu University School of Medicine; Prof. K. Osaka, Dr J. Aida, Dr T. Tuboya, Tohoku University; Dr M. Saito, Nihon Fukushi University; Dr H. Hirai, Iwate University; Dr Y. Shobugawa, Niigata university; Dr K. Suzuki, Aichi Gakuin University; Dr Y. Ichida, Doctoral Institute for Evidence Based Policy; Dr T. Yamamoto, Kanagawa Dental University; Prof. C. Murata, Dr T. Saito, Dr S. Jeong, National Institute for Longevity Sciences; Dr M. Nakade, Tokai Gakuen University; Prof. T Takeda, Seijo University; Prof. N Cable, University College London; Prof. H. Todoroki, Dr K Shirai, University of the Ryukyuus; Mr T Hayashi, Tokai College of Medical Science. Dr A. Tamakoshi, Hokkaido University; Dr J Misawa, Rikkyo University; Dr Y Fujino, University of Occupational and Environmental Health.

Author Contributions

Conceived and designed the experiments: MS NK KK. Performed the experiments: KK the JAGES group. Analyzed the data: MS. Contributed to the writing of the manuscript: MS KK NK AA TO KS.

References

1. Lynch J, Kaplan G (2000) Socioeconomic position. In: Berkman LF, Kawachi I, editors. *Social epidemiology*. New York: Oxford University Press, 13–35.
2. Claussen B, Davey Smith G, Thelle D (2003) Impact of childhood and adulthood socio-economic position on cause specific mortality: the Oslo Mortality Study. Journal of Epidemiology and Community Health, 2003, 57: 40–45.
3. Shaw M, Dorling D, Davey Smith G (2006) Poverty, social exclusion, and minorities. In: Marmot M, Wilkinson R, editors. *Social determinants of health; second edition*. New York: Oxford university press, 196–223.
4. Abe A (2006) Empirical analysis of relative deprivation in Japan using Japanese micro-data. The Journal of Social Policy and Labor Studies (Shakai-seisaku Gakkai Shi). 16: 251–275 (in Japanese with English abstract).
5. Townsend P (1979) *Poverty in the United Kingdom; a survey of household resources and standards of living*. Harmondsworth: Penguin Books.
6. Mack J, Lansley S (1985) *Poor Britain. London*, George Allen and Unwin.
7. Gordon D, Adelman L, Ashworth K, Bradshaw J, Levitas R, et al. (2000) *Poverty and social exclusion in Britain*. Rowntree Foundation.
8. Hiraoka K (2002) *Social inequalities among elderly people in Japan*. Tokyo: University of Tokyo Press. (in Japanese).
9. Bradshaw J, Finch N (2003) Overlaps in dimensions of poverty. Journal of Social Policy, 32(4): 513–525.
10. Whelan CT, Layte R, Maitre B (2003) Persistent income poverty and deprivation in the European Union; an analysis of first three waves of the European Community Household Panel. International Social Policy, 32(1): 1–18.
11. Iwata M, Hamamoto C (2004) Experience of poverty in deflationary depression. In: Higuchi Y, Ota K, the institute for research on household economics, editors. *Women in Heisei depression (Jyosei tachi no Heisei fukyo)*. Nikkei INC, 203–233. (in Japanese).
12. Saunders P (2008) Measuring well-being using non-monetary indicators; deprivation and social exclusion. Family Matters, 78: 8–17.
13. Saunders P, Abe A (2010) Poverty and deprivation in young and old: a comparative study of Australia and Japan. Poverty & Public Policy, 2(1): 67–97.
14. Abe A (2014). Constructing a deprivation scale for Japan; an index to supplement the relative poverty rate. the Quarterly of Social Security Research. 49(4): 360–371. (in Japanese).
15. Saito M, Kondo K, Kondo N, Ojima T, Suzuki K, et al. (2014) Prevalence and characteristics of relative deprivation among older people; from cross-sectional data in JAGES project. the Quarterly of Social Security Research. 50(3): in press. (in Japanese).
16. European Commission (2011) *The social dimension of the Europe 2020 strategy; A report of the social protection committee*. Directorate-General for Employment, Social Affairs and Inclusion.
17. Eames M, Ben-Shlomo Y, Marmot MG (1993) Social deprivation and premature mortality: regional comparison across England. British Medical Journal, 307(6912), 1097–1102.
18. Mac Loon P, Boddy FA (1994) Deprivation and mortality in Scotland, 1981 and 1991. British Medical Journal, 309(6967): 1465–1470.
19. Langford IH, Bentham G (1996) Regional variations in mortality rates in England and Wales: an analysis using multilevel modeling. Social Science & Medicine, 42(6): 897–908.
20. O'Reilly D (2002) Standard indicators of deprivation; Do they disadvantage older people? Age and Ageing, 31(3): 197–202.
21. Nakaya T (2011) Evaluation socio-economic inequalities in cancer mortality by using areal statistics in Japan: a note on the relation between municipal cancer mortality and areal deprivation index. Proceedings of Institute of Statistical Mathematics. 59(2): 239–265. (in Japanese with English abstract).
22. Mac Loon P (1996) Suicide and deprivation in Scotland. British Medical Journal. 312(7030): 543–544.
23. Lawlor DA, Davey Smith G, Patel R, Ebrahim S (2005) Life-course socioeconomic position, area deprivation, and coronary heart disease; findings from the British Women's Heart and Health Study. American Journal of Public Health. 95(1): 91–97.
24. Ellwood RP, Davies GM, Worthington HV, Blinkhorn AS, Taylor GO, et al. (2004) Relationship between area deprivation and the anticaries benefit of an oral health programme providing free fluoride toothpaste to young children. Community Dentistry and Oral Epidemiology, 32(3): 159–165.
25. Bower E, Gulliford M, Steele J, Newton T (2007) Area deprivation and oral health in Scottish adults: a multilevel study. Community Dentistry and Oral Epidemiology, 35(2): 118–129.
26. Walters K, Breeze E, Wilkinson P, Price GM, Bulpitt CJ, et al. (2004) Local area deprivation and urban-rural differences in anxiety and depression among people

older than 75 years in Britain. American Journal of Public Health. 94(10): 1768–1774.

27. Carp FM, Carp A (1981) Age, deprivation, and personal competence; effects on satisfaction. Research on Aging. 3(3): 279–298.
28. Sacker A, Bartley M, Firth D, Fitzpatrick R (2001) Dimensions of social inequality in the health of women in England: occupational, material and behavioral pathways. Social Science and Medicine, 52(5): 763–781.
29. Golant S, La Greca A (1995) The relative deprivation of U.S. elderly households as judged by their housing problems. Journal of Gerontology, 50B(1): S13–S23.
30. Stouffer SA, Suchman EA, Devinney LC, Star SA, Williams RM (1949) *The American Soldier. Volume 1.: Adjustment During Army Life*. Princeton University Press.
31. Runciman WG (1966) *Relative deprivation and social justice: a study of attitudes to social inequality in twentieth century England*. London: Routledge & Kegan Paul.
32. Scase R (1974) Relative deprivation: a comparison of English and Swedish manual workers. Wedderburn.D (eds) *Poverty, inequality, and class structure*. London: Syndics of cambridge university press. 197–216.
33. Crosby FJ (1982) *Relative deprivation and working women*. New York: Oxford University Press.
34. Kosaka K (1986) A model of relative deprivation. Journal of Mathematical Sociology, 12(1): 35–48.
35. Turley RNL (2002) Is relative deprivation beneficial? the effects of richer and poorer neighbors on children's outcomes. Journal of Community Psychology, 30(6): 671–686.
36. Walker I, Smith HJ (2002) *Relative deprivation: specification, development, and integration*. Cambridge: Cambridge University Press.
37. Tougas F, Lagace M, Sablonniere R, Kocum L (2004) A new approach to the link between identity and relative deprivation in the perspective of ageism and retirement. International Journal of Aging and Human Development, 59(1): 1–23.
38. Kondo N, Kawachi I, Hirai H, Kondo K, Subramanian SV, et al. (2009b) Relative deprivation and incident functional disability among older Japanese women and men: prospective cohort study. Journal of Epidemiology & Community Health, 63(6): 461–467.
39. Idler EL, Benyamini Y (1997) Self-rated health and mortality: a review of twenty-seven community studies. Journal of Health Social Behaviour, 38(1): 21–37.
40. Royall DR, Schillerstrom JE, Piper PK, Chiodo LK (2007) Depression and mortality in elders referred for geriatric psychiatry consultation. Journal of the American Medical Directors Association, 8(5): 318–321.
41. Yesavage JA, Brink TL, Rose TL, Lum O, Huang V, et al. (1983) Development and validation of a geriatric depression screening scale: A preliminary report. Journal of Psychiatric Research, 17: 37–49.
42. Sheikh JI, Yesavage JA (1986) Geriatric Depression Scale (GDS): Recent evidence and development of a shorter version. Clinical Gerontologist, 5: 165–173.
43. Murata C, Saito Y, Kondo K, Hirai H (2011) Social support and depression among community living older people. Japanese Journal of Gerontology, 33(1): 15–21. (in Japanese with English abstract).
44. Watanabe M, Imagawa T (2013) Factor structure of short form of the geriatric depression scale (GDS): reliability, validity and cutoff points. the Japanese Journal of Personality, 22(2): 193–197. (in Japanese with English abstract).
45. Abe A (2007) Measuring Social Exclusion in Japan. the Quarterly of Social Security Research. 43(1): 27–40. (in Japanese).
46. Ministry of internal affairs and communications (2009) National Survey of Family Income and Expenditure. (in Japanese). (http://www.stat.go.jp/data/zensho/2009/index.htm. Accessed 2014 Oct 3.).
47. Förster MF (1994) Measurement of low incomes and poverty. OECD labour market and social policy occasional papers, no. 14. doi:10.1787/112854878327.
48. Ichida Y, Kondo K, Hirai H, Hanibuchi T, Yoshikawa G, et al. (2009) Social capital, income inequality and self-rated health in Chita peninsula, Japan: a multilevel analysis of older people in 25 communities. Social Science & Medicine, 69(4): 489–499.
49. Aida J, Hanibuchi T, Nakade M, Hirai H, Osaka K, et al. (2009) The different effects of vertical social capital and horizontal social capital on dental status; A multilevel analysis. Social Science & Medicine, 69(4): 512–518.
50. Krueger AB, Abraham KG, Shapiro C (2012) *Economic report of the president, transmitted to the congress February 2012; together with the annual report of the council of economic advisors*. United States government printing office.
51. National Institute of Population and Social Security Research (2013) *Japanese public statistics data base concerning public assistance* (in Japanese). (http://www.ipss.go.jp/s-info/j/seiho/seiho.asp. Accessed 2014 Oct 3.).
52. Wilkinson R, Marmot M (2003) Social determinants of health: The solid facts (2nd ed.). WHO Regional Office for Europe.
53. Saito M, Kondo N, Kondo K, Ojima T, Hirai H (2012) Gender differences on the impacts of social exclusion on mortality among older Japanese: AGES cohort study. Social Science and Medicine, 75(5): 940–945.
54. Kondo K (2010) *Health inequalities in Japan: An empirical study of the older people*. Melbourne: Trans Pacific Press.

The Efficacy of Paroxetine and Placebo in Treating Anxiety and Depression

Michael A. Sugarman[1]*, Amy M. Loree[1], Boris B. Baltes[1], Emily R. Grekin[1], Irving Kirsch[2]

1 Wayne State University, Department of Psychology, Detroit, Michigan, United States of America, **2** Harvard Medical School, Boston, Massachusetts, United States of America

Abstract

Background: Previous meta-analyses of published and unpublished trials indicate that antidepressants provide modest benefits compared to placebo in the treatment of depression; some have argued that these benefits are not clinically significant. However, these meta-analyses were based only on trials submitted for the initial FDA approval of the medication and were limited to those aimed at treating depression. Here, for the first time, we assess the efficacy of a selective serotonin reuptake inhibitor (SSRI) in the treatment of both anxiety and depression, using a complete data set of all published and unpublished trials sponsored by the manufacturer.

Methods and Findings: GlaxoSmithKline has been required to post the results for all sponsored clinical trials online, providing an opportunity to assess the efficacy of an SSRI (paroxetine) with a complete data set of all trials conducted. We examined the data from all placebo-controlled, double-blind trials of paroxetine that included change scores on the Hamilton Rating Scale for Anxiety (HRSA) and/or the Hamilton Rating Scale for Depression (HRSD). For the treatment of anxiety ($k = 12$), the efficacy difference between paroxetine and placebo was modest ($d = 0.27$), and independent of baseline severity of anxiety. Overall change in placebo-treated individuals replicated 79% of the magnitude of paroxetine response. Efficacy was superior for the treatment of panic disorder ($d = 0.36$) than for generalized anxiety disorder ($d = 0.20$). Published trials showed significantly larger drug-placebo differences than unpublished trials (d's $= 0.32$ and 0.17, respectively). In depression trials ($k = 27$), the benefit of paroxetine over placebo was consistent with previous meta-analyses of antidepressant efficacy ($d = 0.32$).

Conclusions: The available empirical evidence indicates that paroxetine provides only a modest advantage over placebo in treatment of anxiety and depression. Treatment implications are discussed.

Editor: Brett Thombs, McGill University, Canada

Funding: The current study did not have any funding sources. Study design, data collection and analysis, decision to publish, and preparation of the manuscript were all done at the discretion of the study authors.

Competing Interests: The authors have declared that no competing interests exist.

* Email: Mike.Sugarman@wayne.edu

Introduction

Antidepressant medications are prescribed to 8.7% of the US population, making them the third most common class of prescription medications [1]. Antidepressants are approved for the treatment of depression and several other mental disorders, including generalized anxiety disorder [2], panic disorder, social anxiety disorder, obsessive-compulsive disorder, and post-traumatic stress disorder [3]. While several meta-analytic investigations have been conducted examining the efficacy of antidepressants in the treatment of depression, fewer analyses have focused on the efficacy of these drugs in the treatment of other conditions, including anxiety disorders. Moreover, most meta-analyses are conducted only using published studies. However, approximately 40% of the antidepressant trials conducted by pharmaceutical companies are not published [4,5]. Therefore, meta-analyses of antidepressant trials are prone to overestimations of effectiveness due to publication bias.

One strategy for avoiding publication bias is to conduct meta-analyses on data submitted to the Food and Drug Administration (FDA) in the process of obtaining drug approval, as the FDA requires that pharmaceutical companies provide information on all of the trials that they have sponsored [6]. However, analyses of data submitted to the FDA [5,7–9] only include trials conducted prior to approval of the medications. Pharmaceutical companies often conduct additional placebo-controlled double-blind trials after the medications have been approved. Thus, the data submitted to the FDA do not represent the most complete datasets of studies conducted with the medications.

The current study addresses these potential biases by evaluating the efficacy of paroxetine, a selective serotonin reuptake inhibitor (SSRI), across all placebo-controlled double-blind studies conducted by its manufacturer, GlaxoSmithKline, including those conducted following FDA approval. As part of a 2004 lawsuit settlement, GlaxoSmithKline has been required to post online the results of all clinical trials involving its drugs on its Clinical Trial Register [10,11]. Thus, unlike most other antidepressants, all studies of paroxetine can be evaluated without fear of publication bias. A recent meta-analysis reported that paroxetine did not significantly differ in overall efficacy from citalopram, escitalopram, fluoxetine, or sertraline in the treatment of depression [12]. Therefore, findings concerning the efficacy of paroxetine in the treatment of anxiety disorders could possibly generalize to other SSRIs, although further research would be necessary to support that proposition.

The current analysis is the first to evaluate the efficacy of an SSRI in the treatment of anxiety disorders using a complete dataset of sponsored placebo-controlled trials. Paroxetine and other SSRIs have been approved for the treatment of a variety of anxiety disorders, including generalized anxiety disorder, panic disorder, and social anxiety disorder [13–24]. To date, however, only two meta-analyses have investigated the degree to which SSRIs reduce symptoms of anxiety, and both of these meta-analyses focused exclusively on panic disorder [25,26]. One of these studies [25] found a moderate advantage for antidepressants compared to placebo (*Hedge's* $g = 0.41$), and the other study [26] suggested that antidepressants provide a somewhat larger benefit (Mean Effect Size = 0.55). Notably, no meta-analyses have examined anxiety disorders other than panic disorder and none have examined whether SSRIs are differentially effective in treating different types of anxiety disorders. Further, both of these meta-analyses [25,26] observed evidence for publication bias in their analyses and did not have access to a full database of published and unpublished trials, indicating that these figures may be an overestimate of the true effect sizes. The availability of the GlaxoSmithKline Clinical Trial Register provides an opportunity to evaluate the efficacy of an SSRI in the treatment of anxiety disorders without a concern for publication bias.

The availability of a complete dataset of pre-marketing and post-marketing trials also allows for the further examination of antidepressant efficacy in the treatment of depression. Previous meta-analyses of antidepressant data obtained from the FDA have consistently revealed modest differences between drug and placebo, with mean effect sizes ranging from $d = 0.31$ to 0.32 [5,7], and raw score differences in improvement on the Hamilton Rating Scale for Depression (HRSD) [27] ranging from 1.80 to 2.51 points [7,28]. The overall magnitude of the change in placebo-treated individuals duplicated greater than 80% of the antidepressant response [7]. The current study further evaluates the magnitude of benefit between an SSRI medication and placebo in the treatment of depression using the database of trials available through the GlaxoSmithKline Clinical Trial Register.

The goals of the current study are two-fold: 1) to determine the magnitude of benefit for paroxetine compared to placebo in the treatment of anxiety, and 2) to determine the magnitude of benefit for paroxetine compared to placebo in the treatment of depression, utilizing access to a complete database of clinical trials sponsored by the manufacturer. Studies examining antidepressant efficacy in the treatment of anxiety disorders have used a wide range of outcome measures. However, a commonly used measure across double-blind trials of anxiety disorders including generalized anxiety disorder and panic disorder is the Hamilton Rating Scale for Anxiety (HRSA) [29]. Therefore, the current study will focus on the HRSA as an indicator of anxiety-related outcomes. For both HRSA and HRSD analyses, we will analyze available moderator variables to determine which trial variables influence effect sizes in drug and placebo groups.

Methods

Study Retrieval

Data for all trials were obtained through the GlaxoSmithKline Clinical Trial Register [30]. According to the terms of the 2004 lawsuit, this database is required to contain every trial sponsored by GlaxoSmithKline on their medications, including paroxetine. Thus, we do not have concerns of publication bias or selective access to studies. The "result summary" files were downloaded from the website in March 2013. A total of 371 result summaries of studies on paroxetine were downloaded. Each study was evaluated for appropriateness in the current analyses. Trials were included in the current study if they met the following criteria: 1) they were a double-blind randomized intervention study containing a placebo group and at least one group receiving paroxetine; 2) they were conducted within an indicated clinical population with DSM-III or DSM-IV (depending on when the study was conducted) diagnoses of mood and/or anxiety disorders and not on healthy volunteers; 3) they included change on the HRSA and/or the HRSD from pre-treatment to post-treatment amongst their outcome measures; 4) the outcome indices were appropriately matched to the clinical diagnosis (i.e., the HRSA was evaluated in individuals with diagnoses of anxiety disorders and the HRSD was evaluated in individuals with depression); and 5) they did not include individuals who had systematically received additional treatment prior to the randomization to placebo/paroxetine. Examples meeting this last exclusion criterion include trials in which all participants were previously stabilized on another treatment and trials in which all participants simultaneously received treatment in addition to paroxetine.

Additionally, we obtained information regarding the initial approval of paroxetine from the FDA in accordance with the Freedom of Information Act [31]. This initial submission included 16 trials examining the efficacy of paroxetine in the treatment of depression and utilized the HRSD as an outcome measure. These trials have been included in previous meta-analyses of antidepressant data submitted to the FDA [7,8]. We matched these 16 trials to their respective result summary file obtained through the GSK Clinical Trial Register. However, we observed discrepancies in sample sizes for 11 of the 16 studies (ranging from $n = 1$ to $n = 12$ for each group) between the data obtained the FDA and data from the GSK Clinical Trial Register result summaries. In all of these cases, samples were larger in the FDA datasets than in those obtained from the GSK Clinical Trial Register. In the interests of using the most complete datasets and presenting results consistent with previous meta-analyses including these trials, we used the data obtained from the FDA for these 11 trials in our analyses. Further examination revealed that the differences in sample sizes in these trials did not contribute to substantial differences in trial outcome. The overall weighted meta-analytic pre-post effect sizes for both paroxetine and placebo-treated individuals across all trials were essentially identical (within $d = 0.002$) when comparing the two data sources.

Meta-Analytic Data Synthesis

For each outcome index (HRSA and HRSD), we conducted two types of data analysis: 1) an analysis of each trial's arithmetic means for both groups to determine the overall meta-analytic "effect size" [32] as a comparison between the two groups (i.e., the effect size difference between paroxetine and placebo), and 2) each group's change was calculated as the standardized mean difference, dividing the change score by the standard deviation of the change [33]. For trials that included multiple paroxetine groups compared to placebo (e.g., comparing different dosage levels or trials comparing controlled and immediate release tablets), the initial severity and change scores were combined across groups, weighted by the respective sample sizes. All analyses were conducted using the Comprehensive Meta Analysis 2.0 software package (Version 2.2.050, BIOSTAT, Englewood, NJ, USA). All analyses were conducted using both random- and fixed-effects models. Equivalent results (with regard to statistical significance) were observed for both models in almost all analyses; thus, the fixed-effects results are presented here. However, we have made the results of the random-effects models available online for interested readers (see Results S1 and Figures S1–S3). The Q [34] and I^2 [35,36] indices were used to determine the presence or absence of homogeneity and to assess the degree of inconsistency between trials.

Analysis 1 evaluated the effect size magnitude when comparing paroxetine and placebo groups in each trial, determining the benefit of paroxetine over placebo. The effect size was calculated as the difference in the change score between groups divided by the pooled standard deviation. Analysis 2 determined the absolute magnitude of change in both the placebo and paroxetine groups for each trial (i.e., the analyses were conducted separately for each group). This latter analysis allows us to evaluate and compare the magnitude of change for both treatment conditions. For both analyses, the results are presented both in raw metric (as the mean change on the respective Hamilton rating scale) and as a standardized pre-post mean difference (d). The standardized mean difference results account for variation between trials in the standard deviation of the change score [37]. Weights were determined by the sample size times the inverse of the change score variance. Note that in Analysis 1 the meta-analytic weights for each study are determined by the pooled sample size and variance across both paroxetine and placebo groups, and the weights for Analysis 2 are determined for each group separately. Thus, the overall effect sizes for Analysis 1 are slightly different than the results obtained from simply subtracting the placebo from paroxetine effect sizes in Analysis 2.

We examined several moderator variables in both analyses to determine if study characteristics influenced the standardized mean difference within each treatment and/or in the comparison between paroxetine and placebo. For the HRSA, we analyzed the following moderators: 1) Baseline severity of anxiety, as determined by the mean HRSA group score at the beginning of the trial. No previous work has examined whether antidepressant and/or placebo efficacy is superior in more severe cases of anxiety, which might be predicted based on regression to the mean effects. 2) Indication (i.e., whether the individuals in the trial were treated for panic disorder or for generalized anxiety disorder). These analyses were designed to determine if the relative efficacy of paroxetine in the treatment of symptoms of anxiety varied systematically by diagnosis. 3) Length of treatment in weeks. The double-blind trials in these analyses ranged from 8 to 12 weeks; it is possible that longer trials are associated with a larger drug-placebo difference because the drug has more time to exert its effects in longer trials. Although previous studies [7,38] have not found a significant relationship between duration of treatment and antidepressant efficacy in the treatment of depression, no previous analyses have examined this moderator variable for antidepressant efficacy in the treatment of anxiety. 4) Publication status. The current database contains all trials conducted with paroxetine, both published and unpublished; thus, publication bias is not a concern in our outcomes. Previous work [5] has demonstrated that the published literature may represent an overestimate of antidepressant efficacy in the treatment of depression, and the current analysis aimed to determine the magnitude of publication bias in the treatment of anxiety.

For the HRSD, we analyzed the following moderators: 1) Baseline severity of depression, as determined by the mean HRSD group score at the beginning of each trial. Previous analyses [7,39,40] have demonstrated that antidepressant-placebo differences increase with more severe depression. 2) Approval status (i.e., trials submitted to the FDA for the initial approval versus trials conducted post-approval). The 11 trials conducted following FDA approval have not been previously included in meta-analytic investigations. 3) Length of treatment in weeks. 4) Publication status.

Results

Study Selection

A total of 39 trials out of the original sample of 371 studies met inclusion criteria for the current analyses. The trial flow is illustrated in Figure 1. Out of the excluded studies, 121 studies did not evaluate efficacy of the drug (e.g., they evaluated the pharmacokinetics or tolerability of the drug); 153 studies were intervention studies that did not include a placebo group (e.g., they compared multiple doses of the drug, compared paroxetine against other drugs, or were open-label); 28 studies were placebo-controlled intervention studies but did not include the HRSA or HRSD in their outcome measures; 13 trials were extension studies of other trials or evaluated the efficacy of paroxetine for prevention of relapse. In nine studies, paroxetine was not the only treatment included in the intent-to-treat samples (e.g., all participants were previously stabilized on another treatment or received another simultaneous treatment in addition to paroxetine or placebo). Three studies (29060/785, 29060/251, and 29060/874) included change scores for the HRSA but the patients had a primary indication of depression rather than for anxiety disorders and thus these studies were not included. However, two of these studies (29060/251 and 29060/874) included the HRSD as an outcome measure and were included in depression analyses. Four studies included change scores on the HRSD, but the trials were for individuals with obsessive-compulsive disorder (29060/116 and 29060/118) and social phobia (29060/661 and PIR104776). The participants in these studies had low baseline severity scores (mean HRSD scores ranging from 9 to 10) and did not appear to be clinically depressed; thus, these studies were excluded. One study (29060/442) met all criteria but did not include mean change scores on the HRSD and only provided the percentage of "responders" (reduction by ≥50% on the HRSD from pre-treatment to post-treatment) in each group. Thus, we were unable to include this study in the meta-analysis.

Twelve studies were included for the HRSA, comprising 1,835 individuals randomized to paroxetine and 1,550 randomized to placebo. Twenty-seven studies were included for the HRSD, comprising 3,301 individuals randomized to paroxetine and 1,885 randomized to placebo. All studies reported their outcome measures based on "last observation carried forward" methods, meaning that the change scores for individuals who withdrew from the study were calculated based on their final data point. This method helps to control for selective attrition during the studies.

Study Characteristics

Information on all trials is presented in Table 1. The corresponding publication information is provided where applicable. All dosage levels were within the FDA-approved range for the diagnosis. For the 12 trials evaluating change on the HRSA, trial duration ranged between 8 and 12 weeks. Five trials were 8 weeks

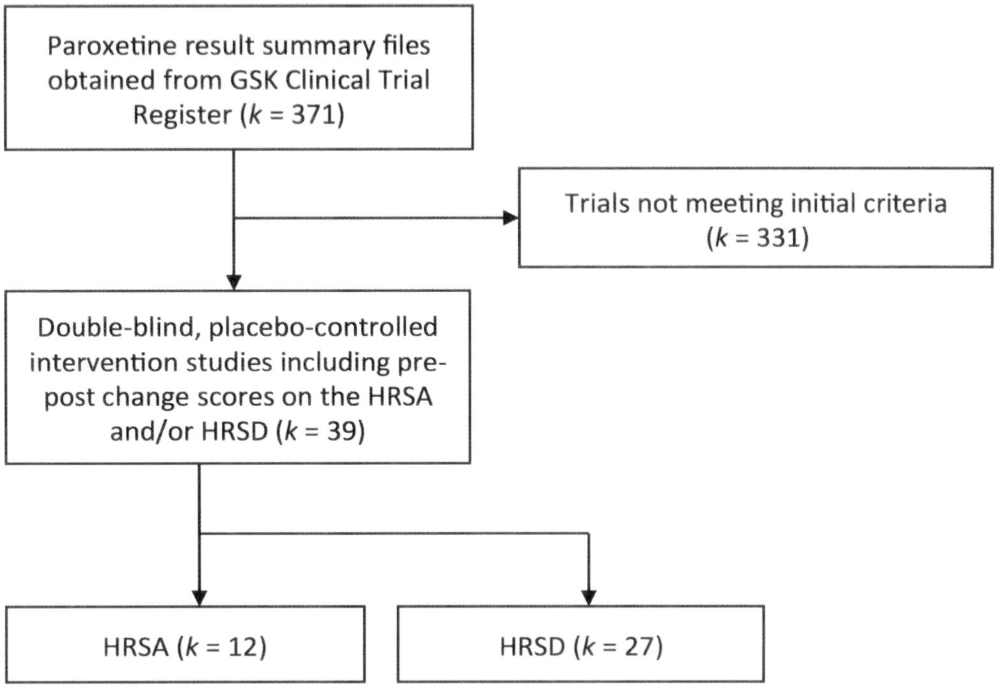

Figure 1. Trial selection Flow chart. GSK = GlaxoSmithKline, HRSA = Hamilton Rating Scale for Anxiety, HRSD = Hamilton Rating Scale for Depression. Please refer to the text for more specific information regarding specific exclusion criteria.

in duration, five were 10 weeks, and two were 12 weeks. Trials were initiated between 1991 and 2003, all following FDA approval of the medication in the treatment of depression. All trials were conducted in adults. Seven trials evaluated panic disorder and five trials evaluated generalized anxiety disorder. Flexible dose adjustment was permitted in 9 of the 12 studies (i.e., the dose of paroxetine and/or placebo could be adjusted during the trial based on therapeutic response). Eight (67%) of the studies were published in peer-reviewed journals.

For the 27 trials that included change on the HRSD as an outcome measure, trial duration ranged between 4 and 12 weeks. One trial was 4 weeks in duration, fifteen were 6 weeks, four were 8 weeks, one was 10 weeks, and six were 12 weeks. Twenty-four trials evaluated change in adults, one trial evaluated change in adolescents, and two trials evaluated change in the elderly. Twenty-six trials evaluated major depressive disorder and one trial evaluated dysthymia. Flexible dose adjustment was permitted in 21 of the 27 trials. Trials were conducted between 1982 and 2009. The trials conducted prior to 1991 ($k = 16$, 59% of trials) were included as part of the original FDA submission, and an additional 11 trials (41% of trials) were conducted following FDA approval, in 1991 or later. Sixteen (59%) of the studies were published in peer-reviewed journals.

Mean Change on the HRSA

Table 2 displays mean baseline severity, mean change, and the standardized mean difference (d) for each of the 12 trials reporting change on the HRSA. Baseline HRSA data were unavailable for two trials. Baseline severity of anxiety ranged from 18.7 to 26.0. The mean drug-placebo difference was 2.31 (95% CI: 1.72,2.91) points on the HRSA with a mean effect size difference of $d = 0.27$ (95% CI: 0.20,0.33). The weighted mean change on the HRSA was 11.11 (95% CI: 10.72,11.50) points for paroxetine and 8.77 (95% 8.35,9.20) points for placebo. The mean pre-post effect size was $d = 1.23$ (95% CI: 1.17,1.30) for paroxetine and $d = 0.96$ (95% CI: 0.90,1.02) for placebo. The differences between groups easily met statistical significance for both the raw change scores on the HRSA ($Z = 7.64$, $p < .001$) and the standardized mean difference ($Z = 7.52$, $p < .001$). The change in the placebo group duplicated 79% of the mean change score and 78% of the standardized mean difference in the paroxetine groups. These percentages are similar to those found for second-generation antidepressants in the treatment of depression [7].

A trend toward heterogeneity was observed for the mean effect size difference between paroxetine and placebo, as demonstrated by the indices of heterogeneity ($Q(11) = 17.63$, $p = .091$, $I^2 = 37.61$ [95% CI: 12.25,55.64]). A wider range of effect sizes was observed within each treatment group (Paroxetine: $Q(11) = 57.27$, $p < .001$, $I^2 = 80.79$ [95% CI: 74.98,85.25]; Placebo: $Q(11) = 65.39$, $p < .001$, $I^2 = 83.18$ [95% CI: 78.29,86.96]). These statistics indicate the necessity for moderator analyses to investigate which trial variables influenced study outcomes. Thus, we conducted moderator analyses with both analytic strategies (i.e., the paroxetine-placebo effect sizes and for paroxetine and placebo groups separately).

HRSA Moderators

The following potential moderators were analyzed: 1) baseline severity of anxiety; 2) indication (i.e., whether the individuals in the trial were treated for panic disorder or for generalized anxiety disorder); 3) length of trial in weeks; and 4) publication status.

There was no significant relationship between baseline anxiety and the paroxetine-placebo effect size difference ($Q(1) = 1.58$, $p = .208$), as shown in Figure 2. A positive relationship was observed between baseline anxiety on the HRSA and effect size for both groups (Paroxetine: $Q(1) = 21.34$, $p < .001$; Placebo: $Q(1) = 23.51$, $p < .001$). These latter effects are consistent with regression to the mean artifact. Baseline severity scores were

Table 1. List of studies.

Protocol Number	Publication	Outcome	Year	Indication	Population	Length	Dosage
29060/108	[18]	HRSA	1991	Panic	Adult	12	Flexible
29060/120	[14]	HRSA	1992	Panic	Adult	10	Fixed
29060/187	[16]	HRSA	1991	Panic	Adult	12	Flexible
29060/223		HRSA	1992	Panic	Adult	10	Flexible
29060/494	[21]	HRSA	1996	Panic	Adult	10	Flexible
29060/495	[21]	HRSA	1996	Panic	Adult	10	Flexible
29060/497	[21]	HRSA	1996	Panic	Adult	10	Flexible
29060/637		HRSA	1998	GAD	Adult	8	Flexible
29060/641	[20]	HRSA	1998	GAD	Adult	8	Fixed
29060/642	[19]	HRSA	1999	GAD	Adult	8	Flexible
29060/791		HRSA	2001	GAD	Adult	8	Flexible
29060A/856		HRSA	2003	GAD	Adult	8	Fixed
29060/01/001		HRSD	1984	Depression	Adult	6	Flexible
29060/02/001	[67,68]	HRSD	1985	Depression	Adult	6	Flexible
29060/02/002	[69,70]	HRSD	1985	Depression	Adult	6	Flexible
29060/02/003	[71]	HRSD	1985	Depression	Adult	6	Flexible
29060/02/004	[72]	HRSD	1985	Depression	Adult	6	Flexible
29060/03/001	[73,74]	HRSD	1985	Depression	Adult	6	Flexible
29060/03/002	[75,76]	HRSD	1985	Depression	Adult	6	Flexible
29060/03/003		HRSD	1985	Depression	Adult	6	Flexible
29060/03/004	[77]	HRSD	1985	Depression	Adult	6	Flexible
29060/03/005	[78]	HRSD	1985	Depression	Adult	6	Flexible
29060/03/006	[79]	HRSD	1985	Depression	Adult	6	Flexible
PAR 09	[80]	HRSD	1985	Depression	Adult	6	Fixed
UK 06	[81]	HRSD	1983	Depression	Adult	4	Fixed
UK 12		HRSD	1983	Depression	Adult	6	Fixed
UK 09		HRSD	1982	Depression	Adult	6	Fixed
PAR 07		HRSD	1986	Depression	Adult	6	Flexible
29060/115		HRSD	1991	Depression	Adult	12	Flexible
29060/128		HRSD	1991	Depression	Adult	12	Flexible
29060/251		HRSD	1992	Depression	Adult	8	Flexible
29060/327		HRSD	1994	Dysthymia	Adult	12	Flexible
29060/329	[82]	HRSD	1994	Depression	Adolescent	8	Flexible
29060/448	[83,84]	HRSD	1996	Depression	Adult	12	Flexible

Table 1. Cont.

Protocol Number	Publication	Outcome	Year	Indication	Population	Length	Dosage
29060/449	[83,84]	HRSD	1996	Depression	Adult	12	Flexible
29060/487	[85]	HRSD	1996	Depression	Elderly	12	Flexible
29060/810	[86]	HRSD	2001	Depression	Adult	8	Fixed
29060/874		HRSD	2003	Depression	Elderly	10	Fixed
112810		HRSD	2009	Depression	Adult	8	Flexible

HRSA = Hamilton Rating Scale for Anxiety. HRSD = Hamilton Rating Scale for Depression. Year: when data collection was initiated. Trials conducted prior to 1991 were submitted for the original FDA approval of the medication. Length: study duration in weeks. GAD = generalized anxiety disorder.

unavailable for two trials (29060/187 [Panic disorder] and BRL29060A/856 [Generalized anxiety disorder]) that were not included in this analysis.

The effect of indication on treatment response (Table 3) was significant. Panic disorder had a significantly larger drug-placebo difference in terms of the standardized mean difference ($Q(1) = 5.09$, $p = .024$) and the raw change score ($Q(1) = 6.77$, $p = .009$). Mean standardized difference was $d = 0.36$ (95% CI: 0.25,0.46) for panic disorder and $d = 0.20$ (95% CI: 0.11,0.29) for generalized anxiety disorder. Raw score differences were 3.24 points (95% CI: 2.32,4.15) for panic disorder and 1.64 points (95% CI: 0.86,2.42) for generalized anxiety disorder. The effect of indication was also significant within each group (Paroxetine: $Q(1) = 24.27$, $p < .001$; Placebo: $Q(1) = 32.97$, $p < .001$). However, the effects were opposite, with generalized anxiety disorder having higher effect sizes and raw change scores on the HRSA for both groups (Paroxetine: $d = 1.38$ [95% CI: 1.29,1.46] and raw change = 11.79 [95% CI: 11.29,12.30] points; Placebo: $d = 1.14$ [95% CI: 1.05,1.22] and raw change = 10.07 [95% CI: 9.49,10.64] points) compared to panic disorder (Paroxetine: $d = 1.07$ [95% CI: 0.98,1.16] and raw change = 10.06 [95% CI: 9.43,10.68] points; Placebo: $d = 0.78$ [95% CI: 0.69,0.86] and raw change = 7.17 [95% CI: 6.53,7.81] points).

Longer trial lengths were significantly associated with larger paroxetine-placebo effect sizes (Intercept = −0.40, Slope = 0.073 [95% CI: 0.023,0.124], $Q(1) = 8.02$, $p = .005$). Within each treatment group, trial length was *inversely* associated with improvement in both groups, and appeared to have a stronger relationship in the placebo group (Paroxetine: Intercept = 2.01, Slope = −0.086 [95% CI: −0.133,−0.038] $Q(1) = 12.51$, $p < .001$; Placebo: Intercept = 2.04, Slope = −0.116 [95% CI: −0.161,−0.072], $Q(1) = 26.54$, $p < .001$). However, this finding is difficult to interpret because it is confounded by differences in study indication. All five trials examining generalized anxiety disorder had a length of eight weeks, and the seven trials examining panic disorder were between 10 and 12 weeks. As described in the previous paragraph, the overall change was larger in both groups for generalized anxiety disorder, which could account for the negative slope within each group, and the drug-placebo difference was larger for panic disorder, which could account for the positive slope in the difference score. Thus, we are unable to make any firm conclusions in this analysis regarding the effect of trial length on anxiolytic response.

There was a significant effect of publication status (Table 3), with larger drug benefits in published trials ($Q(1) = 3.90$, $p = .048$). Published trials ($k = 8$) had a mean drug-placebo effect size of $d = 0.32$ (95% CI: 0.23–0.40), and unpublished trials ($k = 4$) had a mean effect size of $d = 0.17$ (95% CI: 0.06–0.29). This difference appeared to be due to a substantially smaller placebo pre-post effect sizes in published trials (Published: $d = 0.86$ [95% CI: 0.79,0.94], Unpublished: $d = 1.15$ [95% CI: 1.04,1.25], $Q(1) = 18.63$, $p = .001$). The mean pre-post effect size for the paroxetine group was actually marginally smaller for published compared to unpublished trials (Published: $d = 1.19$ [95% CI: 1.12,1.27], Unpublished: $d = 1.32$ [95% CI: 1.21,1.44], $Q(1) = 3.52$, $p = .061$).

Mean Change on the HRSD

Table 4 displays mean baseline severity, mean change, and the standardized mean difference (d) for each of the 27 trials reporting change on the HRSD. Baseline severity scores on the HRSD ranged from 19.0 to 30.5 points, all in the ranges of severe to very severe depression [41]. The weighted mean difference between paroxetine and placebo groups across all studies was 2.51 (95%

Table 2. Baseline scores, mean change, standardized mean change, and sample sizes for all studies reporting change on the Hamilton Rating Scale for Anxiety.

Protocol	Indication	Paroxetine					Placebo				Drug benefit		
		Baseline	Change	*d*	95% CI	*n*	Baseline	Change	*d*	95% CI	*n*	*d*	95% CI
29060/108	Panic	24.3	14.9	2.04	[1.57, 2.51]	58	23.5	10.0	1.62	[1.21, 2.03]	56	0.74	[0.36, 1.12]
29060/120	Panic	18.9	8.4	0.95	[0.77, 1.13]	175	19.7	6.5	0.73	[0.44, 1.02]	60	0.21	[−0.08, 0.50]
29060/187	Panic		10.1	1.10	[0.87, 1.33]	119		5.9	0.59	[0.40, 0.79]	122	0.44	[0.19, 0.70]
29060/223	Panic	20.3	10.2	1.29	[0.94, 1.64]	61	18.7	5.6	0.76	[0.48, 1.04]	65	0.61	[0.25, 0.97]
29060/494	Panic	21.9	10.0	1.08	[0.84, 1.31]	115	20.1	8.0	0.88	[0.67, 1.09]	124	0.22	[−0.04, 0.47]
29060/495	Panic	20.5	9.4	1.03	[0.79, 1.26]	112	20.4	6.6	0.74	[0.54, 0.94]	129	0.31	[0.06, 0.57]
29060/497	Panic	20.5	9.4	0.95	[0.74, 1.16]	128	20.2	6.8	0.75	[0.55, 0.95]	125	0.28	[0.03, 0.52]
29060/637	GAD	26.0	12.4	1.15	[0.96, 1.34]	181	25.9	11.3	1.04	[0.86, 1.22]	183	0.10	[−0.10, 0.31]
29060/641	GAD	23.5	12.3	1.48	[1.33, 1.63]	385	23.9	9.6	1.02	[0.84, 1.20]	180	0.32	[0.14, 0.49]
29060/642	GAD	23.9	11.8	1.32	[1.11, 1.54]	161	23.6	9.5	1.06	[0.86, 1.25]	163	0.26	[0.04, 0.48]
29060/791	GAD	24.4	11.9	1.60	[1.37, 1.84]	163	24.8	10.7	1.44	[1.22, 1.67]	162	0.17	[−0.05, 0.38]
29060A/856	GAD		10.3	1.33	[1.13, 1.53]	177		9.5	1.23	[1.04, 1.43]	181	0.10	[−0.10, 0.31]

GAD = generalized anxiety disorder. Drug benefit denotes the effect size for paroxetine compared to placebo.

CI: 2.06,2.96) points on the HRSD. The weighted mean effect size difference between the two groups was 0.32 (95% CI: 0.26,0.38). The weighted mean change on the HRSD was 11.00 (95% CI: 10.74,11.26) points for paroxetine and 8.37 (95% CI: 8.02,8.72) points for placebo. The mean pre-post effect size was 1.39 (95% CI: 1.34,1.44) for paroxetine, which was significantly greater ($Q(1) = 87.62$, $p < .001$) than the effect size for placebo ($d = 1.03$ [95% CI: 0.97,1.08]). The magnitude of change in the placebo group was equivalent to 76% of the paroxetine change scores on the HRSD and 74% of the standardized mean difference.

Indices of heterogeneity did not indicate statistically significant heterogeneity in the effect size difference between paroxetine and placebo across trials ($Q(26) = 26.54$, $p = .434$, $I^2 = 2.04$ [95% CI: −29.25,25.75]), although we did detect significant heterogeneity within each group (Paroxetine: $Q(26) = 63.21$, $p < .001$, $I^2 = 58.87$ [95% CI: 49.14–66.73]; Placebo: $Q(26) = 80.63$, $p < .001$, $I^2 = 67.75$ [95% CI: 60.63,73.59]). Nevertheless, as planned when designing the study, moderator analyses were conducted for both types of analyses.

HRSD Moderators

We analyzed the following moderators to determine whether the variables could account for variance in effect size across trials: 1) baseline severity of depression; 2) approval status; 3) length of treatment in weeks; and 4) publication status.

Figure 3 displays the relationship between baseline severity of depression on the HRSD and treatment outcome. The benefit of paroxetine over placebo was not significantly related to baseline severity ($Q(1) = 3.01$, $p = .083$), although there was a trend towards a greater benefit at higher baseline severities. The predicted paroxetine-placebo effect size at a baseline severity of HRSD = 19 was $d = 0.20$ (95% CI: 0.03,0.36) and $d = 0.48$ (95% CI: 0.29,0.68) at a baseline severity of HRSD = 30. Greater baseline severity of depression was associated with smaller pre-post effect sizes in both paroxetine ($Q(1) = 15.45$, $p < .001$) and placebo ($Q(1) = 28.23$, $p < .001$) groups. These effects are opposite from those expected based on regression to the mean artifact.

A comparison of the trials submitted for the original FDA approval (pre-approval, $k = 16$) versus trials conducted after approval (post-approval, $k = 11$), shown in Table 5, revealed that the mean paroxetine-placebo effect size did not differ significantly as a function of approval status ($Q(1) = 3.27$, $p = .077$), although there was a trend towards a greater drug-placebo benefit in pre-approval trials (Pre-Approval: $d = 0.41$ [95% CI: 0.30,0.53]; Post-Approval: $d = 0.29$ [95% CI: 0.22,0.36]). However, we observed a significant effect within both groups, with larger mean standardized differences in the post-approval trials (Table 5). For paroxetine, the mean effect size for pre-approval trials was $d = 1.24$ (95% CI: 1.15,1.33), compared to $d = 1.45$ (95% CI: 1.39,1.50) for post-approval ($Q(1) = 14.43$, $p < .001$). For placebo, the mean effect sizes were $d = 0.77$ (95% CI: 0.67,0.87) and $d = 1.14$ (95% CI: 1.07,1.21) for the pre- and post-approval trials, respectively ($Q(1) = 35.01$, $p < .001$).

An examination of the effect of trial duration on efficacy (Figure 4) revealed that the benefit of paroxetine over placebo was not significantly associated with trial duration ($Q(1) = 1.30$, $p = .254$). Likewise, the response to paroxetine did not significantly differ as a function of study length ($Q(1) = 2.62$, $p = .105$), although the mean change in the placebo group was significantly larger in longer studies ($Q(1) = 13.74$, $p < .001$).

The weighted mean difference between paroxetine and placebo was not significantly different between published and unpublished trials (Table 5; $Q(1) = 1.50$, $p = .221$). Published trials ($k = 16$) had a weighted mean effect size of $d = 0.36$ (95% CI: 0.27,0.44) and

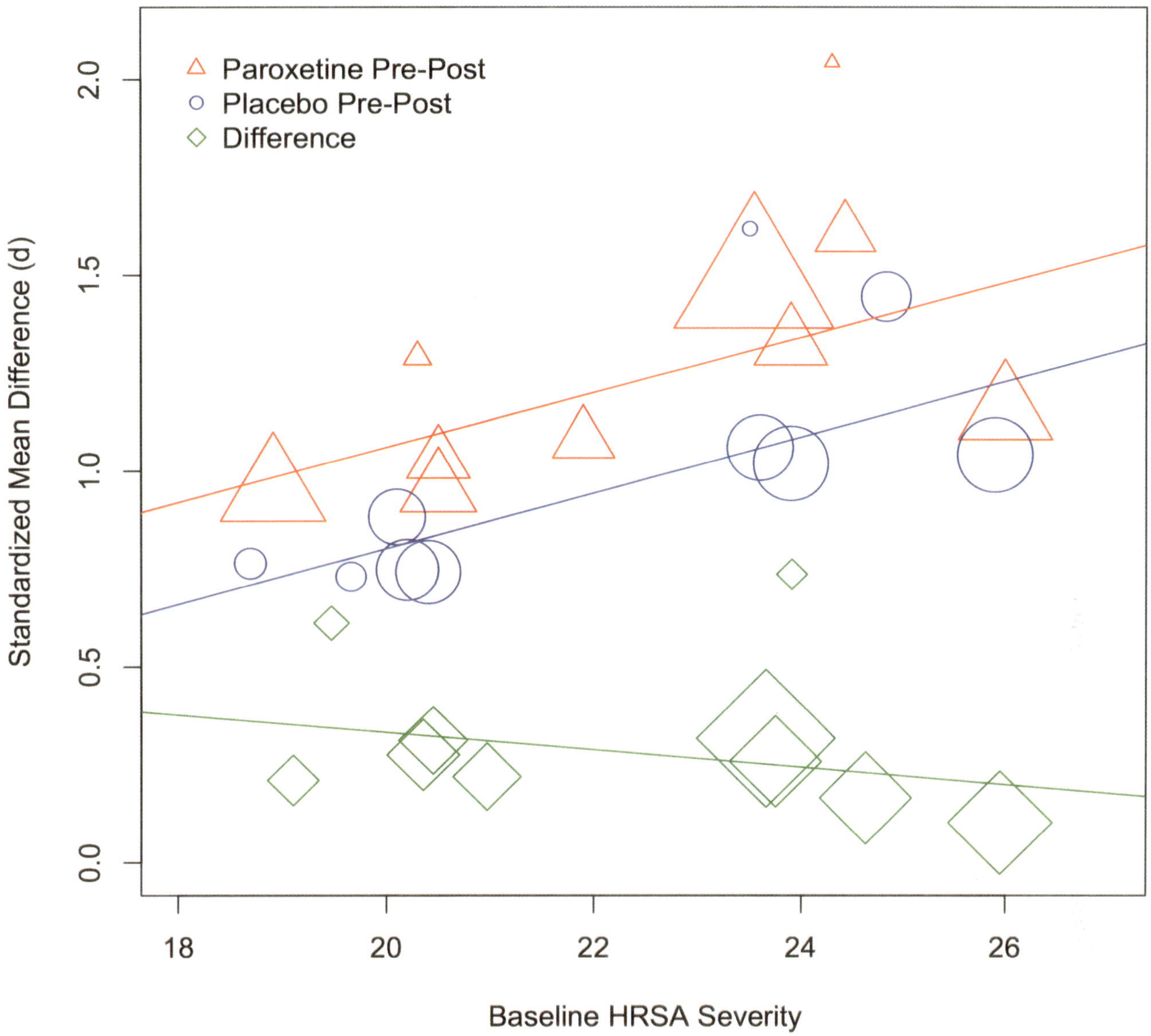

Figure 2. Baseline severity of anxiety and the mean change on the Hamilton Rating Scale for Anxiety (HRSA). The size of the marker reflects the relative weight of the study in the meta-analysis.

unpublished trials ($k=11$) had an effect size of $d=0.28$ (95% CI: 0.20,0.37).

Comparison of Change on the HRSA and HRSD

A comparison of the standardized mean difference between the change on the two scales indicated that the paroxetine-placebo effect size did not significantly differ between the HRSA and the HRSD (HRSA: $d=0.27$ [95% CI: 0.20,0.33], HRSD: $d=0.32$ [95% CI: 0.26,0.38], $Q(1)=1.41$, $p=.235$). The mean pre-post effect size for paroxetine treatment was significantly larger ($Q(1)=14.55$, $p<.001$) for the HRSD ($d=1.39$ [95% CI: 1.34,1.44], $k=27$) than for the HRSA ($d=1.23$ [95% CI: 1.17,1.30], $k=12$). A non-significant trend ($Q(1)=2.38$, $p=.123$) was observed in the placebo group for larger pre-post effect sizes on the HRSD ($d=1.03$ [95% CI: 0.97,1.08]) than on the HRSA ($d=0.96$ [95% CI: 0.90,1.02]).

Discussion

The current analysis is the first evaluation of the efficacy of an SSRI medication in the treatment of multiple anxiety disorders, and the first to utilize a complete database of published and unpublished trials sponsored by the drug's manufacturer. Our results indicated that paroxetine presented a modest benefit over placebo in the treatment of anxiety and depression, with mean change score differences of 2.3 and 2.5 points on the HRSA and HRSD, respectively. The standardized mean difference of paroxetine over placebo was $d=0.27$ and $d=0.32$ for the treatment of anxiety and depression, respectively. Put another way, the average symptom reduction for an individual treated with paroxetine fell at the 61st percentile for individuals who received placebo for anxiety, and at the 63rd percentile for individuals who received placebo for depression. The difference of $d=0.32$ in the treatment of depression is consistent with previous meta-analyses of antidepressant efficacy [5,7]. The mean treatment response did

Table 3. Moderator effects in trials examining change on the Hamilton Rating Scale for Anxiety.

Indication		**Effect Size**	**95% CI**	*Q*(1)	*p*
Paroxetine - Placebo	Panic	0.36	[0.25, 0.46]	5.09	*.024*
	GAD	0.20	[0.11, 0.29]		
Paroxetine	Panic	1.07	[0.98, 1.16]	24.27	*<.001*
	GAD	1.38	[1.29, 1.46]		
Placebo	Panic	0.78	[0.69, 0.86]	32.97	*<.001*
	GAD	1.14	[1.05, 1.22]		
Publication Status		**Effect Size**	**95% CI**	***Q*(1)**	***p***
Paroxetine - Placebo	Published	0.32	[0.23, 0.40]	3.90	*.048*
	Unpublished	0.17	[0.06, 0.29]		
Paroxetine	Published	1.19	[1.12, 1.27]	3.52	.061
	Unpublished	1.32	[1.21, 1.44]		
Placebo	Published	0.86	[0.79, 0.94]	18.63	*<.001*
	Unpublished	1.15	[1.04, 1.25]		

GAD = generalized anxiety disorder.

not significantly differ between treatment of anxiety and treatment of depression. We demonstrated that individuals given placebo exhibited 79% of the magnitude of change compared to paroxetine. We also provided further support for the large magnitude of the changes in placebo groups in the treatment of depression (76% compared to paroxetine).

Several moderator variables were significantly associated with pre-post effect sizes for paroxetine and placebo on both the HRSA and the HRSD. For anxiety, we found that higher baseline severity was unrelated to drug-placebo differences, although higher severity was associated with greater changes in both paroxetine and placebo groups. Efficacy was superior in the treatment of panic disorder compared to generalized anxiety disorder; however, the overall response to both paroxetine and placebo was larger for generalized anxiety disorder. Samples with higher baseline severities were associated with lower changes in both paroxetine and placebo groups in the treatment of depression, an effect that is especially peculiar given that it is opposite to that predicted by regression toward the mean. Longer treatment was associated with larger pre-post placebo effect sizes in the treatment of depression. The increase in the symptom reduction in the placebo group in longer trials for the treatment of depression is especially interesting, given the widespread belief that placebo effects are short lived.

The magnitude of change in the placebo group was greater than 75% of the paroxetine response in the treatment of both anxiety and depression. Large effect sizes in placebo groups have been reported in the treatment of other conditions as well. However, these changes compared to the drug effect sizes do not appear to be as large as those observed in antidepressant trials in the treatment of depression and anxiety. For example, a review of the placebo effect compared to active medications (including antidepressants and anticonvulsants) in the treatment of pain associated with fibromyalgia revealed that the mean change in placebo groups accounted for 45% of the drug response [44]. This same review found that pain reduction in the placebo groups compared to the drug response in individuals with painful peripheral diabetic neuropathy was 62% [44]. Similar meta-analytic reviews have found that mean change in placebo groups replicates about 40% of drug responses in global symptom reduction during treatment of irritable bowel syndrome [45,46]. In a meta-analysis of change in placebo compared to drug groups in the treatment of symptoms of chronic fatigue syndrome, the mean placebo effect replicated only 20% of the drug response [47]. Thus, the replication of greater than 75% of the drug response indicates that the magnitude of the placebo effect is especially large in the treatment of anxiety and depression.

Given the similar efficacy between paroxetine and other second-generation antidepressants in the treatment of depression [7,12,48], it is possible that a similar magnitude of placebo effect sizes are present in the treatment of anxiety disorders with other antidepressants. However, further research will be necessary to support this proposition. The current analysis indicates that the published literature represents an overestimate of the true efficacy of paroxetine in the treatment of anxiety.

Although the differences between drug and placebo are statistically significant, whether antidepressants produce clinically significant benefits has been a topic of debate in recent years. However, to date there has been no consensus regarding what constitutes a clinically significant benefit. In their 2004 guidelines for the treatment of depression, the National Institute of Health and Clinical Excellence (NICE) proposed a mean drug-placebo standardized mean difference (SMD) ≥ 0.50 or a difference of at least three points on the HRSD as criteria for clinical significance [43]. Based on these criteria, the mean antidepressant benefit in a previous meta-analysis of trials submitted to the FDA [7] was clinically significant only in the most severe cases of depression (baseline HRSD ≥ 28). In a subsequent revision of their guidelines for the treatment of depression [42], NICE replaced the term "clinical significance" with "clinical importance." Although they did not specify their criteria for determining whether an effect was clinically important, their comparisons of SSRI-placebo differences in HRSD scores were the same as in the earlier guidelines, and the same conclusions regarding "clinical importance" were reached as had been reached with respect to "clinical significance" in 2004. Specifically, the overall difference between SSRIs and placebo (SMD = 0.34) was described as "unlikely to be of clinical importance" (pg. 317). According to these criteria, the mean

Table 4. Baseline scores, mean change, standardized mean change, and sample sizes for all studies reporting change on the Hamilton Rating Scale for Depression.

Protocol	Approval	Paroxetine					Placebo					Drug Benefit	
		Baseline	Change	*d*	95% CI	*n*	Baseline	Change	*d*	95% CI	*n*	*d*	95% CI
29060/01/001	Pre	28.0	13.5	1.66	[0.99, 2.33]	24	27.4	10.5	1.30	[0.71, 1.89]	24	0.37	[−0.20, 0.94]
29060/02/001	Pre	26.6	12.3	1.27	[0.89, 1.65]	51	25.9	6.8	0.70	[0.40, 1.01]	53	0.57	[0.18, 0.97]
29060/02/002	Pre	25.0	10.9	1.24	[0.78, 1.69]	36	24.9	5.8	0.65	[0.27, 1.04]	34	0.60	[0.12, 1.08]
29060/02/003	Pre	28.6	9.7	0.93	[0.50, 1.35]	33	28.9	7.2	0.69	[0.29, 1.08]	33	0.24	[−0.24, 0.73]
29060/02/004	Pre	28.9	12.7	1.87	[1.29, 2.44]	36	27.3	7.6	1.12	[0.70, 1.54]	38	0.76	[0.29, 1.24]
29060/03/001	Pre	24.9	10.8	1.60	[1.11, 2.09]	40	24.8	4.7	0.69	[0.33, 1.06]	38	0.92	[0.45, 1.39]
29060/03/002	Pre	24.9	8.0	1.14	[0.72, 1.55]	40	25.6	6.2	0.88	[0.51, 1.26]	40	0.26	[−0.18, 0.70]
29060/03/003	Pre	25.7	9.9	1.18	[0.76, 1.59]	41	27.0	10.0	1.19	[0.78, 1.60]	42	−0.01	[−0.44, 0.42]
29060/03/004	Pre	27.6	10.4	1.32	[0.86, 1.78]	37	27.0	6.7	0.85	[0.46, 1.24]	37	0.48	[0.02, 0.95]
29060/03/005	Pre	26.1	10.0	1.00	[0.60, 1.39]	40	26.8	4.1	0.41	[0.08, 0.73]	42	0.60	[0.16, 1.05]
29060/03/006	Pre	29.7	9.1	1.10	[0.69, 1.52]	39	28.7	3.0	0.36	[0.02, 0.71]	37	0.76	[0.29, 1.23]
PAR 09	Pre	25.2	9.1	1.28	[1.15, 1.41]	403	24.5	8.2	1.14	[0.78, 1.51]	51	0.12	[−0.17, 0.41]
UK 06	Pre	23.7	6.0	0.97	[0.38, 1.57]	19	24.2	6.2	0.83	[0.31, 1.35]	22	−0.03	[−0.64, 0.58]
UK 12	Pre	22.8	9.1	1.23	[0.57, 1.88]	19	22.3	6.7	0.86	[0.00, 1.73]	10	0.34	[−0.43, 1.11]
UK 09	Pre	26.8	8.8	0.80	[0.26, 1.35]	20	25.5	4.5	0.49	[0.01, 0.97]	21	0.45	[−0.17, 1.07]
PAR 07	Pre	30.5	13.1	1.20	[0.37, 2.03]	13	28.3	10.9	0.99	[0.19, 1.79]	12	0.22	[−0.57, 1.00]
29060/115	Post		10.6	1.23	[1.07, 1.39]	272		9.1	1.09	[0.85, 1.33]	113	0.18	[−0.04, 0.40]
29060/128	Post	25.6	11.8	1.34	[1.19, 1.48]	350	25.7	9.1	1.05	[0.84, 1.26]	136	0.31	[0.11, 0.51]
29060/251	Post	24.5	10.2	1.33	[1.08, 1.57]	120	24.4	8.3	1.07	[0.85, 1.30]	123	0.26	[0.01, 0.51]
29060/327	Post		7.3	1.14	[0.85, 1.42]	79		4.8	0.75	[0.51, 1.00]	83	0.40	[0.09, 0.71]
29060/329	Post	19.0	10.7	1.39	[1.09, 1.68]	90	19.0	9.1	1.16	[0.89, 1.44]	87	0.21	[−0.08, 0.51]
29060/448	Post	23.2	11.9	1.45	[1.25, 1.65]	206	23.4	9.9	1.22	[0.96, 1.48]	101	0.25	[0.01, 0.48]
29060/449	Post	23.8	12.7	1.54	[1.35, 1.74]	218	23.5	10.2	1.24	[0.99, 1.49]	110	0.30	[0.07, 0.53]
29060/487	Post	22.2	12.2	1.68	[1.46, 1.89]	206	22.1	9.5	1.28	[1.02, 1.54]	107	0.37	[0.14, 0.61]
29060/810	Post	23.3	12.0	1.68	[1.50, 1.86]	294	23.8	10.0	1.37	[1.14, 1.60]	142	0.28	[0.08, 0.49]
29060/874	Post	22.5	11.4	1.42	[1.27, 1.57]	334	22.4	8.9	1.10	[0.91, 1.28]	178	0.32	[0.14, 0.50]
112810	Post	22.7	12.7	1.69	[1.50, 1.89]	241	22.6	10.4	1.28	[1.07, 1.48]	171	0.30	[0.10, 0.49]

"Approval" column designates whether the study was submitted as part of the original approval submission to the FDA or whether it was conducted following FDA approval in 1991 or later. Drug benefit denotes the effect size for paroxetine compared to placebo.

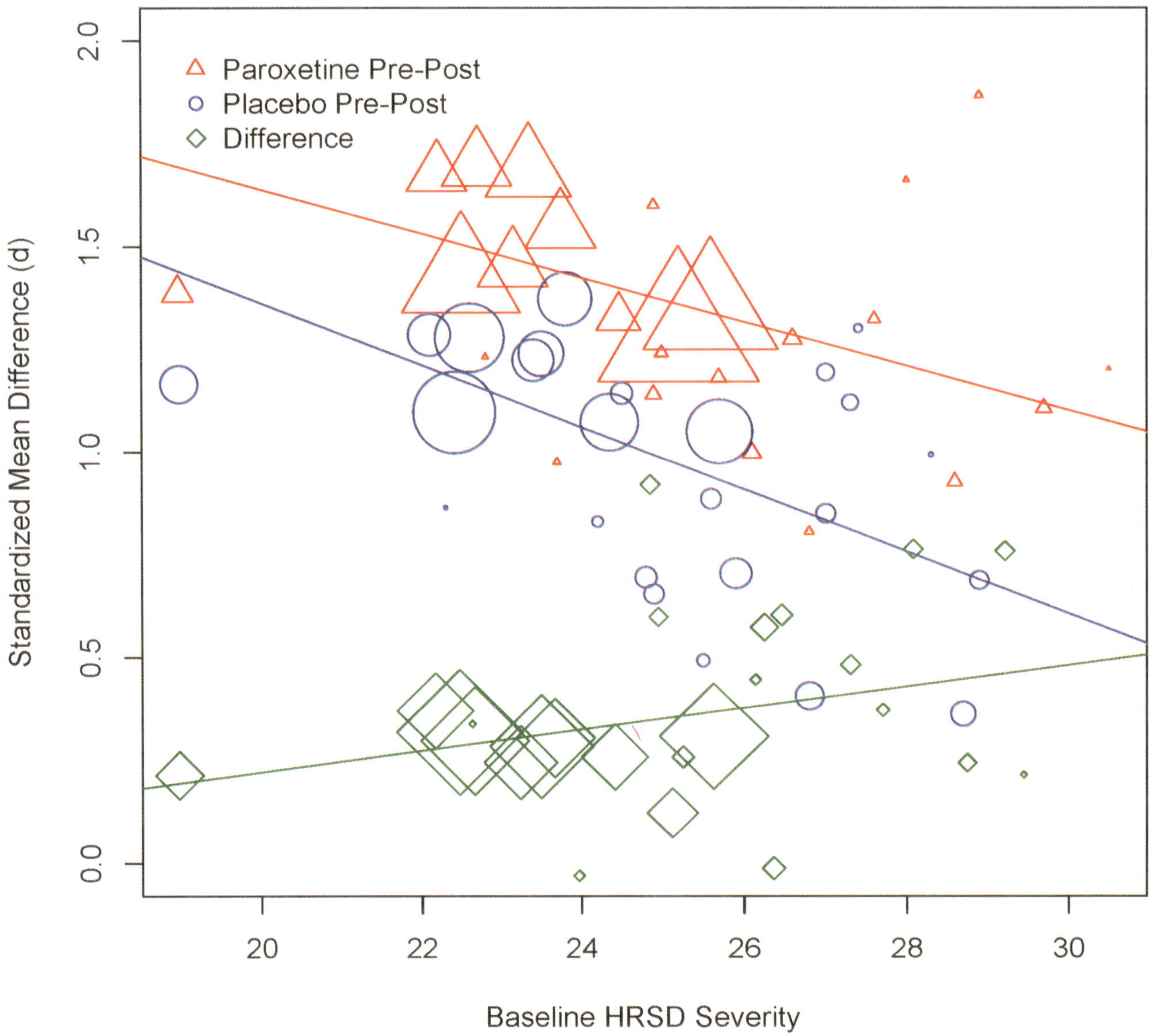

Figure 3. Baseline severity of depression and the mean change on the Hamilton Rating Scale for Depression (HRSD). The size of the marker reflects the relative weight of the study in the meta-analysis.

difference between paroxetine and placebo in the current analyses fell short of clinical significance for the treatment of both anxiety and depression.

The NICE criteria have been criticized for being arbitrary and lacking empirical justification [49]. However, a recent analysis of raw data from 43 antidepressant trials [50] compared HRSD change scores with clinician ratings of improvement on the Clinical Global Impressions Scale (CGI) [51] to establish the clinical relevance of HRSD scores. They found that change of three points or less on the HRSD corresponded to a clinician rating of "No Change" on the CGI. That is, changes of three points or less did not correspond to a clinically detectable change according to this clinician-rated measure. Thus, the drug-placebo differences that have been observed in the current and previous antidepressant meta-analyses [7,28], while statistically significant, appear to be of marginal clinical significance.

These findings have important clinical implications. The obvious alternative for the treatment of both anxiety and depression is psychotherapy intervention. However, direct comparisons of acute phase treatment for pharmacotherapy and psychotherapy in the treatment of major depression generally have yielded no significant differences between the treatment modalities [52–54]. Fewer clinical trials have directly compared antidepressants and psychotherapy in the treatment of anxiety disorders, although the available literature indicates similar comparability between antidepressants and psychotherapy. For example, one study [55] found that that acute phase cognitive-behavioral therapy yields comparable efficacy to imipramine in the treatment of panic disorder. Another study [56] found comparable 12-week efficacy between sertraline and cognitive-behavioral therapy in the treatment of childhood anxiety disorders. Overall, antidepressants, psychotherapy, and placebo all yield substantial changes in symptomatology, and are superior to no-treatment control groups [9]. Thus, in terms of treatment, the specific type of intervention may be less important than simply getting patients involved in some sort of active therapy program [53].

Table 5. Moderator effects in trials examining change on the Hamilton Rating Scale for Depression.

Pre- vs. Post-Approval		Effect Size	95% CI	Q(1)	p
Paroxetine - Placebo	Pre-Approval	0.41	[0.30, 0.53]	3.27	.071
	Post-Approval	0.29	[0.22, 0.36]		
Paroxetine	Pre-Approval	1.24	[1.15, 1.33]	14.43	<.001
	Post-Approval	1.45	[1.39, 1.50]		
Placebo	Pre-Approval	0.77	[0.67, 0.87]	35.01	<.001
	Post-Approval	1.14	[1.07, 1.21]		
Publication Status		**Effect Size**	**95% CI**	**Q(1)**	**p**
Paroxetine - Placebo	Published	0.36	[0.27, 0.44]	1.50	.221
	Unpublished	0.28	[0.20, 0.37]		
Paroxetine	Published	1.41	[1.35, 1.48]	1.45	.229
	Unpublished	1.35	[1.28, 1.43]		
Placebo	Published	0.99	[0.91, 1.07]	1.46	.227
	Unpublished	1.06	[0.98, 1.15]		

Pre-approval and Post-approval refer to whether the trial was included as part of the original approval submission to the FDA ($k = 16$) or whether it was conducted following FDA approval in 1991 or later ($k = 11$).

When given two seemingly equivalent alternatives with regard to symptom reduction, the decision may come down to patient preference and to the safety profile associated with the treatment. A meta-analysis of patient preferences when given the choice between psychological and pharmacologic treatment [57] revealed that 75% of patients prefer psychological intervention across 30 studies comprising individuals seeking treatment for depression or anxiety disorders. Paroxetine and other SSRIs have also been associated with a number of adverse events during treatment. Greater than 70% of patients report treatment-emergent symptoms of sexual dysfunction including reduced desire, arousal, and/or orgasm dysfunction, compared to less than 10% of individuals who received placebo [58]. Other adverse reported effects include drowsiness and weight gain, observed in greater than 7% of patients taking SSRIs [59]. Infrequent but severe symptoms such as serotonin syndrome [60] and increased suicidal ideation in younger adults [61,62] have also been reported. Additionally, abrupt withdrawal can result in a discontinuation syndrome in 66% of patients taking paroxetine, including symptoms of dizziness, worsened mood, agitation, headache, and nausea [63]. It is also notable that the frequency of adverse events many be underestimated in the clinical literature, as patients with depression are far more likely to self-report side effects on questionnaires than report them to physicians as is typical during clinical trials [64].

Although meta-analyses have indicated comparable efficacy between antidepressants and psychotherapy during acute stage treatment, their comparability is not as clear for long-term treatment. One study [54] found that individuals who had received "bona fide" psychotherapy from trained professionals displayed greater symptom reduction compared to those who had received SSRI treatment at post-acute phase follow-up ranging from 18 to 40 weeks ($d = 0.29$, $k = 6$). Another meta-analysis [52] of long-term naturalistic follow-up between individuals who were randomized to either acute-phase pharmacotherapy or psychotherapy in the treatment of depression across 11 studies revealed an advantage for psychotherapy at an average follow-up length of 15 months. Moreover, length of follow-up was a significant moderator such that the advantage of psychotherapy over medication was superior at longer follow-up intervals. The authors suggest that psychotherapy offers a "prophylactic effect" resulting in its long-term superiority over medications [52]. In an additional analysis of nine studies, Imel et al. [52] demonstrated that acute-phase discontinued psychotherapy was as efficacious as continued pharmacotherapy at an average follow-up interval of 14 months. That is, short-term psychotherapy (between 7 and 24 sessions) provided an equivalent long-term benefit to continuous medication usage. These findings can help to explain why antidepressants are frequently used for chronic treatment; more than 60% of individuals who take antidepressants have done so for longer than 2 years, and greater than 30% use them for 5 years or more [65]. In sum, the drawbacks to antidepressant usage and their modest benefit compared to placebo should be seriously considered before they are chosen as the primary treatment for depression or anxiety.

A limitation of the current work is that the trial database was limited to studies sponsored by GlaxoSmithKline, and does not include any additional trials that may have been conducted by independent researchers. Additionally, it is possible that GlaxoSmithKline omitted some of the outcome indices from the trial summaries posted online. A further limitation of the current analysis is that baseline severity and change were evaluated with the mean values for each group. An analysis including baseline values and response at the individual patient level would afford more power in determining a more precise estimate for the relative benefit of paroxetine over placebo at differing levels of baseline severity. The standard result summaries provided by the GlaxoSmithKline Clinical Trial Register provide baseline values and change scores only at the group level. These result summary documents also provided limited information regarding the ways in which the trials were conducted, which hindered our ability to conduct a thorough analysis for study quality. However, it appears that clinical trial sponsors are recognizing the importance of the availability of patient-level data. Several sponsors, including GlaxoSmithKline, have committed to posting patient-level study results online at Clinical Study Data Request [66]. According to

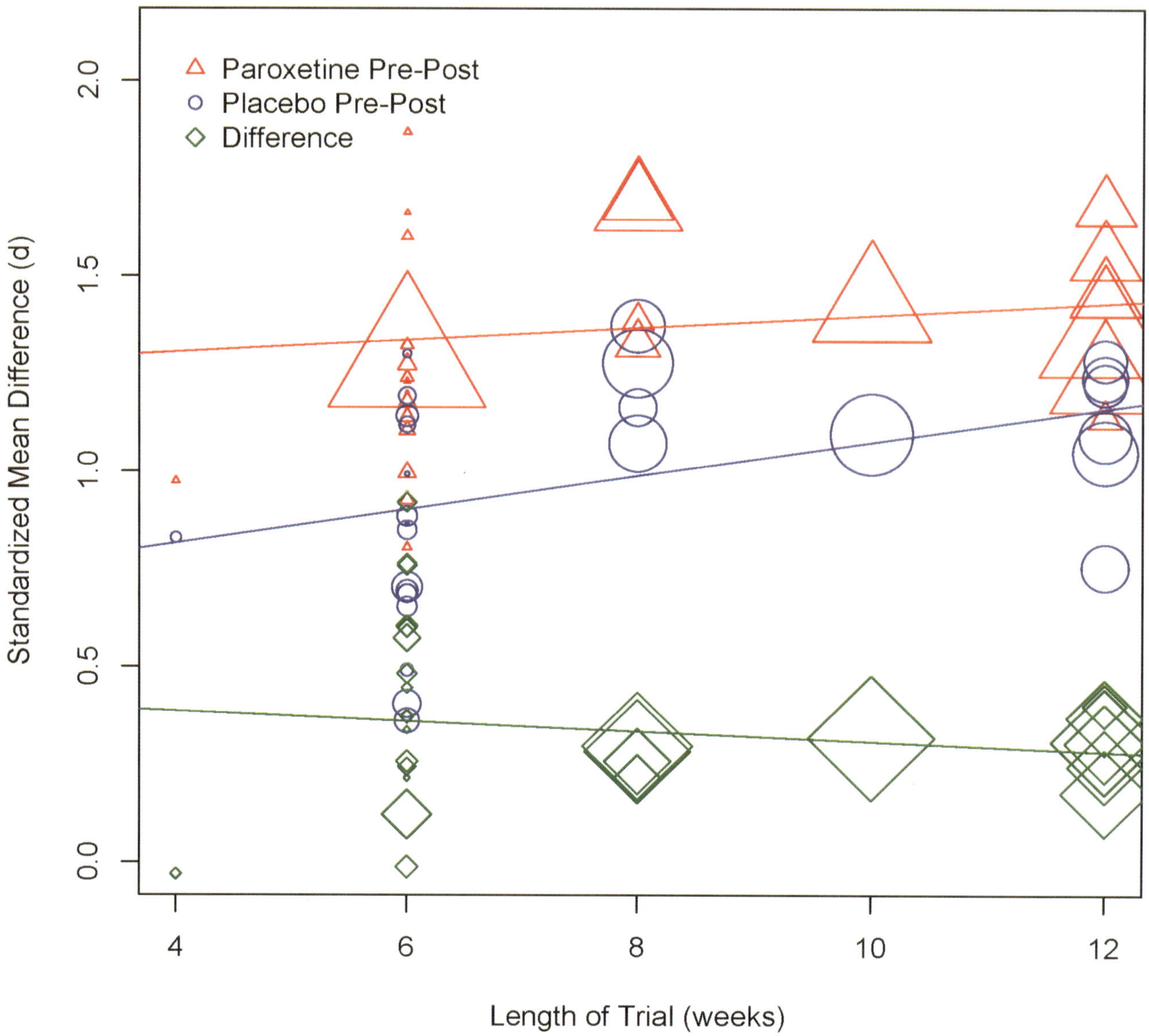

Figure 4. Trial duration (in weeks) and the mean change on the Hamilton Rating Scale for Depression (HRSD). The size of the marker reflects the relative weight of the study in the meta-analysis.

this site, GlaxoSmithKline plans to have data for all studies conducted after December 2000 freely available some time in 2015, with further studies available upon request. This site may be a valuable resource for future meta-analyses of drug efficacy.

A recent study conducted a patient-level analysis examining the relationship between baseline severity and antidepressant efficacy in the treatment of depression [39]. This study analyzed individuals from six double-blind, placebo-controlled studies of paroxetine and imipramine and found that the drug-placebo difference was greater than three points on the HRSD only at baseline severity levels of 25 and above. In fact, for individuals with mild or moderate depression (HRSD ≤ 18), the drug benefit was less than one point on the HRSD. This finding is concerning given that among Americans aged 12 years or older, approximately 19% and 28% of individuals with mild and moderate depression, respectively, take antidepressants [65].

In conclusion, paroxetine provides only a modest benefit over placebo in treating symptoms of anxiety based on the available evidence. In addition, the current study supports previous work [7] indicating that paroxetine treatment presents only a modest benefit over placebo in the treatment of depression.

Supporting Information

Checklist S1 PRISMA checklist.

Figure S1 Baseline severity of anxiety and the mean change on the Hamilton Rating Scale for Anxiety (HRSA). The size of the marker reflects the relative weight of the study in the meta-analysis. Random effects assumptions were used in the analyses. The relationship between baseline severity and effect size was marginally significant for paroxetine ($p = .069$) and statistically significant for placebo ($p = .020$), but not for the difference between paroxetine over placebo ($p = .401$).

Figure S2 Baseline severity of depression and the mean change on the Hamilton Rating Scale for Depression (HRSD). The size of the marker reflects the relative weight of the study in the meta-analysis. Random effects assumptions were used in the analyses. The relationship between baseline severity and effect size was statistically significant for paroxetine ($p = .029$) and for placebo ($p = .004$), but not for the difference between paroxetine over placebo ($p = .094$).

Figure S3 Trial duration (in weeks) and the mean change on the Hamilton Rating Scale for Depression (HRSD). The size of the marker reflects the relative weight of the study in the meta-analysis. Random effects assumptions were used in the analyses. The relationship between trial length and effect size was not statistically significant for paroxetine ($p = .126$), but was statistically significant for placebo ($p = .017$). The relationship was not statistically significant for the difference between paroxetine over placebo ($p = .297$).

Results S1 Contains Table S1 and Table S2.

Author Contributions

Conceived and designed the experiments: MAS AML BBB ERG IK. Performed the experiments: MAS AML. Analyzed the data: MAS AML BBB ERG IK. Wrote the paper: MAS AML BBB ERG IK.

References

1. National Center for Health Statistics (2013) Health, United States, 2012: With special feature on emergency care. Hyattsville, MD: Centers for Disease Control and Prevention. 489 p.
2. Baldwin D, Woods R, Lawson R, Taylor D (2011) Efficacy of drug treatments for generalised anxiety disorder: Systematic review and meta-analysis. BMJ 10.1136/bmj.d1199.
3. Ravindran LN, Stein MB (2010) The pharmacologic treatment of anxiety disorders: A review of progress. J Clin Psychiatry 10.4088/JCP.10r06218blu.
4. Melander H, Ahlqvist-Rastad J, Meijer G, Beermann B (2003) Evidence b(i)ased medicine–selective reporting from studies sponsored by pharmaceutical industry: Review of studies in new drug applications. BMJ 10.1136/bmj.326.7400.1171.
5. Turner EH, Matthews AM, Linardatos E, Tell RA, Rosenthal R (2008) Selective publication of antidepressant trials and its influence on apparent efficacy. N Engl J Med 10.1056/NEJMsa065779.
6. Center for Drug Evaluation and Research (1996) Guidance for industry: Guideline for the format and content of the summary for new drug and antibiotic applications. Rockville, MD: U.S. Department of Health, Education, and Welfare. Food and Drug Administration. Available: http://www.fda.gov/downloads/Drugs/GuidanceComplianceRegulatoryInformation/Guidances/ucm072058.pdf. Accessed 31 October 2013.
7. Kirsch I, Deacon BJ, Huedo-Medina TB, Scoboria A, Moore TJ, et al. (2008) Initial severity and antidepressant benefits: A meta-analysis of data submitted to the Food and Drug Administration. PLoS Med 10.1371/journal.pmed.0050045.
8. Kirsch I, Moore TJ, Scoboria A, Nicholls SS (2002) The emperor's new drugs: An analysis of antidepressant medication data submitted to the US Food and Drug Administration. Prevention & Treatment 10.1037/1522-3736.5.1.523a.
9. Kirsch I, Sapirstein G (1998) Listening to Prozac but hearing placebo: A meta-analysis of antidepressant medication. Prevention and Treatment 10.1037/1522-3736.1.1.12a.
10. Harris G (2004) Maker of Paxil to release all trial results. New York: New York Times. Available: http://www.nytimes.com/2004/08/26/business/26CND-DRUG.html. Accessed 31 October 2013.
11. Meier B (2004) Glaxo begins posting drug trial results. New York: New York Times. Available: http://www.nytimes.com/2004/09/01/business/01registry.html?_r=0. Accessed 31 October 2013.
12. Gartlehner G, Hansen RA, Morgan LC, Thaler K, Lux L, et al. (2011) Comparative benefits and harms of second-generation antidepressants for treating major depressive disorder: An updated meta-analysis. Ann Intern Med 10.7326/0003-4819-155-11-201112060-00009.
13. Baldwin D, Bobes J, Stein DJ, Scharwachter I, Faure M (1999) Paroxetine in social phobia/social anxiety disorder. Randomised, double-blind, placebo-controlled study. Paroxetine Study Group. Br J Psychiatry 10.1192/bjp.175.2.120.
14. Ballenger JC, Wheadon DE, Steiner M, Bushnell W, Gergel IP (1998) Double-blind, fixed-dose, placebo-controlled study of paroxetine in the treatment of panic disorder. Am J Psychiatry 155: 36–42.
15. Lecrubier Y, Bakker A, Dunbar G, Judge R (1997) A comparison of paroxetine, clomipramine and placebo in the treatment of panic disorder. Collaborative Paroxetine Panic Study Investigators. Acta Psychiatr Scand 10.1111/j.1600-0447.1997.tb00388.x.
16. Lepola U, Bergtholdt B, St Lambert J, Davy KL, Ruggiero L (2004) Controlled-release paroxetine in the treatment of patients with social anxiety disorder. J Clin Psychiatry 65: 222–229.
17. Liebowitz MR, Stein MB, Tancer M, Carpenter D, Oakes R, et al. (2002) A randomized, double-blind, fixed-dose comparison of paroxetine and placebo in the treatment of generalized social anxiety disorder. J Clin Psychiatry 10.4088/JCP.v63n0113.
18. Oehrberg S, Christiansen PE, Behnke K, Borup AL, Severin B, et al. (1995) Paroxetine in the treatment of panic disorder. A randomised, double-blind, placebo-controlled study. Br J Psychiatry 10.1192/bjp.167.3.374.
19. Pollack MH, Zaninelli R, Goddard A, McCafferty JP, Bellew KM, et al. (2001) Paroxetine in the treatment of generalized anxiety disorder: Results of a placebo-controlled, flexible-dosage trial. J Clin Psychiatry 62: 350–357.
20. Rickels K, Zaninelli R, McCafferty J, Bellew K, Iyengar M, et al. (2003) Paroxetine treatment of generalized anxiety disorder: A double-blind, placebo-controlled study. Am J Psychiatry 10.1176/appi.ajp.160.4.749.
21. Sheehan DV, Burnham DB, Iyengar MK, Perera P (2005) Efficacy and tolerability of controlled-release paroxetine in the treatment of panic disorder. J Clin Psychiatry 66: 33–40.
22. Stein MB, Liebowitz MR, Lydiard RB, Pitts CD, Bushnell W, et al. (1998) Paroxetine treatment of generalized social phobia (social anxiety disorder): A randomized controlled trial. JAMA 10.1001/jama.280.8.708.
23. Wagner KD, Berard R, Stein MB, Wetherhold E, Carpenter DJ, et al. (2004) A multicenter, randomized, double-blind, placebo-controlled trial of paroxetine in children and adolescents with social anxiety disorder. Arch Gen Psychiatry 10.1001/archpsyc.61.11.1153.
24. GlaxoSmithKline (2013) Paxil Medication Guide. Research Triangle Park, NC: GlaxoSmithKline. 49 p.
25. Mitte K (2005) A meta-analysis of the efficacy of psycho- and pharmacotherapy in panic disorder with and without agoraphobia. J Affect Disord 10.1016/j.jad.2005.05.003.
26. Otto MW, Tuby KS, Gould RA, McLean RY, Pollack MH (2001) An effect-size analysis of the relative efficacy and tolerability of serotonin selective reuptake inhibitors for panic disorder. Am J Psychiatry 158: 1989–1992.
27. Hamilton M (1960) A rating scale for depression. J Neurol Neurosurg Psychiatry 10.1136/jnnp.23.1.56.
28. Khin NA, Chen YF, Yang Y, Yang P, Laughren TP (2011) Exploratory analyses of efficacy data from major depressive disorder trials submitted to the US Food and Drug Administration in support of new drug applications. J Clin Psychiatry 10.4088/JCP.10m06191.
29. Hamilton M (1959) The assessment of anxiety states by rating. Br J Med Psychol 10.1111/j.2044-8341.1959.tb00467.x.
30. GlaxoSmithKline (2014) GSK Clinical Study Register. Brentford, UK: GlaxoSmithKline. Available: http://www.gsk-clinicalstudyregister.com. Accessed 10 February 2014.
31. Freedom of Information Act (FOIA) (1994 & Supp. II 1996) Freedom of Information Act (FOIA). 5 US Congress. 552.
32. Lipsey MW, Wilson DB (2001) Practical meta-analysis (applied social research methods). Thousand Oaks, CA: Sage Publications.
33. Gibbons RD, Hedeker DR, Davis JM (1993) Estimation of effect size from a series of experiments involving paired comparisons. Journal of Educational and Behavioral Statistics 10.2307/1165136.
34. Hedges LV, Olkin I (1985) Statistical methods for meta-analysis. New York, NY: Academic Press. 369 p.
35. Higgins JPT, Thompson SG (2003) Measuring inconsistency in meta-analyses. BMJ 10.1136/bmj.327.7414.557.
36. Higgins JP, Thompson SG (2002) Quantifying heterogeneity in a meta-analysis. Stat Med 10.1002/sim.1186.
37. Bond CF Jr, Wiitala WL, Richard FD (2003) Meta-analysis of raw mean differences. Psychol Methods 10.1037/1082-989X.8.4.406.
38. Khan A, Kolts RL, Thase ME, Krishnan KR, Brown W (2004) Research design features and patient characteristics associated with the outcome of antidepressant clinical trials. Am J Psychiatry 10.1176/appi.ajp.161.11.2045.
39. Fournier JC, DeRubeis RJ, Hollon SD, Dimidjian S, Amsterdam JD, et al. (2010) Antidepressant drug effects and depression severity: A patient-level meta-analysis. JAMA 10.1001/jama.2009.1943.
40. Montgomery SA, Kasper S (2007) Severe depression and antidepressants: Focus on a pooled analysis of placebo-controlled studies on agomelatine. Int Clin Psychopharmacol 10.1097/YIC.0b013e3280c56b13.
41. American Psychiatric Association Task Force for the Handbook of Psychiatric Measures (2000) Handbook of Psychiatric Measures. Washington, DC: American Psychiatric Publishing. 864 p.

42. National Center for Health & Clinical Excellence (2010) Depression: The treatment and management of depression in adults (updated edition). London: The British Psychological Society and The Royal College of Psychiatrists. 705 p.
43. National Institute for Clinical Excellence (2004) Depression: Management of depression in primary and secondary care. London: National Institute for Clinical Excellence. 670 p.
44. Hauser W, Bartram-Wunn E, Bartram C, Reinecke H, Tolle T (2011) Systematic review: Placebo response in drug trials of fibromyalgia syndrome and painful peripheral diabetic neuropathy-magnitude and patient-related predictors. Pain 10.1016/j.pain.2011.01.050.
45. Patel SM, Stason WB, Legedza A, Ock SM, Kaptchuk TJ, et al. (2005) The placebo effect in irritable bowel syndrome trials: A meta-analysis. Neurogastroenterol Motil 10.1111/j.1365-2982.2005.00650.x.
46. Dorn SD, Kaptchuk TJ, Park JB, Nguyen LT, Canenguez K, et al. (2007) A meta-analysis of the placebo response in complementary and alternative medicine trials of irritable bowel syndrome. Neurogastroenterol Motil 10.1111/j.1365-2982.2007.00937.x.
47. Cho HJ, Hotopf M, Wessely S (2005) The placebo response in the treatment of chronic fatigue syndrome: A systematic review and meta-analysis. Psychosom Med 10.1097/01.psy.0000156969.76986.e0.
48. Kroenke K, West SL, Swindle R, Gilsenan A, Eckert GJ, et al. (2001) Similar effectiveness of paroxetine, fluoxetine, and sertraline in primary care: A randomized trial. JAMA 10.1001/jama.286.23.2947.
49. Moller HJ (2008) Isn't the efficacy of antidepressants clinically relevant? A critical comment on the results of the metaanalysis by Kirsch et al. 2008. Eur Arch Psychiatry Clin Neurosci 10.1007/s00406-008-0836-5.
50. Leucht S, Fennema H, Engel R, Kaspers-Janssen M, Lepping P, et al. (2013) What does the HAMD mean? J Affect Disord 10.1016/j.jad.2012.12.001.
51. Busner J, Targum SD (2007) The clinical global impressions scale: applying a research tool in clinical practice. Psychiatry (Edgmont) 4: 28–37.
52. Imel ZE, Malterer MB, McKay KM, Wampold BE (2008) A meta-analysis of psychotherapy and medication in unipolar depression and dysthymia. J Affect Disord 10.1016/j.jad.2008.03.018.
53. Khan A, Faucett J, Lichtenberg P, Kirsch I, Brown WA (2012) A systematic review of comparative efficacy of treatments and controls for depression. PLoS One 10.1371/journal.pone.0041778.
54. Spielmans GI, Berman MI, Usitalo AN (2011) Psychotherapy versus second-generation antidepressants in the treatment of depression: a meta-analysis. J Nerv Ment Dis 10.1097/NMD.0b013e31820caefb.
55. Barlow DH, Gorman JM, Shear MK, Woods SW (2000) Cognitive-behavioral therapy, imipramine, or their combination for panic disorder: A randomized controlled trial. JAMA 10.1001/jama.283.19.2529.
56. Walkup JT, Albano AM, Piacentini J, Birmaher B, Compton SN, et al. (2008) Cognitive behavioral therapy, sertraline, or a combination in childhood anxiety. N Engl J Med 10.1056/NEJMoa0804633.
57. McHugh RK, Whitton SW, Peckham AD, Welge JA, Otto MW (2013) Patient preference for psychological vs pharmacologic treatment of psychiatric disorders: a meta-analytic review. J Clin Psychiatry 10.4088/JCP.12r07757.
58. Serretti A, Chiesa A (2009) Treatment-emergent sexual dysfunction related to antidepressants: a meta-analysis. J Clin Psychopharmacol 10.1097/JCP.0b013e3181a5233f.
59. Cascade E, Kalali AH, Kennedy SH (2009) Real-World Data on SSRI Antidepressant Side Effects. Psychiatry (Edgmont) 6: 16–18.
60. Boyer EW, Shannon M (2005) The serotonin syndrome. N Engl J Med 10.1056/NEJMra041867.
61. Carpenter DJ, Fong R, Kraus JE, Davies JT, Moore C, et al. (2011) Meta-analysis of efficacy and treatment-emergent suicidality in adults by psychiatric indication and age subgroup following initiation of paroxetine therapy: A complete set of randomized placebo-controlled trials. J Clin Psychiatry 10.4088/JCP.08m04927blu.
62. Stone M, Laughren T, Jones ML, Levenson M, Holland PC, et al. (2009) Risk of suicidality in clinical trials of antidepressants in adults: analysis of proprietary data submitted to US Food and Drug Administration. BMJ 10.1136/bmj.b2880.
63. Rosenbaum JF, Fava M, Hoog SL, Ascroft RC, Krebs WB (1998) Selective serotonin reuptake inhibitor discontinuation syndrome: a randomized clinical trial. Biol Psychiatry 10.1016/S0006-3223(98)00126-7.
64. Zimmerman M, Galione JN, Attiullah N, Friedman M, Toba C, et al. (2010) Underrecognition of clinically significant side effects in depressed outpatients. J Clin Psychiatry 10.4088/JCP.08m04978blu.
65. Pratt LA, Brody DJ, Gu Q (2011) Antidepressant use in persons aged 12 and over: United States, 2005–2008. NCHS Data Brief 76: 1–8.
66. ideaPoint (2014) Clinical Study Data Request Site. Quincy, MA: ideaPoint, Inc. Available: https://clinicalstudydatarequest.com. Accessed 9 May 2014.
67. Rickels K, Amsterdam J, Clary C, Fox I, Schweizer E, et al. (1989) A placebo-controlled, double-blind, clinical trial of paroxetine in depressed outpatients. Acta Psychiatr Scand Suppl doi:10.1111/j.1600-0447.1989.tb07188.x.
68. Rickels K, Amsterdam J, Clary C, Fox I, Schweizer E, et al. (1992) The efficacy and safety of paroxetine compared with placebo in outpatients with major depression. J Clin Psychiatry 53(Suppl): 30–32.
69. Claghorn J (1992) A double-blind comparison of paroxetine and placebo in the treatment of depressed outpatients. Int Clin Psychopharmacol 10.1097/00004850-199206004-00006.
70. Claghorn JL (1992) The safety and efficacy of paroxetine compared with placebo in a double-blind trial of depressed outpatients. J Clin Psychiatry 53(Suppl): 33–35.
71. Smith WT, Glaudin V (1992) A placebo-controlled trial of paroxetine in the treatment of major depression. J Clin Psychiatry 53(Suppl): 36–39.
72. Kiev A (1992) A double-blind, placebo-controlled study of paroxetine in depressed outpatients. J Clin Psychiatry 53(Suppl): 27–29.
73. Feighner JP, Boyer WF (1989) Paroxetine in the treatment of depression: A comparison with imipramine and placebo. Acta Psychiatr Scand Suppl 10.1111/j.1600-0447.1989.tb07190.x.
74. Feighner JP, Boyer WF (1992) Paroxetine in the treatment of depression: A comparison with imipramine and placebo. J Clin Psychiatry 53(Suppl): 44–47.
75. Cohn JB, Crowder JE, Wilcox CS, Ryan PJ (1990) A placebo- and imipramine-controlled study of paroxetine. Psychopharmacol Bull 26: 185–189.
76. Cohn JB, Wilcox CS (1992) Paroxetine in major depression: A double-blind trial with imipramine and placebo. J Clin Psychiatry 53(Suppl): 52–56.
77. Shrivastava RK, Shrivastava SH, Overweg N, Blumhardt CL (1992) A double-blind comparison of paroxetine, imipramine, and placebo in major depression. J Clin Psychiatry 53(Suppl): 48–51.
78. Peselow ED, Filippi AM, Goodnick P, Barouche F, Fieve RR (1989) The short- and long-term efficacy of paroxetine HCl: A. Data from a 6-week double-blind parallel design trial vs. imipramine and placebo. Psychopharmacol Bull 25: 267–271.
79. Fabre LF (1992) A 6-week, double-blind trial of paroxetine, imipramine, and placebo in depressed outpatients. J Clin Psychiatry 53(Suppl): 40–43.
80. Dunner DL, Dunbar GC (1992) Optimal dose regimen for paroxetine. J Clin Psychiatry 53(Suppl): 21–26.
81. Miller SM, Naylor GJ, Murtagh M, Winslow G (1989) A double-blind comparison of paroxetine and placebo in the treatment of depressed patients in a psychiatric outpatient clinic. Acta Psychiatr Scand Suppl 10.1111/j.1600-0404.1989.tb01773.x.
82. Keller MB, Ryan ND, Strober M, Klein RG, Kutcher SP, et al. (2001) Efficacy of paroxetine in the treatment of adolescent major depression: A randomized, controlled trial. J Am Acad Child Adolesc Psychiatry 10.1097/00004583-200107000-00010.
83. Golden RN (2003) Efficacy and tolerability of controlled-release paroxetine. Psychopharmacol Bull (Suppl 1): 176–186.
84. Golden RN, Nemeroff CB, McSorley P, Pitts CD, Dube EM (2002) Efficacy and tolerability of controlled-release and immediate-release paroxetine in the treatment of depression. J Clin Psychiatry 63: 577–584.
85. Rapaport MH, Schneider LS, Dunner DL, Davies JT, Pitts CD (2003) Efficacy of controlled-release paroxetine in the treatment of late-life depression. J Clin Psychiatry 64: 1065–1074.
86. Trivedi MH, Pigotti TA, Perera P, Dillingham KE, Carfagno ML, et al. (2004) Effectiveness of low doses of paroxetine controlled release in the treatment of major depressive disorder. J Clin Psychiatry 65: 1356–1364.

Characteristics of Effective Collaborative Care for Treatment of Depression

Peter A. Coventry[1]*, Joanna L. Hudson[2], Evangelos Kontopantelis[3], Janine Archer[4], David A. Richards[5], Simon Gilbody[6], Karina Lovell[4], Chris Dickens[5], Linda Gask[1], Waquas Waheed[7], Peter Bower[3]

1 Collaboration for Leadership in Applied Health Research and Care, Centre for Primary Care and Manchester Academic Health Science Centre, University of Manchester, Manchester, United Kingdom, **2** Health Psychology Section, Psychology Department, Institute of Psychiatry, King's College London, London, United Kingdom, **3** NIHR School for Primary Care Research, Centre for Primary Care and Manchester Academic Health Science Centre, University of Manchester, Manchester, United Kingdom, **4** School of Nursing, Midwifery & Social Work, University of Manchester, Manchester, United Kingdom, **5** Institute of Health Service Research, University of Exeter Medical School, University of Exeter, Exeter, United Kingdom, **6** Mental Health Research Group, Department of Health Sciences and Hull York Medical School, University of York, York, United Kingdom, **7** Lancashire Care NHS Foundation Trust, Preston, United Kingdom

Abstract

Background: Collaborative care is a complex intervention based on chronic disease management models and is effective in the management of depression. However, there is still uncertainty about which components of collaborative care are effective. We used meta-regression to identify factors in collaborative care associated with improvement in patient outcomes (depressive symptoms) and the process of care (use of anti-depressant medication).

Methods and Findings: Systematic review with meta-regression. The Cochrane Collaboration Depression, Anxiety and Neurosis Group trials registers were searched from inception to 9th February 2012. An update was run in the CENTRAL trials database on 29th December 2013. Inclusion criteria were: randomised controlled trials of collaborative care for adults $\geq$18 years with a primary diagnosis of depression or mixed anxiety and depressive disorder. Random effects meta-regression was used to estimate regression coefficients with 95% confidence intervals (CIs) between study level covariates and depressive symptoms and relative risk (95% CI) and anti-depressant use. The association between anti-depressant use and improvement in depression was also explored. Seventy four trials were identified (85 comparisons, across 21,345 participants). Collaborative care that included psychological interventions predicted improvement in depression (β coefficient -0.11, 95% CI -0.20 to -0.01, $p=0.03$). Systematic identification of patients (relative risk 1.43, 95% CI 1.12 to 1.81, $p=0.004$) and the presence of a chronic physical condition (relative risk 1.32, 95% CI 1.05 to 1.65, $p=0.02$) predicted use of anti-depressant medication.

Conclusion: Trials of collaborative care that included psychological treatment, with or without anti-depressant medication, appeared to improve depression more than those without psychological treatment. Trials that used systematic methods to identify patients with depression and also trials that included patients with a chronic physical condition reported improved use of anti-depressant medication. However, these findings are limited by the observational nature of meta-regression, incomplete data reporting, and the use of study aggregates.

Editor: Phillipa J. Hay, University of Western Sydney, Australia

Funding: This study was funded by a Research and Capability Funding grant awarded by the NIHR Collaboration for Leadership in Applied Health Research and Care for Greater Manchester (ref:RCF_R10_PC). The funders had no role in study design, data collection and analysis, decision to publish, or preparation of the manuscript.

Competing Interests: The authors have been/are involved in the conduct of trials of collaborative care in the United Kingdom funded by the Medical Research Council and the National Institute for Health Research.

* Email: peter.a.coventry@manchester.ac.uk

Introduction

Major depressive disorder accounted for 8.2% of years living with disability in 2010, making it the second leading direct cause of global disease burden [1]. People with depression and a chronic physical disease have worse health status than people with depression alone or people with any combination of chronic physical disease without depression [2].

Significant advances have occurred in primary care in recent years to improve the management of chronic disease, principally by introducing structured disease management programmes that draw on the Chronic Care Model [3]. The chronic care model promotes a more proactive, planned and population-based approach to disease management and has been instrumental in transforming ambulatory care in primary care [4]. The concept and components of the chronic care model are fully specified here: http://www.improvingchroniccare.org/. Depression shares with other chronic diseases many features that can be addressed by the chronic care model, such as multiple recurrent episodes [5], where successful management hinges on regular monitoring, care coordination, enhancing providers' expertise, and supporting patients to self-manage. Interventions that include at least one component of the chronic care model have been shown to improve clinical outcomes and the process of care for people with chronic disease, including depression [6].

'Collaborative care' is the most promising chronic care model-based strategy for improving care of depression. While the make-up of collaborative care interventions for treatment of depression vary, they typically include a multi-professional approach to patient care, structured management, scheduled patient follow-ups, and enhanced inter-professional communication [7]. A recent Cochrane review that included 79 randomised controlled trials (RCTs) and 24,308 participants conclusively showed that collaborative care is more effective than usual care for both depression and anxiety after treatment, and up to two years later [8]. There is also ample evidence that these benefits are cost effective [9].

However, while some authors suggest that there is now sufficient evidence about effectiveness and that research should now shift to implementation [10], collaborative care is a complex intervention and there is significant variation in the exact nature of the intervention between trials, as well as differences in patient populations, contexts, comparators, and design. A number of these factors have already been shown to be related to estimates of effect: setting (i.e. country), recruitment of patients using systematic or population health approaches (e.g. disease registers), using case managers with a mental health background, and regular clinical supervision of case managers [11]. There has since been considerable international expansion of collaborative care outside of the United States and extension of this care model to populations with depression and chronic physical disease. We have therefore used meta-regression with a comprehensive and updated data set of randomised controlled trials of collaborative care to identify factors associated with improvement in patient outcome (i.e. depressive symptoms) and/or the process of care (i.e. anti-depressant use). The results will be used to distinguish which features of collaborative care effectively improve patient outcomes and/or the process of care and which do not.

Methods

This systematic review and meta-regression is reported in accordance with the Preferred Reporting Items for Systematic Reviews and Meta-Analyses Statement (see Figure 1 and Checklist S1) [12].

Information sources

The Cochrane Collaboration Depression, Anxiety and Neurosis Group (CC-DAN) trials registers (including both the references register and the studies register) were searched from inception to 9th February 2012. The CC-DAN registers include Randomised Controlled Trials indexed in MEDLINE, EMBASE, PsycINFO, CENTRAL, World Health Organisation's trials portal (ICTRP), Clinicaltrials.gov, and CINAHL. Details of the search strategy used can be found in Archer et al [8]. The CENTRAL search used in the Cochrane review by Archer et al [8] was updated on 29th December 2013 (see Methods S1 for search strategy). For the purposes of an update the comprehensive coverage of the CENTRAL database makes exhaustive searching of individual bibliographic databases unnecessary [13]. All reference lists of included studies and previously published reviews were checked.

Characteristics of collaborative care and conceptual model to be tested

For the purposes of this review we used a definition of collaborative care derived from a systematic review of complex interventions for managing depression in primary care [7]. Collaborative care consists of four key criteria: multi-professional approach to patient care, structured management, scheduled patient follow-ups, and enhanced inter-professional communication (Table 1).

A key innovation arising from collaborative care is the introduction of a non-medical case or care manager who works with a medical practitioner and under the supervision of a mental health specialist to deliver and coordinate psychological treatment, and to monitor progress with psychological and/or pharmacological treatment [14]. While chronic disease management interventions that include one or more features of patient or provider education, feedback, and reminders can lead to improved disease control and adherence to guidelines [15] enhanced roles in primary care for case managers are seen as central to the provision of effective and integrated interventions for depression [16]. Based on current understanding about how the intervention might work and based on previous knowledge about mechanisms of change and active ingredients of collaborative care we tested 10 factors (study covariates) that could potentially moderate patient and process outcomes (Table 2).

Eligibility criteria

Studies were included in this meta-analysis and meta-regression if they:

1) Were RCTs or clustered RCTs of collaborative care delivered in primary care settings or community settings. Primary care was defined as a person's first and ongoing contact point for health care [17].
2) Included adults over the age of 18 with a primary diagnosis of depression or mixed anxiety and depressive disorder according to clinical diagnosis or research assessment (observer interview or validated self-report measure). No restrictions on severity or chronicity of depression were made.
3) Compared the effectiveness of collaborative care with standard or enhanced usual care.

Standard usual care was defined as care routinely provided by primary care providers to patients with depression or mixed anxiety and depressive disorder. This could include onward referral to mental health teams or feedback on participants' depressive status if specified in the protocol.

Enhanced usual care was defined as care where any one or more of the following were present:

i. The patient received additional resources (i.e. educational leaflets, lists of locally available resources, letter from research team with self-help advice) OR the patient had access to enhanced care systems (i.e. consultation-liaison, enhanced referral systems to psychology services, case reviews between health professionals, equal contact time with a health professional, medication management, patient-primary care provider electronic messaging system, person-

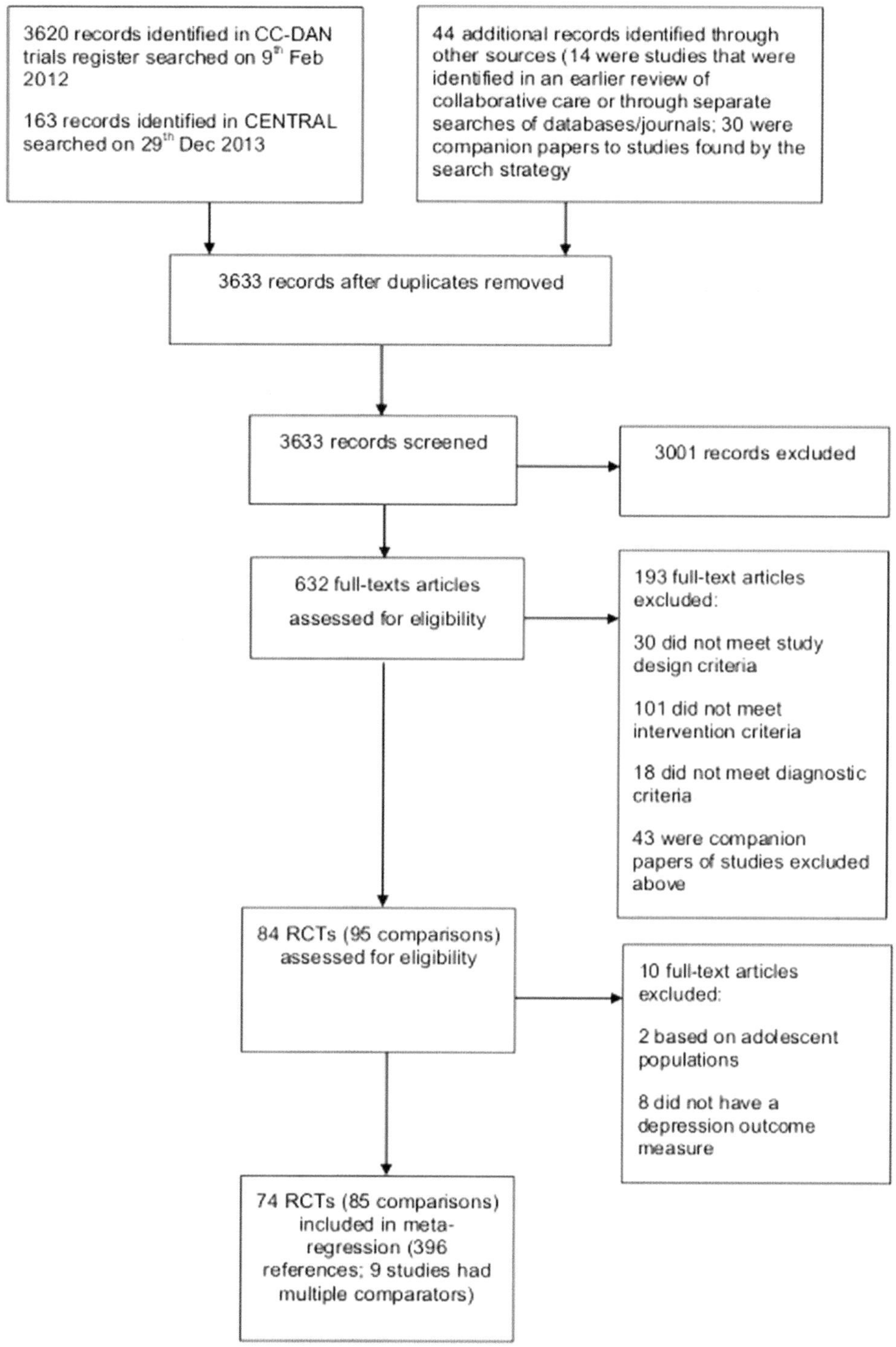

Figure 1. PRISMA Flow Diagram.

alised patient treatment plans from the principal investigator).

ii. Didactic training for the primary care provider.

iii. Primary care providers were supplied with manualised treatment algorithms or evidence based guidelines.

iv. Primary care providers received educational materials other than evidence based guidelines (e.g. educational DVD).

4) Measured change in self-reported or observer rated depression scores as a continuous or dichotomous measure (e.g. ≥ 50% decrease in symptom scores from baseline or remission)

AND/OR

Measured change in use of anti-depressant medication (e.g. proportion of patients taking medication or proportion of patients adhering appropriately to predefined criteria/guidelines), based on self-report or administrative records data.

Table 1. Key characteristics of collaborative care.

A multi-professional approach to patient care
A general practitioner (GP) or family physician and at least one other health professional (e.g. nurse, psychologist, psychiatrist, pharmacist) were involved with patient care, usually acting as a case or care manager to coordinate and/or deliver care for the depressed person
A structured management plan
Evidence based guidelines or treatment protocols. Interventions could include both pharmacological (e.g. antidepressant medication) and non-pharmacological interventions (e.g. patient screening, patient and provider education, counselling, cognitive behaviour therapy)
Scheduled patient follow-ups
An organised approach to patient follow-up that could include one or more scheduled telephone or in-person follow-up appointments to provide specific interventions, facilitate treatment adherence, or monitor symptoms or adverse effects
Enhanced inter-professional communication
Mechanisms to facilitate communication between professionals caring for the depressed person: team meetings, case-conferences, individual consultation/supervision, shared medical records, patient-specific written or verbal feedback between care-givers

Study selection

We identified eligible studies included in the Cochrane review of collaborative care for depression and anxiety [8] and also from eligible studies identified by the updated search of the CENTRAL trials database. Three authors (JH, PB, PC) independently screened non-overlapping subsets of studies against the inclusion criteria for this meta-regression.

Data extraction

Intervention content. Characteristics of collaborative and usual care intervention groups were independently extracted verbatim and coded using a standardised data extraction form and coding manual, specifically tailored to the content of collaborative care interventions (Methods S2).

Patient and process outcomes. The primary patient outcome was reduction in depressive symptoms as measured by observer or patient self-report. Outcomes were extracted for all reported follow-up time points (e.g. six months, twelve months). Most studies reported outcomes at six months follow-up and our analysis was therefore restricted to this time point to maximise both consistency and the number of studies included in the meta-regression. If eligible studies ($n = 9$) reported outcomes at follow-ups beyond six months we used short term follow-up data closest in time to six months. Where the studies reported two comparisons versus a control group, sample sizes were halved to avoid double counting.

To allow both continuous and dichotomous outcomes to be included in the same meta-regression, we translated dichotomous outcomes into standardised mean differences and standard errors using the *metaeff* Stata command [18].

Collaborative care improves the process of depression care, and use of anti-depressant medications may be a key driver for depressive outcomes. Anti-depressant use as a dichotomous process outcome was extracted; we used risk ratios with log-transformations applied [19].

When studies applied cluster randomisation procedures we accounted for increased Type I error rates by applying the "effective sample sizes" procedure outlined in the Cochrane Handbook [20]. An intraclass correlation coefficient (ICC) of 0.02 [21] was used and sensitivity analyses were performed to explore the impact of adjustments for clustering using an ICC of 0.00 and 0.05 [22]. We also used study sample sizes as a proxy for publication bias [23]. We explored using meta-regression whether there was an inverse relationship between study sample sizes and reported effect sizes. Allocation concealment, an important feature of trials known to reduce risk of bias, was assessed using a binary measure [24].

Analysis

Stata's (Version 12 for Windows) *metan* [25] and *metareg* [26] commands were used to calculate an overall effect size estimate of collaborative care on depressive symptoms and anti-depressant medication use. Consistent with the recommendations of Thompson and Higgins [27], ten covariates were hypothesised to have an effect on these outcomes *a priori* (See Table 2) [11]. In contrast to Bower et al [11] we revised the conceptualisation of enhanced usual care to include an ordinal measure of enhanced usual care in place of primary care provider training (See Methods S2 for the coding and scoring of enhanced usual care).

We used a DerSimonian-Laird [28] random-effects model to calculate the overall effect of collaborative care, accounting for estimated heterogeneity. To quantify the estimated heterogeneity we used the I^2 index, which represents the percentage of estimated between-study variability in the total variability [29]. By convention I^2 values of 25% are considered low, 50% moderate, and 75% high [20]. The main analysis used random-effects meta-regression to estimate a regression coefficient with 95% CIs between study level covariates and outcomes for:

i) Meta-regression model one (multivariable): study level covariates as predictors of depressive symptoms.
ii) Meta-regression model two (multivariable): study level covariates as predictors of anti-depressant use.
iii) Meta-regression model three (univariable; mechanisms of change): anti-depressant use as a predictor of depressive symptoms. This model tested whether use of anti-depressant medication predicted the treatment effect on depressive symptoms.

We explored the potential for confounding or collinearity across the 10 covariates using logistic regression analyses to perform pairwise comparisons. Shared variance between each pair was low (≤ 0.14), indicating that there is a very small risk of measured confounding or collinearity in our measured variables. To retain statistical power we identified covariates for testing in the multivariable meta-regression models by initially performing a series of separate univariable meta-regression analyses, using a significance criterion of $p \leq 0.10$. The $p \leq 0.10$ threshold was chosen to avoid prematurely discounting potentially important

Table 2. Study level covariates (N = 85 comparisons).

Characteristic	**Description**	**N**
Country		
US	Study setting	60
Non-US	Study setting	25
Recruitment method		
Systematic identification	Patients were referred into the study if they were: i) identified from a clinical database as having depression or ii) screened positive for depression on an outcome measure and/or diagnostic clinical interview	69
Referral by clinicians	Patients were referred into the study by their clinician	16
Patient sample		
Anti-depressant medication NOT inclusion criteria	Participants did not have to be on or willing to take anti-depressant medication as part of the study's inclusion criteria	62
Anti-depressant medication part of inclusion criteria	Participants had to be currently taking or willing to take anti-depressant medication as part of the study's inclusion criteria	23
Chronic physical health condition		
Present	Participants with a chronic physical health condition were actively recruited as part of the study's inclusion criteria	19
Absent	Participants with a chronic physical health condition were NOT actively recruited as part of the study's inclusion criteria	66
Case manager professional background		
Mental health professional	Trained in mental health disciplines outside of the context of the trial (i.e. psychologist, psychiatric nurse, social worker)	47
Non-mental health professional	No extensive training in mental health other than that provided by the trial	38
Intervention content		
Medication management	Intervention included a medication management plan to ensure optimal levels of adherence to pharmacotherapy. This does not represent degree of adherence (i.e. anti-depressant use).	38
Psychological or both	Intervention included a recognised psychological treatment model (i.e. behavioural activation, problem solving) either on its own or combined with medication.	47
Number of sessions		
Continuous variable	Based on number of planned sessions in the first six months. If the number of sessions differed based on the treatment modality offered (i.e. participants could choose between medication management or psychological therapy) then a mean score was calculated.	
Supervision frequency		
Ad hoc	No regular patterns of supervision.	29
Scheduled	Supervision occurred on a regular basis (i.e. weekly).	52
Not applicable	Applies to studies whose collaborative care intervention included only the primary care provider but the case manager was a certified mental health practitioner (e.g. psychiatrist, psychologist, psychotherapist).	4
Enhanced usual care		
Ordinal variable (based on summed score, 0 4)	See description provided in Methods S2	
Allocation concealment		
Low risk of bias	Coded according to Cochrane risk of bias tool	39
High risk of bias	Coded according to Cochrane risk of bias tool	4

explanatory variables. Table 2 summarises all ten study level covariates included in both meta-regression models one and two.

Results

Characteristics of included studies

Seventy four trials met our inclusion criteria for the meta-regression (including 85 relevant comparisons, across 21,345 participants); 84 comparisons had data on depressive symptoms (across 21,284 participants), and 59 comparisons had data on anti-depressant use (across, 14, 465 participants). See Figure 1.

Of the 85 comparisons included in the meta-regression 25 (29%) were conducted outside the United States; only 4% were conducted in low to middle income countries (Table S1). Nineteen (22%) comparisons specifically recruited patients with chronic physical disease. As stated in the methods section trials had to meet the four criteria for collaborative care to be included in the review. Key factors that differentiated the type of interventions tested in the meta-regression were case manager background and content of the structured management plan. In 47 (55%) comparisons the case manager was a mental health practitioner, and in 38 (45%) comparisons case managers were drawn from a variety of non-mental health backgrounds. In 39 (46%) comparisons the

Table 3. Characteristics of collaborative care.

Author	Multi-professional approach to patient care		Structured management plan	Number of scheduled follow-ups	Enhanced inter professional communication	
	Medical professional	Case manager background			CM liaison with PCP	Supervision frequency
Adler 2004	Doctor	Non-mental health practitioner	Medication management	6	Shared note system	Scheduled
Araya 2003	Doctor	Mental health practitioner	Both	9	Shared note system	Ad hoc
Bartels 2004	Doctor	Mental health practitioner	Medication management	Not reported	Multiple methods	Not reported
Blanchard 1995	Doctor	Mental health practitioner	Both	12	Verbal	Ad hoc
Bogner 2008	Mixed	Mental health practitioner	Medication management	5	Liaison method	Scheduled
Bogner 2010	Mixed	Non-mental health practitioner	Medication management	5	Liaison method	Scheduled
Bogner 2012	Doctor	Non-mental health practitioner	Medication management	5	Verbal	Ad hoc
Bruce 2004	Doctor	Mental health practitioner	Both	15	Liaison method	Scheduled
Buszewicz 2011	Doctor	Non-mental health practitioner	Both	4	Verbal	Ad hoc
Capoccia 2004	Doctor	non-mental health practitioner	Medication management	10	Shared note system	Scheduled
Chaney 2011	Doctor	Non-mental health practitioner	Medication management	5	Multiple methods	Scheduled
Chew-Graham 2007	Doctor	Mental health practitioner	Both	11	Multiple methods	Scheduled
Ciechanowski 2004	Doctor	Mental health practitioner	Psychological therapy	9	Other	Scheduled
Ciechanowski 2010	Specialist	Mental health practitioner	Psychological therapy	9	Other	Scheduled
Cole 2006	Doctor	Non-mental health practitioner	Both	24	Liaison method	Ad hoc
Datto 2003	Doctor	Mental health practitioner	Medication management	6	Written communication	Scheduled
Davidson 2013	Doctor	Mental health practitioner	Both	11	Verbal	Scheduled
Dietrich 2004	Doctor	Mental health practitioner	Medication management	6	Written communication	Scheduled
Dwight-Johnson 2005	Doctor	Mental health practitioner	Both	7	Multiple methods	Scheduled
Dwight-Johnson 2010	Doctor	Mental health practitioner	Both	12	Liaison method	Scheduled
Dwight-Johnson 2011	Specialist	Mental health practitioner	Psychological therapy	8	Liaison method	Scheduled
Ell 2007	Doctor	Mental health practitioner	Both	12	Liaison method	Ad hoc
Ell 2008	Specialist	Mental health practitioner	Both	21	Multiple methods	Scheduled
Ell 2010	Doctor	Mental health practitioner	Both	18	Liaison method	Scheduled
Finley 2003	Doctor	Non-mental health practitioner	Medication management	8	Multiple methods	Scheduled
Fortney 2007	Doctor	Non-mental health practitioner	Medication management	26	Shared note system	Scheduled
Fritsch 2007	Doctor	Non-mental health practitioner	Medication management	6	Other	Ad hoc
Gensichen 2009	Doctor	Non-mental health practitioner	Both	13	Written communication	Ad hoc

Table 3. Cont.

Author	Multi-professional approach to patient care		Structured management plan	Number of scheduled follow-ups	Enhanced inter professional communication	
	Medical professional	Case manager background			CM liaison with PCP	Supervision frequency
Gjerdingen 2008	Doctor	Mental health practitioner	Medication management	12	Written communication	Ad hoc
Hedrick 2003	Doctor	Mental health practitioner	Both	Not reported	Shared note system	Scheduled
Huffman 2011	Doctor	Mental health practitioner	Medication management	4	Liaison method	Scheduled
Huijbregts 2013	Doctor	Non-mental health practitioner	Both	12	Share note system	Scheduled
Hunkeler 2000	Doctor	Non-mental health practitioner	Both	14	Liaison method	Scheduled
Katon 1995a	Doctor	Mental health practitioner	Both	2	Multiple methods	Not reported
Katon 1995b	Doctor	Mental health practitioner	Both	2	Multiple methods	Not reported
Katon 1996a	Doctor	Mental health practitioner	Both	10	Multiple methods	Scheduled
Katon 1996b	Doctor	Mental health practitioner	Both	10	Multiple methods	Scheduled
Katon 1999	Doctor	Mental health practitioner	Medication management	3	Multiple methods	Not reported
Katon 2001	Doctor	Mental health practitioner	Both	4	Multiple methods	Scheduled
Katon 2004	Doctor	Non-mental health practitioner	Both	7	Multiple methods	Scheduled
Katon 2010	Doctor	Non-mental health practitioner	Both	Not reported	Liaison method	Scheduled
Katzelnick 2000	Doctor	Non-mental health practitioner	Medication management	3	Multiple methods	Ad hoc
Kroenke 2010	Doctor	Non-mental health practitioner	Medication management	4	Other	Scheduled
Landis 2007	Doctor	Mental health practitioner	Medication management	9	Liaison method	Scheduled
Lobello 2010	Doctor	Non-mental health practitioner	Medication management	3	Written communication	Ad hoc
Ludman 2007a	Doctor	Non-mental health practitioner	Medication management	3	Multiple methods	Scheduled
Ludman 2007b	Doctor	Non-mental health practitioner	Both	15	Multiple methods	Scheduled
Ludman 2007c	Doctor	Non-mental health practitioner	Both	25	Multiple methods	Scheduled
Mann 1998	Doctor	Non-mental health practitioner	Medication management	Not reported	Multiple methods	Ad hoc
McCusker 2008	Doctor	Mental health practitioner	Psychological therapy	5	Written communication	Ad hoc
McMahon 2007	Doctor	Mental health practitioner	Medication management	6	Liaison method	Scheduled
Menchetti 2013	Doctor	Non-mental health practitioner	Both	Not reported	Verbal	Scheduled
Morgan 2013	Doctor	Non-mental health practitioner	Both	2	Written communication	Ad hoc
Oslin 2003	Doctor	Mental health practitioner	Medication management	8	Liaison method	Scheduled
Patel 2010	Doctor	Non-mental health practitioner	Both	Not reported	Liaison method	Ad hoc
Piette 2011	Doctor	Mental health practitioner	Psychological therapy	15	Multiple methods	Scheduled

Table 3. Cont.

Author	Multi-professional approach to patient care		Structured management plan	Number of scheduled follow-ups	Enhanced inter professional communication	
	Medical professional	Case manager background			CM liaison with PCP	Supervision frequency
Pyne 2011	Specialist	Non-mental health practitioner	Medication management	Not reported	Shared note system	Scheduled
Richards 2008a	Doctor	Mental health practitioner	Both	10	Multiple methods	Scheduled
Richards 2008b	Doctor	Mental health practitioner	Both	10	Multiple methods	Scheduled
Richards 2012	Specialist	Mental health practitioner	Both	12	Liaison method	Scheduled
Rojas 2007	Doctor	Non-mental health practitioner	Both	8	Not reported	Ad hoc
Rollman 2009	Doctor	Non-mental health practitioner	Both	10	Multiple methods	Scheduled
Ross 2008	Doctor	Mental health practitioner	Medication management	5	Liaison method	Ad hoc
Rost 2002a	Doctor	Non-mental health practitioner	Medication management	6	Written communication	Ad hoc
Rost 2002b	Doctor	Non-mental health practitioner	Medication management	6	Written communication	Ad hoc
Rubenstein 2006	Doctor	Non-mental health practitioner	Medication management		Other	Ad hoc
Simon 2000a	Doctor	Mental health practitioner	Medication management	3	Multiple methods	Scheduled
Simon 2000b	Doctor	Mental health practitioner	Medication management	3	Multiple methods	Scheduled
Simon 2004a	Doctor	Mental health practitioner	Both	3	Multiple methods	Scheduled
Simon 2004b	Doctor	Mental health practitioner	Both	11	Multiple methods	Scheduled
Simon 2011	Doctor	Mental health practitioner	Medication management	4	Shared note system	Scheduled
Smit 2005a	Doctor	Mental health practitioner	Both	4	Written communication	Ad hoc
Smit 2005b	Doctor	Mental health practitioner	Both	4	Written communication	Ad hoc
Smit 2005c	Doctor	Mental health practitioner	Both	8	Written communication	Ad hoc
Strong 2008	Doctor	Non-mental health practitioner	Both	13	Multiple methods	Scheduled
Swindle 2003	Doctor	Mental health practitioner	Medication management	4	Liaison method	Ad hoc
Uebelacker 2011	Doctor	Non-mental health practitioner	Both	8	Written communication	Scheduled
Unutzer 2002	Doctor	Mental health practitioner	Both	15	Shared note system	Scheduled
Vera 2010	Doctor	Mental health practitioner	Medication management	Not reported	Liaison method	Scheduled
Vlasveld 2011	Specialist	Non-mental health practitioner	Both	9	Liaison method	Ad hoc
Wells 2000a	Doctor	Non-mental health practitioner	Medication management	8	Written communication	Ad hoc
Wells 2000b	Doctor	Mental health practitioner	Psychological therapy	Not reported	Written communication	Ad hoc
Wilkinson 2003	Doctor	Non-mental health practitioner	Medication management	5	Not reported	Ad hoc
Williams 2007	Mixed	Non-mental health practitioner	Medication management	7	Liaison method	Scheduled

Table 3. Cont.

Author	Multi-professional approach to patient care		Structured management plan	Number of scheduled follow-ups	Enhanced inter professional communication	
	Medical professional	Case manager background			CM liaison with PCP	Supervision frequency
Yeung 2010	Doctor	Non-mental health practitioner	Medication management	8	Other	Scheduled

CM = case manager; PCP = primary care provider.

intervention included both psychological therapy and antidepressant medication management; 40 (47%) included medication management alone; and 6 (7%) included psychological therapy alone. Table 3 describes characteristics of collaborative care used in the included trials. A reference list of included trials is presented in Results S1.

Meta-analysis of the effect of collaborative care on depressive symptoms and anti-depressant use

Compared with usual care, collaborative care was associated with improvements in depressive symptoms (standardised mean difference, SMD −0.28, 95% CI −0.33 to −0.23; $I^2 = 62.2\%$, 95% CI 52.2% to 70.1%; Figure S1) and increased anti-depressant use (relative risk, RR 1.53, 95% CI 1.40 to1.68; $I^2 = 80.8\%$, 95% CI 75.8% to 84.8%; Figure S2).

Meta-regression model one: predictors of depressive symptoms

The results of the univariable analyses of study-level and patient-aggregate covariates on depressive symptoms are shown in Table 4 and the multivariable analyses are shown in Table 5. Four covariates were identified for inclusion in the multivariable meta-regression model: recruitment by systematic identification using either interviews, outcome measures or electronic medical records (study-level; ß −0.16, 95% CI −0.30 to −0.02), people with a chronic physical condition as an inclusion criterion (study-level; ß −0.17, 95% CI −0.28 to −0.05), psychological interventions, alone or with medication (study-level; ß −0.13, 95% CI −0.23 to −0.03), and scheduled supervision (study-level; ß −0.12, 95% CI −0.23 to −0.02). In the multivariable model only psychological intervention remained as a statistically significant predictor of depressive symptoms (study-level; ß −0.11, 95% CI −0.20 to −0.01). Studies that included psychological interventions (alone or with medication) reported greater improvements in depressive outcomes, compared with those studies that included medication management alone.

The beta coefficient reported for the multivariable predictors of depressive symptoms can be back-transformed from an SMD to a mean difference under certain assumptions for the variance of the effect [30]. We only proceeded to back-transform to the patient health questionnaire-9, for which we observed similar within variability across studies reporting on the same scale, and the beta was equivalent to a decrease of 0.67 (95% CI −1.23 to 0.06). The multivariable model reduced the I^2 statistic from 62.2% (95% CI 52.2% to 70.1%) to 47.8% (95% CI 32.6 to 59.6).

Meta-regression model two: predictors of anti-depressant use

The results of the univariable analyses of study level covariates on antidepressant medication use are shown in Table 6 and multivariable analyses are shown in Table 7. Two study level covariates were identified for inclusion in the multivariable meta-

Table 4. Univariable predictors on depressive symptoms (N = 84).

Variable		Regression Coefficient (95% CI)	SE	P	I^2 (95% CI)
Dichotomous or categorical					
Country	Non-US (vs US)	−0.04 (−0.16 to 0.07)	.06	.47	62.4 (52.5 to 70.3)
Recruitment method	Systematic (vs GP referral)	−0.16 (−0.30 to −0.02)	.07	.03	60.8 (50.3 to 69.1)
Patient sample	Medication inclusion criteria (vs not inclusion criteria)	0.08 (−0.04 to 0.20)	.06	.21	62.3 (52.3 to 70.2)
Chronic physical health condition	Present (vs absent)	−0.17 (−0.28 to −0.05)	.06	.01	58.9 (47.7 to 67.7)
Case manager background	Mental health (vs non-mental health)	0.03 (−0.07 to 0.14)	.05	.53	62.5 (52.6 to 70.3)
Intervention content	Psychological intervention or both (vs medication only)	−0.13 (−0.23 to −0.03)	.05	.01	56.8 (44.9 to 66.1)
Supervision frequency	Scheduled (vs ad hoc)	−0.12 (−0.23 to −0.02)	.05	.02	53.7 (40.7 to 63.9)
	Not applicable (vs ad hoc)	0.10 (−0.13 to 0.33)	.12	.38	
Allocation concealment	High risk (vs low risk)	0.06 (−0.03 to 0.16)	.05	.20	62.0 (51.9 to 70.0)
Continuous					
Enhanced usual care*¶		0.02 (−0.03 to 0.08)	.03	.37	62.0 (51.9 to 70.0)
Number of sessions*¶		−0.01 (−0.02 to 0.00)	.01	.26	50.7 (35.5 to 62.3)

*N of 74 comparisons.
¶model intercepts (constants) not reported.

Table 5. Multivariable predictors of depressive symptoms (N = 84).

Variable	Regression Coefficient (95% CI)	SE	P
Recruitment method (Systematic)	−0.12 (−0.26 to 0.02)	.07	.10
Chronic physical health condition (Present)	−0.10 (−0.22 to 0.02)	.06	.11
Intervention content (Psychological intervention or both)	−0.11 (−0.20 to −0.01)	.05	.03
Supervision frequency (Scheduled)*	−0.08 (−0.19 to 0.02)	.05	.13
Supervision frequency (Not applicable)*	0.06 (−0.15 to 0.28)	.11	.57
Intercept (constant)	−0.05 (−0.20 to 0.10)	.08	.53

I^2 = 47.8% (95% CI 32.6 to 59.6).
*Compared with the reference category, ad hoc supervision.

regression model: studies that recruited participants using systematic identification (RR 1.55, 95% CI 1.22 to 1.97) and studies that included participants with a chronic physical condition (RR 1.45, 95% CI 1.16 to 1.83). In the multivariable meta-regression model studies that recruited participants systematically (RR 1.43, 95% CI 1.12 to 1.81) and included participants with a chronic physical condition (RR 1.32, 95% CI 1.05 to 1.65) remained statistically significant predictors of anti-depressant use. Studies including participants who were systematically identified and those with a chronic physical condition adhered more to their anti-depressant medications. The multivariable model reduced the I^2 statistic from 80.8% (95% CI 75.8% to 84.8%) to 75.2% (95% CI 68.1% to 80.7%).

Sensitivity analyses using intraclass correlation coefficients of 0.00 and 0.05 for cluster trials did not impact greatly on the multivariable meta-regression findings (see Results S2 and Results S3). The subgroup analysis exploring the relationship between sample size and effect size for both depressive symptoms and medication use was statistically non-significant, thus decreasing the likelihood that our findings are susceptible to publication bias (Results S4).

Meta-regression model three: the effect of change in anti-depressant use on depressive symptoms

Increased anti-depressant use was not associated with improvement in depressive symptoms (ß −0.13, 95% CI −0.27 to 0.004, p = 0.06).

Discussion

Overall, collaborative care successfully improves both patient outcomes and the process of care for depression. Studies that included psychological interventions, (alone or with medication management), as part of collaborative care were associated with greater improvements in depressive symptoms compared with studies that only included medication management alone. Use of antidepressants was increased in studies that included participants with a chronic physical health condition and in studies that recruited participants through a process of systematic identification.

Strengths and limitations

Our analyses were based on a priori decisions about covariates likely to moderate the treatment effect of collaborative care [11] and included the largest and most comprehensive dataset about

Table 6. Univariable predictors of antidepressant use (N = 59).

Variable		Relative risk (95% CI)	SE	P	I^2 (95% CI)
Dichotomous or categorical					
Country	Non-US (vs US)	0.89 (0.71 to 1.13)	.11	.34	80.1 (74.8 to 84.3)
Recruitment method	Systematic (vs GP referral)	1.55 (1.22 to 1.97)	.19	<.001	77.3 (71.0 to 82.2)
Patient sample	Medication inclusion criteria (vs not inclusion criteria)	0.85 (0.68 to 1.07)	.10	.16	80.6 (75.5 to 84.6)
Chronic physical health condition	Present (vs absent|)	1.45 (1.16 to 1.83)	.17	.001	78.2 (72.2 to 82.9)
Case manager background	Mental health (vs non-mental health)	1.06 (0.85 to 1.31)	.12	.61	80.9 (75.9 to 84.9)
Intervention content	Psychological intervention or both (vs medication only)	0.92 (0.74 to 1.14)	.10	.44	81.1 (76.2 to 85.0)
Supervision frequency	Scheduled (vs ad hoc)	1.03 (0.82 to 1.29)	.12	.83	81.3 (76.4 to 85.2)
	Not applicable (vs ad hoc)	0.94 (0.44 to 2.02)	.37	.87	
Allocation concealment	High risk (vs low risk)	0.89 (0.72 to 1.09)	.09	.25	80.9 (75.9 to 84.9)
Continuous					
Enhanced usual care		0.93 (0.85 to 1.03)	.05	.17	81.0 (76.0 to 84.9)
Number of sessions*¶		0.99 (0.97 to 1.01)	.01	.54	78.2 (71.9 to 83.1)

*N of 53 comparisons.
¶model intercepts (constants) not reported.

Table 7. Multivariable predictors of antidepressant use (N = 59).

Variable	Relative risk (95% CI)	SE	P
Recruitment method (systematic)	1.42 (1.12 to 1.81)	.17	.004
Chronic physical health condition (Present)*	1.32 (1.05 to 1.65)	.15	.02
Intercept (constant)	1.08 (0.88 to 1.32)	.11	.46

I^2 = 75.2% (95% CI 68.1% to 80.7%).
*Compared with the reference category, physical health condition absent.

collaborative care. By searching extensively, we were able to include almost twice as many trials as previous reviews, and this substantially enhanced our ability to quantify and explore heterogeneity with a greater level of statistical power, thus reducing the chance of spurious findings [31]. In addition, the large number of studies gives us more confidence in the asymptotic meta-analysis methods employed [32], even if the study effects are not normally distributed [33]. The high levels of estimated heterogeneity are a positive finding since it appears heterogeneity levels are being consistently underestimated in meta-analyses [34]. Although there is a link between meta-analysis size and heterogeneity levels and we would expect to detect high levels given the size of our review [34], as we do, the large between-study variability implies that there might be other study or patient-level variables that could explain some of it (e.g. depression severity, ethnicity of patients, fidelity to intervention, quality of case manager training, and level of engagement in psychological treatment).

Additionally, meta-regression can be weakened by other statistical considerations and poor reporting. For example, we were not able to include demographic variables in the regression models due to a lack of variability, and we were unable to model a dose response relationship between treatment effects and case management sessions because most trials did not report data about the frequency, intensity, and duration of psychological treatments. We contacted authors for this information but this process did not overcome this limitation pointing to the need for more comprehensive reporting about the delivery of treatments in psychological therapy trials. More severely depressed patients are more responsive to psychological [35] and pharmacological interventions [36] but we were unable to replicate these analyses in trials of collaborative care because depression severity was inconsistently reported; contacting authors did not overcome this issue. Failure to include these covariates may have biased our results [37]. This limitation also highlights the need for more consistent and comprehensive reporting about the content of complex mental health interventions and efforts to strengthen reporting and specification of complex behaviour change are a step forward to overcoming this limitation [38].

In the absence of individual patient data we had to rely on analyses of mean study effects which are prone to bias ('ecological fallacy': deducing for an individual from a group mean), which are difficult to interpret since the relationships within- and between-studies might differ, making evidence from such analyses inconclusive [27]. In addition, we could not use a single structural equation model to properly account for mediating and moderating effects and the relationships between antidepressant use and depressive symptoms.

Most trials included in this review only reported short-term follow-up limiting opportunities to conduct sensitivity analyses of moderators of long term effectiveness of collaborative care. The absence of long term follow-up data among the group of trials included in this review resembles the findings of Deshauer et al., who screened more than 2000 records for classic placebo-controlled RCTs of selective serotonin reuptake inhibitors and identified only six studies with follow-up of 6 months or greater [39]. There is a clear need to build longer term follow-up into trials of treatment of depression given that depression is episodic and the ultimate goal of treatment is to bring about sustained recovery. Additionally, most trials did not report if the trial population included patients with comorbid chronic physical health conditions, further reducing the number of comparisons entered into the regression models. Furthermore, it is reasonable to assume that all studies that included older adults will have included patients with unreported comorbidity, potentially rendering comparisons of collaborative care in chronic physical health conditions redundant. However, our analysis suggests that presence of a chronic physical health condition as a study inclusion criteria remained a key moderator of medication adherence irrespective of the presence of unreported comorbidities, suggesting that this issue has substantive significance, and does not represent confounding.

We analysed ten theoretically plausible covariates that might determine the effectiveness of collaborative care on both depressive symptoms and medication use using an initial p value of 0.10. Assuming statistical independence then approximately one in ten of our tests was susceptible to type I error but we did not adjust for multiple testing. However, we felt justified in this approach. Although adopting a more conservative approach to hypothesis testing using multiplicity adjustments would have decreased our chances of making a Type I error, we would have also increased our chances of Type II errors (i.e. false negatives), and thus rejected important predictors of the effectiveness of collaborative care outcomes [40].

Comparisons with the previous meta-regression analysis

A novel finding of our meta-regression is that including psychological therapy, either alone or with antidepressant medication, conferred additional benefit, at least for depressive symptoms. Compared with previous analyses [11] we included a greater number of trials (+50) in our analysis which means that our analysis is the first to be powered to detect this finding. In addition, we showed that studies that systematically identified patients were important moderators of anti-depressant medication use. This finding may also be due to increased statistical power generated by our meta-regression. Additionally, we also showed that the presence of a chronic physical condition moderated use of anti-depressant medications – trials that included patients with chronic physical conditions reported increased use of anti-depressant medication. This patient characteristic was not explored in the previous meta-regression.

Contrary to the findings of a previous meta-regression [11], case-manager background did not predict reduction in depressive symptoms. Despite improvements there are still shortages of psychologists and psychotherapists, especially in low and middle-income countries [41], but case management of depression in the context of collaborative care might not need be delivered by a mental health professional. Indeed there is emerging evidence, mainly from the United States, that nurse-led collaborative care is more effective than usual care for treating depression in people with chronic physical disease [42], suggesting that non-mental health trained primary care nurses are as well placed as mental health professionals to work as case managers for certain types of patients. However, where case managers are drawn from non-mental health professions there may need to be more emphasis on ensuring that there are satisfactory arrangements in place for regular specialist supervision.

Clinical supervision of psychological therapists can positively affect the process of treatment, leading to greater confidence, self-awareness, and competence among therapists [43], and, in the context of brief psychological treatment, possibly improved patient outcomes [44]. Our initial univariable analysis adds weight to previous findings [11] that compared with ad hoc supervision the availability of scheduled case manager supervision from a mental health specialist predicted improved depressive symptom outcomes. This finding has important implications for patient benefit given that large scale epidemiological studies have shown that depression is under-treated because of inadequate anti-depressant medication management by health care providers, along with poor clinical supervision and patient follow-up [45]. Inadequate anti-depressant treatment of depression is more pronounced in people with chronic physical conditions [46]. Recurrence of symptoms is also common, but patients who continue treatment with anti-depressants reduce the risk of recurrence by 70% compared with those who discontinue treatment [47], although it is not clear whether reduction in relapse represents true long term efficacy or avoidance of relapse precipitated by antidepressant withdrawal [48]. Additionally, few patients respond to an initial 20 mg dose of citalopram and only about 40% of patients achieve remission after receiving the full therapeutic dosage of an anti-depressant medication [49]. Furthermore, up to 20% of patients remain depressed after completing an initial phase of treatment [50]. Regular supervision within collaborative care could thus help to overcome therapeutic impasse by supporting case managers to identify and manage patients who do not initially respond to or discontinue treatment by facilitating changes to anti-depressant dosage, augmentation of medication with another therapy, or recommending switching to another treatment.

Implications for policy and practice

Our findings show that structured management plans that included psychological interventions either as a standalone therapy or in combination with antidepressant medication predicted reductions in depressive symptoms more so than collaborative care that only offered patients anti-depressant medication. While the additional effects associated with psychological treatment were small this result does highlight the importance of patient choice in the delivery of health care for depression. Across a diverse range of psychiatric conditions and health care settings patients have reported a 3-fold preference for psychological treatment over pharmacological treatment, underscoring the need to link treatment strategies to patient preference [51].

We showed that certain types of patients appear to be better at taking anti-depressant medications than others. In the absence of collaborative care depression is under-treated with anti-depressant medication in older adults with chronic physical conditions [46]. However, our findings show that this patient group showed improved levels of anti-depressant use compared with those without chronic physical conditions. It may be that patients with depression and chronic physical conditions are primed to respond well to structured management programmes that include anti-depressant medication because they are well versed in using medications to self-manage their chronic illness. However the burden of treatment for patients with complex, chronic physical and mental comorbidities may reduce their capacity to collaborate in their care [52].

Novel to this review was our finding that compared with recruitment by clinicians, trials that systematically identified patients were associated with increased use of anti-depressant medication. This finding goes beyond methodological considerations about how to effectively recruit patients into mental health trials. Patients referred to mental health services by clinicians tend to be patients with most to gain as they may be more severely depressed. However, the fact that we found that systems based approaches to patient identification predicted increased use of anti-depressant medication highlights the fact that population approaches to disease management can identify different types of patients who may have additional capacity to benefit, further underlining the importance of structured approaches to depression care.

Future work and conclusion

Given the premise that collaborative care is an organisational framework within which different combinations of psychological and pharmacological interventions can be used a key unanswered question relates to how interventions can be tailored, adjusted, or changed to meet the needs of patients. Most collaborative care trials have only measured adherence to anti-depressants but not frequency of changes to medication dosage or augmentation of medication with another therapy. Given that use of anti-depressant medication might be a proxy for why collaborative care is effective it is critical that future trials include process measures that can evaluate adjustment and augmentation of medication similar to those used in the Teamcare trial [53]. Additionally, meta-analysis using individual rather than study-level data would increase opportunities to detect differential treatment effects across individuals in randomised trials, and allows for more complex modelling of the association of treatment effects and patient characteristics [54].

In conclusion, these results update and expand on a previous analysis of factors that differentiate collaborative care trials that improve patient outcomes and/or the process of care from those that do not. Psychological therapy is an active ingredient in collaborative care with or without anti-depressant medication, emphasising the importance of building flexible collaborative care models that include different combinations of pharmacological and non-pharmacological therapies that meet patients' treatment preferences. Furthermore, patients systematically identified and those with chronic physical conditions are likely to adhere more to pharmacological treatments. Using systems based approaches to identify patients with depression highlights the importance of borrowing elements from chronic disease management models to improve the process of depression care.

Supporting Information

Figure S1 Forest plot of effect of collaborative care on depressive symptoms. *Meta-analysis of individual trial and* *pooled effects. Random effects model used. 95% CI = 95% confidence intervals.*

Figure S2 Forest plot of effect of collaborative care on antidepressant use. *Meta-analysis of individual trial and pooled effects. Random effects model used. 95% CI = 95% confidence intervals.*

Table S1 Characteristics of included studies.

Methods S1 Central Search Strategy.

Methods S2 Meta-regression coding manual.

Checklist S1 PRISMA Checklist.

Results S1 Reference list of included studies.

Results S2 Sensitivity analysis: Cluster Intraclass correlation coefficient of 0.00.

Results S3 Sensitivity analysis: Cluster Intraclass correlation coefficient of 0.05.

Results S4 Sensitivity analysis: Relationship between sample size and effect size.

Acknowledgments

PC is the guarantor of this work and, as such, had full access to all the data in the study and takes responsibility for the integrity of the data and the accuracy of the data analysis.

Author Contributions

Conceived and designed the experiments: PC JH EK PB. Analyzed the data: JH EK PC PB JA. Wrote the paper: PC JH EK PB. Edited the manuscript: WW LG SG DR CD KL JA.

References

1. Ferrari AJ, Charlson FJ, Norman RE, Patten SB, Freedman G, et al. (2013) Burden of Depressive Disorders by Country, Sex, Age, and Year: Findings from the Global Burden of Disease Study 2010. PLoS Med 10: e1001547.
2. Moussavi S, Chatterji S, Verdes E, Tandon A, Patel V, et al. (2007) Depression, chronic diseases, and decrements in health: results from the World Health Surveys. Lancet 370: 851–858.
3. Wagner EH, Austin BT, Michael Von K (1996) Organizing Care for Patients with Chronic Illness. The Milbank Quarterly 74: 511–544.
4. Bodenheimer T, Wagner EH, Grumbach K (2002) Improving primary care for patients with chronic illness. JAMA 288: 1775–1779.
5. Furukawa TA, Yoshimura R, Harai H, Imaizumi T, Takeuchi H, et al. (2009) How many well vs. unwell days can you expect over 10 years, once you become depressed? Acta Psychiatrica Scandinavica 119: 290–297.
6. Tsai AC, Morton SC, Mangione CM, Keeler EB (2005) A meta-analysis of interventions to improve care for chronic illnesses. American Journal of Managed Care 11: 478–488.
7. Gunn J, Diggens J, Hegarty K, Blashki G (2006) A systematic review of complex system interventions designed to increase recovery from depression in primary care. BMC Health Serv Res 6: 88.
8. Archer J, Bower P, Gilbody S, Lovell K, Richards D, et al. (2012) Collaborative care for depression and anxiety problems. Cochrane Database Syst Rev 10: CD006525.
9. Gilbody S, Bower P, Whitty P (2006) Costs and consequences of enhanced primary care for depression: systematic review of randomised economic evaluations. Br J Psychiatry 189: 297–308.
10. Katon W, Unutzer J (2006) Collaborative care models for depression: time to move from evidence to practice. Arch Intern Med 166: 2304–2306.
11. Bower P, Gilbody S, Richards D, Fletcher J, Sutton A (2006) Collaborative care for depression in primary care. Making sense of a complex intervention: systematic review and meta-regression. Br J Psychiatry 189: 484–493.
12. Liberati A, Altman DG, Tetzlaff J, Mulrow C, Gotzsche PC, et al. (2009) The PRISMA Statement for Reporting Systematic Reviews and Meta-Analyses of Studies That Evaluate Health Care Interventions: Explanation and Elaboration. Annals of Internal Medicine 151: W-65.
13. Royle P, Waugh N (2005) A simplified search strategy for identifying randomised controlled trials for systematic reviews of health care interventions: a comparison with more exhaustive strategies. BMC Medical Research Methodology 5: 23.
14. Korff MV, Goldberg D (2001) Improving outcomes in depression. BMJ 323: 948–949.
15. Weingarten SR, Henning JM, Badamgarav E, Knight K, Hasselblad V, et al. (2002) Interventions used in disease management programmes for patients with chronic illnesswhich ones work? Meta-analysis of published reports. BMJ 325: 925.
16. Gilbody S, Whitty P, Grimshaw J, Thomas R (2003) Educational and organizational interventions to improve the management of depression in primary care: a systematic review. JAMA 289: 3145–3151.
17. Boerma WG, Verhaak PF (1999) The general practitioner as the first contacted health professional by patients with psychosocial problems: a European study. Psychol Med 29: 689–696.
18. Kontopantelis E, Reeves D (2009) METAEFF: Stata module to perform effect sizes calculations for meta-analyses. Statistical Software Components.
19. Lipsey MW, Wilson D (2001) Practical Meta-Analysis. Thousand Oaks: Sage Publictions Inc.
20. Higgins JPT, Green S (2011) Cochrane Handbook for Systematic Reviews of Interventions Version 5.1.0: Cochrane Collaboration.
21. Adams G, Gulliford MC, Ukoumunne OC, Eldridge S, Chinn S, et al. (2004) Patterns of intra-cluster correlation from primary care research to inform study design and analysis. Journal of clinical epidemiology 57: 785–793.
22. Donner A, Klar N (2002) Issues in the meta-analysis of cluster randomized trials. Statistics in medicine 21: 2971–2980.
23. Pereira TV, Horwitz RI, Ioannidis JA (2012) Empirical evaluation of very large treatment effects of medical interventions. JAMA 308: 1676–1684.
24. Hewitt C, Hahn S, Torgerson DJ, Watson J, Bland JM (2005) Adequacy and reporting of allocation concealment: review of recent trials published in four general medical journals. BMJ 330: 1057–1058.
25. Harris R, Bradburn M, Deeks J, Harbord R, Altman D, et al. (2008) metan: fixed- and random-effects meta-analysis. Stata Journal 8: 3–28.
26. Harbord RM, Higgins JPT (2008) Meta-regression in Stata. Stata Journal 8: 493–519.
27. Thompson SG, Higgins JP (2002) How should meta-regression analyses be undertaken and interpreted? Stat Med 21: 1559–1573.
28. DerSimonian R, Laird N (1986) Meta-analysis in clinical trials. Controlled clinical trials 7: 177–188.
29. Higgins JP, Thompson SG (2002) Quantifying heterogeneity in a meta-analysis. Stat Med 21: 1539–1558.
30. Kontopantelis E, Reeves D (2009) MetaEasy: A Meta-Analysis Add-In for Microsoft Excel. Journal of Statistical Software 30.
31. Peduzzi P, Concato J, Kemper E, Holford TR, Feinstein AR (1996) A simulation study of the number of events per variable in logistic regression analysis. J Clin Epidemiol 49: 1373–1379.
32. Brockwell SE, Gordon IR (2001) A comparison of statistical methods for meta-analysis. Statistics in medicine 20: 825–840.
33. Kontopantelis E, Reeves D (2012) Performance of statistical methods for meta-analysis when true study effects are non-normally distributed: A simulation study. Statistical methods in medical research 21: 409–426.
34. Kontopantelis E, Springate DA, Reeves D (2013) A Re-Analysis of the Cochrane Library Data: The Dangers of Unobserved Heterogeneity in Meta-Analyses. PLoS One 8: e69930.
35. Driessen E, Cuijpers P, Hollon SD, Dekker JJ (2010) Does pretreatment severity moderate the efficacy of psychological treatment of adult outpatient depression? A meta-analysis. J Consult Clin Psychol 78: 668–680.
36. Kirsch I, Deacon BJ, Huedo-Medina TB, Scoboria A, Moore TJ, et al. (2008) Initial severity and antidepressant benefits: a meta-analysis of data submitted to the Food and Drug Administration. PLoS Med 5: e45.
37. Negassa A, Hanley JA (2007) The effect of omitted covariates on confidence interval and study power in binary outcome analysis: a simulation study. Contemp Clin Trials 28: 242–248.
38. Michie S, Richardson M, Johnston M, Abraham C, Francis J, et al. (2013) The Behavior Change Technique Taxonomy (v1) of 93 Hierarchically Clustered Techniques: Building an International Consensus for the Reporting of Behavior Change Interventions. Annals of Behavioral Medicine 46: 81–95.
39. Deshauer D, Moher D, Fergusson D, Moher E, Sampson M, et al. (2008) Selective serotonin reuptake inhibitors for unipolar depression: a systematic review of classic long-term randomized controlled trials. Canadian Medical Association Journal 178: 1293–1301.

40. Rothman KJ (1990) No adjustments are needed for multiple comparisons. Epidemiology 1: 43–46.
41. Saraceno B, van Ommeren M, Batniji R, Cohen A, Gureje O, et al. (2007) Barriers to improvement of mental health services in low-income and middle-income countries. The Lancet 370: 1164–1174.
42. Ekers D, Murphy R, Archer J, Ebenezer C, Kemp D, et al. (2013) Nurse-delivered collaborative care for depression and long-term physical conditions: A systematic review and meta-analysis. J Affect Disord 149: 14–22.
43. Milne D, James I (2000) A systematic review of effective cognitive-behavioural supervision. British Journal of Clinical Psychology 39: 111–127.
44. Bambling M, King R, Raue P, Schweitzer R, Lambert W (2006) Clinical supervision: Its influence on client-rated working alliance and client symptom reduction in the brief treatment of major depression. Psychotherapy Research 16: 317–331.
45. Salisbury C, Johnson L, Purdy S, Valderas JM, Montgomery AA (2011) Epidemiology and impact of multimorbidity in primary care: a retrospective cohort study. British Journal of General Practice 61: e12–e21.
46. Kendrick T, Dowrick C, McBride A, Howe A, Clarke P, et al. (2009) Management of depression in UK general practice in relation to scores on depression severity questionnaires: analysis of medical record data. BMJ 338: b750.
47. Dickens C, Katon W, Blakemore A, Khara A, McGowan L, et al. (2012) Does depression predict the use of urgent and unscheduled care by people with long term conditions? A systematic review with meta-analysis. Journal of Psychosomatic Research 73: 334–342.
48. El-Mallakh R, Briscoe B (2012) Studies of Long-Term Use of Antidepressants. CNS Drugs 26: 97–109.
49. Mathur R, Hull SA, Badrick E, Robson J (2011) Cardiovascular multimorbidity: the effect of ethnicity on prevalence and risk factor management. British Journal of General Practice 61: e262–e270.
50. Bower P, Macdonald W, Harkness E, Gask L, Kendrick T, et al. (2011) Multimorbidity, service organization and clinical decision making in primary care: a qualitative study. Family Practice 28: 579–587.
51. RK M, SW W, AD P, JA W, MW O (2013) Patient preference for psychological vs pharmacologic treatment of psychiatric disorders: a meta-analytic review. Journal of Clinical Psychiatry 74: 595–602.
52. May C, Montori VM, Mair FS (2009) We need minimally disruptive medicine. BMJ 339: b2803.
53. Katon WJ, Lin EH, Von Korff M, Ciechanowski P, Ludman EJ, et al. (2010) Collaborative care for patients with depression and chronic illnesses. N Engl J Med 363: 2611–2620.
54. Riley RD, Lambert PC, Abo-Zaid G (2010) Meta-analysis of individual participant data: rationale, conduct, and reporting. BMJ 340: c221.

The Effects of Short-Term Synaptic Depression at Thalamocortical Synapses on Orientation Tuning in Cat V1

Aylin Cimenser[1,2]*, Kenneth D. Miller[3,4,5]

1 Harvard Medical School, Boston, Massachusetts, United States of America, 2 Department of Physics, Boston University, Boston, Massachusetts, United States of America, 3 Center for Theoretical Neuroscience, College of Physicians and Surgeons, Columbia University, New York, New York, United States of America, 4 Department of Neuroscience, College of Physicians and Surgeons, Columbia University, New York, New York, United States of America, 5 Swartz Program in Theoretical Neuroscience, College of Physicians and Surgeons, Columbia University, New York, New York, United States of America

Abstract

We examine the effects of short-term synaptic depression on the orientation tuning of the LGN input to simple cells in cat primary visual cortex (V1). The total LGN input has an untuned component as well as a tuned component, both of which grow with stimulus contrast. The untuned component is not visible in the firing rate responses of the simple cells. The suppression of the contribution of the untuned input component to firing rate responses is key to establishing orientation selectivity and its invariance with stimulus contrast. It has been argued that synaptic depression of LGN inputs could contribute to the selective suppression of the untuned component and thus contribute to the tuning observed in simple cells. We examine this using a model fit to the depression observed at thalamocortical synapses *in-vivo*, and compare this to an earlier model fit based on *in-vitro* observations. We examine the tuning of both the conductance and the firing rate induced in simple cells by the net LGN input. We find that depression causes minimal suppression of the untuned component. The primary effect of depression is to cause the contrast response curve to saturate at lower contrasts without differentially affecting the tuned vs. untuned components. This effect is slightly weaker for *in-vivo* vs. *in-vitro* parameters. Thus, synaptic depression of LGN inputs does not appreciably contribute to the orientation tuning of V1 simple cells.

Editor: Li I. Zhang, University of Southern California, United States of America

Funding: This study was supported by R01-EY11001 (http://report.nih.gov) to KM and by the Gatsby Charitable Foundation through the Gatsby Initiative in Brain Circuitry at Columbia University (http://www.gatsby.org.uk/en/Neuroscience.aspx). The funders had no role in study design, data collection and analysis, decision to publish, or preparation of the manuscript.

Competing Interests: The authors have declared that no competing interests exist.

* Email: aylin@nmr.mgh.harvard.edu

Introduction

Much of the stimulus selectivity of simple cells in layer 4 of cat primary visual cortex (V1), including their tuning for stimulus orientation, can be understood from the feedforward input they receive along with cellular and synaptic nonlinearities [1–27]. Factors that may play a role in determining orientation tuning include the pattern of inputs the cells receive from the lateral geniculate nucleus (LGN) of the thalamus [5]; feedforward inhibition driven by LGN inputs [20,24,26]; suppression of voltage variability with increasing stimulus contrast, which changes the cell's input/output function [17,19]; and synaptic depression [27,28]. Intracortical excitation affects the gain of simple-cell responses but does not seem to alter the orientation tuning induced by these other factors [6,7] (see also in rodents: [29,30]).

The arrangement of LGN inputs alone cannot account for orientation tuning. The net input driven by a simple cell's LGN cells can be decomposed into an orientation-untuned component and a tuned component, which for a drifting grating stimulus correspond respectively to the mean and the temporal modulation of the input [20,24]. Both components increase with contrast, so that the peak LGN input (mean plus modulation) in response to a high-contrast stimulus at the null orientation (orthogonal to the preferred) should be higher than that for a low-contrast preferred stimulus [20,26]. Yet most V1 cells respond little to a high-contrast null stimulus while responding robustly to a low-contrast preferred stimulus [17,31–33].

Two factors appear to suppress null relative to preferred responses. First, voltage responses to a null stimulus are weaker, relative to preferred, than predicted from the arrangement of LGN inputs. A null stimulus evokes depolarization that grows with contrast, but even at the highest contrast this depolarization is rarely if ever larger than the preferred-orientation voltage response at low (4%) contrast (Fig. 5A of [17]). Recurrent amplification of preferred responses may contribute to this. Considering LGN input alone, at any given contrast the mean LGN-induced input should be equal for the null and the preferred orientations [20]. Experimentally, the LGN-input-induced mean voltage response to the null is estimated to be only about 70% of that to the preferred (Fig. S3B of [19]). Second, the firing rate to a null stimulus is strongly suppressed relative to this voltage response, typically remaining slightly suppressed relative to spontaneous firing across all stimulus contrasts, so that the ratio of preferred to null firing rate strongly increases with stimulus contrast [17,31]. The suppression of null spiking response is largely explained by an observed reduction in voltage variability with increasing contrast, which causes the mean null voltage response to remain a constant number of standard deviations of the voltage noise below spike threshold, keeping spiking probability (the firing rate) constant across contrasts [17,19].

It has been argued that synaptic depression at geniculocortical synapses could suppress null voltage response and, along with the arrangement of LGN inputs, explain orientation tuning [28]. Here we reexamine this issue, using a model fit to the weaker synaptic depression seen *in-vivo* [34] as well as one fit to the stronger depression seen *in-vitro* [35].

Materials and Methods

We modeled the spatial arrangement of the relay cells in LGN that connect to a V1 simple cell as in previous studies [20]. We used measured LGN firing rates and included synaptic depression, either fit by us to *in-vivo* experimental studies [34] as described below, or using a previous fit [23] to an *in-vitro* experimental study [35]. We modeled the tuning of the total LGN input – the total LGN-evoked excitatory conductance – to a V1 simple cell under three conditions: 1. No depression at thalamocortical synapses, 2. Depression, using *in-vivo* fit parameters 3. Depression, using *in-vitro* fit parameters. We also modeled the tuning of simple-cell firing rates that would be elicited by these conductances. We focused only on tuning, ignoring response amplitude (that is, we present tuning curves normalized to the response at the preferred orientation and maximal contrast studied), because tuning but not amplitude seems to be determined simply by feedforward input and its processing at the synapse and the postsynaptic cell, independently of intracortical excitation [6,7,29,30] (excepting possible effects of intracortical excitation on voltage variability, which influences spike rate tuning, but this effect is incorporated in our spiking model as discussed further below).

Determining the LGN firing rate

To determine orientation tuning curves at varying contrasts, we used LGN firing rates from experimental data (Dataset S1) that is kindly provided to us by Chong Weng and Jose-Manuel Alonso (SUNY). These data consist of the responses of seven LGN X-cells to drifting sinusoidal gratings in anesthetized cat LGN. The temporal frequency of the gratings was 1.6 Hz and the spatial frequency of the grating was.28 cycles/degree. The sinusoidal gratings were presented at contrasts: 3%, 6%, 12%, 24%, 48%, 72% and 96%.

We took the firing rate for a given LGN cell in response to a grating of a given contrast to be given by the cell's cycle-averaged peri-stimulus time histogram (PSTH; the average firing rate as a function of time across one cycle of the drifting grating) for gratings of that contrast, averaged over 300 stimulus cycles. The phase of the PSTH for a grating of a given orientation was matched to the phase of the grating as it passed over the cell's receptive field center (locations of LGN receptive field centers are described below). We also compared the performance of a linear rectified model fit to the PSTH, constructed as follows. Rectified sinusoids of the form $|B+Asin(2\pi ft)|_+$ were constructed, where B was the background firing rate, taken to be the mean firing rate at 3% contrast; f was the temporal frequency of the stimulus; A was the amplitude; and $|x|_+=x,\ x>0;\ |x|_+=0$ otherwise. The amplitude, A, was adjusted so that the rectified sinusoid and the cycle-averaged PSTH had the same Fourier amplitude at the stimulus frequency.

The LGN firing rates used in fitting the depression model are described below, in the Materials and Methods subsection "Fitting the synaptic depression model".

Constructing LGN spike trains

For a given time-dependent firing rate of an LGN cell, spike timings were constructed from an inhomogeneous Poisson process with an absolute refractory period of $t_{ref}=1$ msec (or a homogeneous Poisson process in the case of background firing, when firing rates are not changing in time). The problem of generating spike trains with a specified refractory period was first studied by [36] and further analysis was done by [37–41]. For an absolute refractory period, the correction is simple: if the firing rate at time t is $r(t)$, then the average fraction of trials that exhibit refractoriness at t is $\int_{t-t_{ref}}^{t} r(t')dt'$. Thus, if the firing rate when not refractory – the "free firing rate" – is $q(t)$, then the observed firing rate is equal to the free firing rate times the percentage of time not refractory:

$$r(t)=q(t)\ (1-\int_{t-t_{ref}}^{t} r(t')dt'). \tag{1}$$

We used a discretized version of this formula, given $r(t)$ from the data, to compute $q(t)$; computed the next spike time after the last refractory period from an inhomogeneous Poisson process with rate\$q(t)$; and set spike probability to zero for $t_{ref}=1$ msec after each spike. Note that when the firing rate is a constant, the free firing rate can be written as:

$$\frac{1}{q}=\frac{1}{r}-t_{ref}. \tag{2}$$

For fitting the model to the data of Boudreau and Ferster [34], we used bins of 0.1 msec duration. For the remaining analysis, we estimated the firing rates using bins of 1 msec duration.

Spatial Organization of LGN

The LGN was constructed with four overlying sheets [42] as in [20]. Each sheet covered the same $6.8°\times6.8°$ area of the visual field. A sheet consisted of two lattices with 30×30 ON cells and 30×30 OFF cells. The two lattices were offset by one-half of the lattice spacing. A cell's receptive field center location corresponded to its lattice position.

Connections of relay cells in LGN to a simple cell in V1

A simple cell receptive field was modeled as a Gabor function [5,43]: a sinusoidal oscillation of 0.8 cycles/degree multiplied by Gaussian envelopes parallel to and perpendicular to the direction of oscillation. We used the "broadly tuned" receptive field parameters of [20]: letting x and y be the directions parallel and perpendicular to the oscillation, respectively, the Gaussians in the Gabor had standard deviations $\sigma_x=.24°$ and $\sigma_y=.41°$. This results in a receptive field with 1.85 subfields (defined as the ratio of the length of the Gaussian parallel to the oscillation to one half-cycle of the oscillation, where the length of a Gaussian is defined as the distance between the points where it takes 5% of its peak value). The orientation of the receptive field was aligned with the

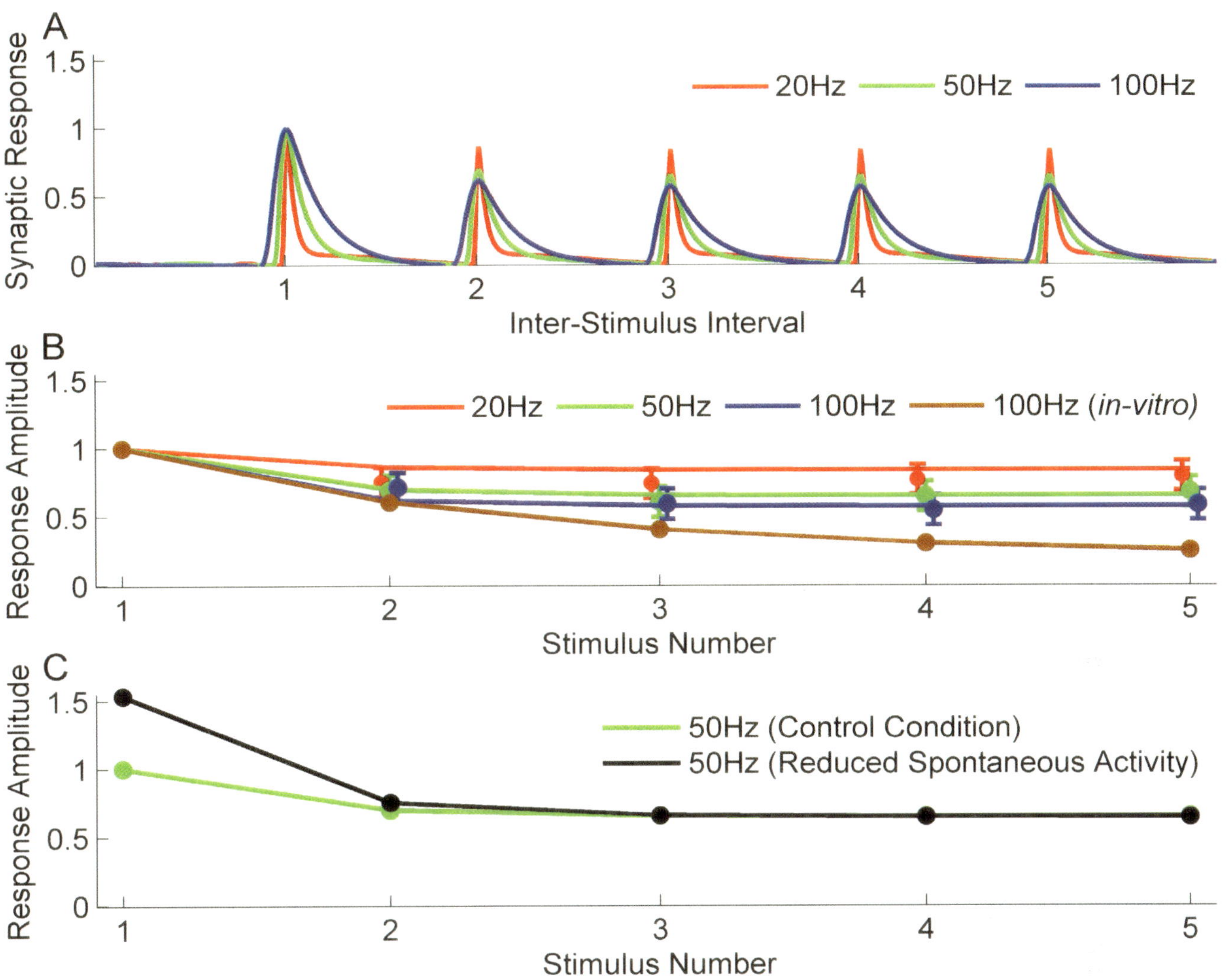

Figure 1. Results from our model of synaptic depression at visual thalamocortical synapses *in-vivo*, based on the model of Dittman and Regehr (1998). A) Model behavior: Dynamics of the normalized PSP's evoked in response to stimulation of a model synapse with different frequencies. Average responses are shown to delivery of 20 Hz, 50 Hz and 100 Hz trains of electrical stimuli to LGN following the background activity. The response is normalized to equal 1 at 90% of the peak value (see Materials and Methods). Note that peaks are aligned and the response to the first stimulus is identical to all three frequencies. The *x-axis* is scaled so that inter-stimulus interval is shown as equal at all frequencies. In units of time, inter-stimulus intervals are 50 msec, 20 msec and 10 msec for the red, green and blue curves. B) Comparison with experimental data: Smooth curves show model response amplitudes (90% of peak value from panel A) as a function of stimulus number at stimulation frequencies of 20 (red), 50 (green) and 100 (blue) Hz. Mean *in-vivo* response amplitudes measured by Boudreau and Ferster [34] are indicated by colored dots; error bars show the size of the data points in their figures, which they state are larger than the error bars and thus serve as an upper bound of the experimental error bars. For comparison, results obtained by using *in-vitro* depression parameters ($f-\tau$ model) are shown for the case of 100 Hz stimulation (brown circles and line). C) Effect of increased intraocular pressure. Green: control response to 50 Hz stimulation, identical to green line in (B). Black: responses when background LGN firing rates were reduced before stimulation from a mean value of 11.8 Hz for control condition to a mean value of 4.1 Hz, modeling effects of increase in intraocular pressure (see Materials and Methods). The response to the first stimulus when the LGN firing rates were low is 1.5 times the value when the LGN firing rates were high. The corresponding ratio from Boudreau and Ferster [34] is 1.45±0.11.

LGN grid. The Gabor function was chosen to be symmetric about the center of the receptive field.

We determined the thalamocortical connection strengths to the model simple cell from this Gabor function receptive field stochastically as in [20]. This gives a time-invariant strength g^j for the connection from the jth LGN neuron to the cortical cell. In addition, each strength is modulated by a time-varying factor $w^j(t)$ determined by synaptic depression, as explained below. The time dependence of the AMPA conductances for the jth synapse were modeled as differences of simple exponentials for each presynaptic spike, weighted by the value of the depression factor $w^j(t)$ at the time of the spike:

$$g^j_{AMPA}(t) = \sum_{\{t_i\}<t} w^j(t_i)\left(e^{(t-t_i)\big/\tau^{fall}_{AMPA}} - e^{-(t-t_i)\big/\tau^{rise}_{AMPA}} \right) \quad (3)$$

with corresponding time constants $\tau^{rise}_{AMPA} = .25$ msec, $\tau^{fall}_{AMPA} = 1.75$ msec [20], where $\{t_i\} < t$ represents the presynaptic spike timings, $t_1, t_2, ..,$ up to time t. The time course of NMDA conductances was also modeled with exponentials, except that the decay of NMDA conductance was modeled as a double exponential with a fast and a slow time constant:

$$g^j_{NMDA}(t) = \sum_{\{t_i\}<t} w^j(t_i)\left(f_{fast}\cdot e^{-(t-t_i)/\tau^{fall}_{NMDA,fast}} + (1-f_{fast})\cdot e^{-(t-t_i)/\tau^{fall}_{NMDA,slow}} - e^{-(t-t_i)/\tau^{rise}_{NMDA}}\right) \quad (4)$$

The values were chosen from [22] as $\tau^{rise}_{NMDA}=5.5$ msec, $\tau^{fall}_{NMDA,fast}=63$ msec, $\tau^{fall}_{NMDA,slow}=200$ msec and $f_{fast}=88\%$. Voltage dependence of the NMDA conductance was ignored. The total conductance evoked by the jth synapse was: $g^j_{TOTAL}(t)=g^j\left((1-\alpha)\frac{g^j_{AMPA}(t)}{\int \tilde{g}^j_{AMPA}(t)dt}+\alpha\frac{g^j_{NMDA}(t)}{\int \tilde{g}^j_{NMDA}(t)dt}\right)$ where $\tilde{g}^j_{AMPA}(t)$ is $g^j_{AMPA}(t)$ evaluated with a single presynaptic spike and $w^j=1$, and similarly for $\tilde{g}^j_{NMDA}(t)$. $\alpha=80\%$ is the ratio of NMDA to AMPA conductances.

Distribution of transmission delays from LGN to cortex

Boudreau and Ferster [34] classified cortical cells with response latencies less than 2.3 msec as monosynaptic cells, and provided a distribution of these response latencies. Reasoning that the difference in response latencies reflects differences in transmission delays between LGN and cortex, we randomly picked the transmission delay between a given LGN neuron and the model cortical neuron from the distribution mentioned above. This is accomplished by shifting the contribution to the PSP from an individual LGN neuron by the corresponding delay, and ensures that the response latency of the model cortical neuron is equal to the average latency of the monosynaptic cells studied in Boudreau and Ferster.

Modeling synaptic depression

Depression is modeled as a factor $w(t)$ for each synapse that varies between 0 and 1, reflecting the degree of depression.

In-vivo: Depression was modeled with a calcium-dependent recovery time as suggested in previous studies [44]. The idea behind this model is that as calcium accumulates, the time constant for recovery becomes smaller, thereby speeding up the process of recovery from depression. In mathematical terms, between two spikes, the change in Calcium concentration, $Ca(t)$, is given as:

$$\tau_{Ca}\frac{dCa(t)}{dt} = Ca_{rest} - Ca(t) \quad (5)$$

and the change in release ready sites, $N(t)$, is given as:

$$-\frac{dN(t)}{dt} = (N(t)-N_0)\frac{k_{\max}}{1+K_N Ca_0/Ca(t)}. \quad (6)$$

During a spike, the change in Calcium concentration is:

$$Ca(t_+) = Ca(t_-) + Ca_0 \quad (7)$$

and the change in release ready sites is:

$$N(t_+) = (1-p_o)N(t_-). \quad (8)$$

Here, t_- represents the time just before a spike and t_+ represents the time just after a spike. Ca_0 is the increase in calcium concentration after each spike. N_0 is the total number of ready sites. Initially, all the sites are release ready, $N(t_0-)=N_0$, and after each spike, a fraction p_0 of the release ready sites are used. The synaptic strength associated with a spike at time t is proportional to $p_0 N(t_-)$, so $w(t)=N(t_-)/N_0$.

Defining $\tilde{K}_N \equiv K_N Ca_0/Ca(t)$, experimental data suggests that small changes in Ca_0 lead to measurable changes in $\tilde{K}_N$ [44]. In order to allow the model to reproduce this behavior, K_N should be on the order of 1. We chose $K_N=1$. Defining $k_0 \equiv \frac{k_{\max}}{1+Ca_0/Ca_{rest}}$ and solving the above equations in between spikes, with t representing the time just after the last spike and $t'>t$ the time being solved for, the dynamics of the calcium concentration can be written as:

$$Ca(t') = Ca_{rest} + (Ca(t) - Ca_{rest})\exp(-(t'-t)/\tau_{Ca}) \quad (9)$$

while the available release ready sites can be written as:

$$N(t') = N_0 - (N_0 - N(t))\exp(-k_0(t'-t)) \left(\frac{Ca_0 + Ca(t)}{Ca_0 + Ca_{rest} + (Ca(t) - Ca_{rest})\exp(-(t'-t)/\tau_{Ca})}\right)^{-\tau_{Ca}(k_{\max}-k_0)} \quad (10)$$

In-vitro: We used the "$f-\tau$" model of synaptic depression [45,46]. Between spikes, w recovers toward 1 with time constant τ: $\tau\frac{dw}{dt}=1-w$. At each spike, a fraction $(1-f)$ of the synaptic resources are used: $w\to fw$. The depression parameter associated with a spike is equal to w just before the spike. In agreement with Boudreau and Ferster [34], we were not able to fit the *in-vivo* data with an $f-\tau$ model within the error bars given in Fig. 1A. As a comparison to the model described above fit to *in-vivo* data, we used the $f-\tau$ model with parameters that were fit in previous work [23] to *in-vitro* paired-pulse experiments in cat V1 slices [35]. These parameters are $f=.563$, $\tau=99$ msec.

Quantifying the PSP amplitude

To fit the *in-vivo* depression model to the data of Boudreau and Ferster [34], we equate the relative amplitude of the conductance in our model with the relative PSP amplitude. This is based on the fact that, if the synaptic conductance is small relative to the background conductance, then a scaling of the synaptic conductance vs. time by a factor just scales the potential vs. time by the same factor. As in Ref. [34], depression is characterized by PSP amplitudes relative to the first amplitude in a train. To quantify the relative PSP amplitude in our model, we follow the procedures in the experiments of Boudreau and Ferster [34]. These authors observed that the incremental amplitude of the responses to individual stimuli in each train were superimposed on slow trends. To remove the slow trends, we first interpolate (by using spline interpolation; MATLAB; Mathworks, Natick, MA) the total LGN input (as conductance) measured at each stimulus onset and subtract the fit from the original total LGN input. Then, we define the amplitude of the cortical PSP to the first stimulus as the magnitude of the conductance at 90% of the peak relative to the baseline, where baseline is defined as the average response over $0.7-1.2$ msec after stimulus onset, as in Boudreau and Ferster [34]. Subsequent PSP amplitudes are measured at the same time relative to stimulus onset as the first PSP amplitude.

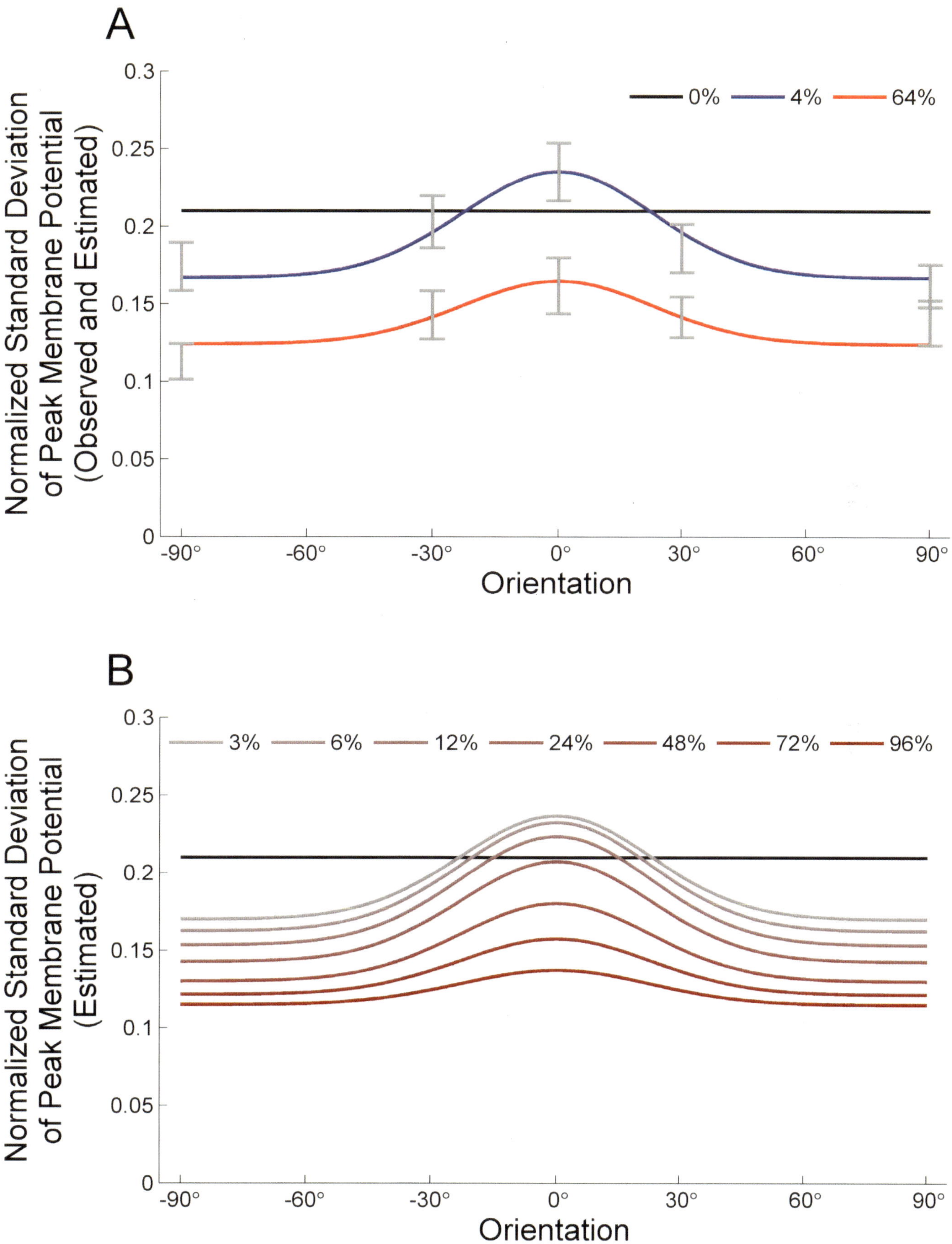
A
0%
4%
64%
Normalized Standard Deviation of Peak Membrane Potential (Observed and Estimated)
0.3
0.25
0.2
0.15
0.1
0.05
0
-90°
-60°
-30°
0°
30°
60°
90°
Orientation
B
3%
6%
12%
24%
48%
72%
96%
Normalized Standard Deviation of Peak Membrane Potential (Estimated)
Orientation

Figure 2. Tuning of the standard deviation of the peak membrane potential normalized to the mean peak membrane potential at 64% contrast preferred orientation. A) Data from Finn et al. [17] (data points and error bars) and our fits to them (smooth curves). Observed normalized standard deviation for the background (0% contrast) is 0.21. For 4% and 64% contrasts observed values are shown as error bars at orientations $-90°$,$-30°$,$0°$,$30°$ and $90°$. Estimated normalized standard deviation values are shown as smooth curves that are fit to the data by considering a single function, $f(contrast,orientation)$, (Eq. 12), which is constrained to give observed experimental values (see Materials and Methods). $f(contrast,orientation)$ is shown here for 0% contrast (black curve), 4% contrast (blue curve) and 64% contrast (red curve). B) The estimated normalized standard deviation values, *f(contrast, orientation)*, that we use in our simulations for contrasts 0%, 3%, 6%, 12%, 24%, 48%, 72% and 96%.

Fitting the synaptic depression model

Boudreau and Ferster [34] allowed the system to recover for periods of 1.75 sec between successive trains of stimuli. However, even with recovery between successive trains of stimuli, spontaneous activity can cause synaptic depression and affect the response of the cortical neurons to stimulation. In order to study this effect, Boudreau and Ferster used increased intraocular pressure as a means to reduce spontaneous LGN activity and studied its effect on response properties of cortical neurons. They reported that LGN spontaneous rates were 11.8 ± 2.9 spikes/sec in the control condition and 4.1 ± 1.4 spikes/sec in the condition of increased intraocular pressure.

We replicated these experiments in our simulations as follows: For each set of depression parameters, all of the LGN neurons in the model were made to fire spontaneously for a period of 1.75 sec. Following this, stimulus trains at 20, 50 or 100 Hz were presented (all of the LGN neurons fire synchronously, but note they have varying transmission delays as described above), and the resulting PSP's in the cortical neuron were monitored. Each simulation leads to estimates of the train of cortical PSP amplitudes (quantified as discussed previously) at the corresponding stimulus frequency. For the control condition, we took the spontaneous firing rates of the LGN cells to be 11.8 spikes/sec. To model the effect of reduced spontaneous activity, we again allowed the LGN neurons to fire with a background rate of 11.8 spikes/sec for a period of 1.75 sec and then with a background rate of 4.1 spikes/sec for 5 sec, as in the experiments. At the end of this period, a stimulus train was presented at 50 Hz, and the resulting PSP's in the cortical neuron were monitored. We compared the cortical PSP amplitudes from the control conditions (20, 50 and 100 Hz) and the first PSP amplitude from the reduced spontaneous activity case with the experimental data. For the reduced spontaneous activity case, Boudreau and Ferster [34] reported that the first PSP amplitude increased by $44.9\pm0.11\%$ (mean$\pm$stan-standard error) relative to control, and that subsequent PSP amplitudes were not significantly different from control. Their standard error corresponds to an error bar of ±0.11 in the relative units of our Fig. 1. For the control condition, Boudreau and Ferster referred to error bars that were smaller than their displayed data points (their Fig. 4D); their data points had a radius of 0.11 in the same relative units. We use this value of 0.11 in relative units for all error bars in our Fig. 1B and for the error bar (not shown in our Fig. 1C) for the first PSP for the reduced spontaneous activity. We searched the parameter space for p_o within $0<p_o<1$, $k_{\max}$ within $0<k_{\max}<100$, $k_0/k_{\max}$ within $0<k_0/k_{\max}<1$, and τ_{Ca} within $0\text{msec}<\tau_{Ca}<20\text{msec}$, and determined parameters that agreed with the experimental data (produced values within error bars for all data points). We chose from among those the values $p_o=0.85$, $k_{\max}=84\,\text{sec}^{-1}$, $k_0/k_{\max}=0.03$ and $\tau_{Ca}=3msec$, which were the parameters giving the minimum value for the maximum absolute error over the 5 stimulus trains for the spontaneous case (at 20, 50 and 100 Hz) and the first stimulus for the control case.

Estimating the firing rate of a simple cell

To determine whether spike threshold might alter or amplify tuning effects of synaptic depression, we estimated the tuning of firing rate that would be induced by the LGN inputs. To do so, we make the simplifying assumption that voltage is linear in the excitatory conductance. For large voltage excursions, voltage response can be sublinear in the excitatory conductance [47], but the assumption of linearity can be justified for two reasons (i) From resting potential to spike threshold, i.e $\sim$20 mV, the relationship can be reasonably approximated as linear [47]. (ii) To the degree that voltage response is sublinear in the excitatory conductance, the problem with tuning will get worse, i.e. the difference between null and preferred responses will be weaker, so linearity is a conservative assumption for purposes of our study, which focuses on whether synaptic depression can enhance the difference between null and preferred responses.

Given the assumption that voltage response is linear in the conductance, we estimate the normalized firing rate of simple cells from the LGN input using the results of Finn et al [17]. These authors found that the firing rate of simple cells is related to mean membrane potential and its standard deviation across trials through the following power law relationship.

$$R(v_m,v_s)=constant\ x\ |v_m+k*v_s|_+^{\ p} \tag{11}$$

Here, $|x|_+=x,x>0;=0$, otherwise. v is the membrane potential relative to the resting potential, $v_m=mean(v)$, $v_s=std(v)$, $k=0.68$ and p was found by fitting Fig. 7B of [17] to Eq. 11, giving the exponent $p=3.62$.

Supplementary Fig. 1C of [17] (replotted in our Fig. 2A, data points with error bars) shows the tuning of the normalized standard deviation of the peak voltages for three contrasts (0%, 4% and 64%) and five orientations ($-90°$, $-30°$, $0°$, $30°$, $90°$), averaged over 52 simple cells in cat V1. For each cell, the preferred orientation was set to $0°$, and the tuning curve was normalized by the cell's peak voltage at 64% contrast at the preferred orientation. To estimate the standard deviation values for other values of contrast, c, and orientation, o, we first fit the data (Supplementary Fig. 1C of [17]) to a smooth function that we found could well fit the data, given by.

$$f(c,o)=f_{background}+(a_1c^{1/4}-a_2c^{1/2})\exp(-(o/o_s)^2/2)-a_3c^{1/4} \tag{12}$$

Here, $f_{background}\equiv f(c=0,o)$ corresponds to the value at zero contrast, $f_{background}=0.21$ [17]. We fit the remaining constants: $a_1=0.26$, $a_2=0.24$, $a_3=0.096$ and $o_s=23°$. This function is shown as the smooth curves in Fig. 2A which are fits to the data of Supplementary Fig. 1C of [17]. The curves fall within the experimentally reported range. Next, we estimated the standard deviations at contrasts (3%, 6%, 12%, 24%, 48%, 72% and 96%; curves for these contrasts shown in Fig. 2B) and orientations ($-90°$ to $90°$ with $10°$ intervals) to use in our simulations as follows: For each contrast c and orientation o, we generated many trials of simple cell responses and determined the mean, c_m, and standard deviation, c_s, of the conductance response at each time across the

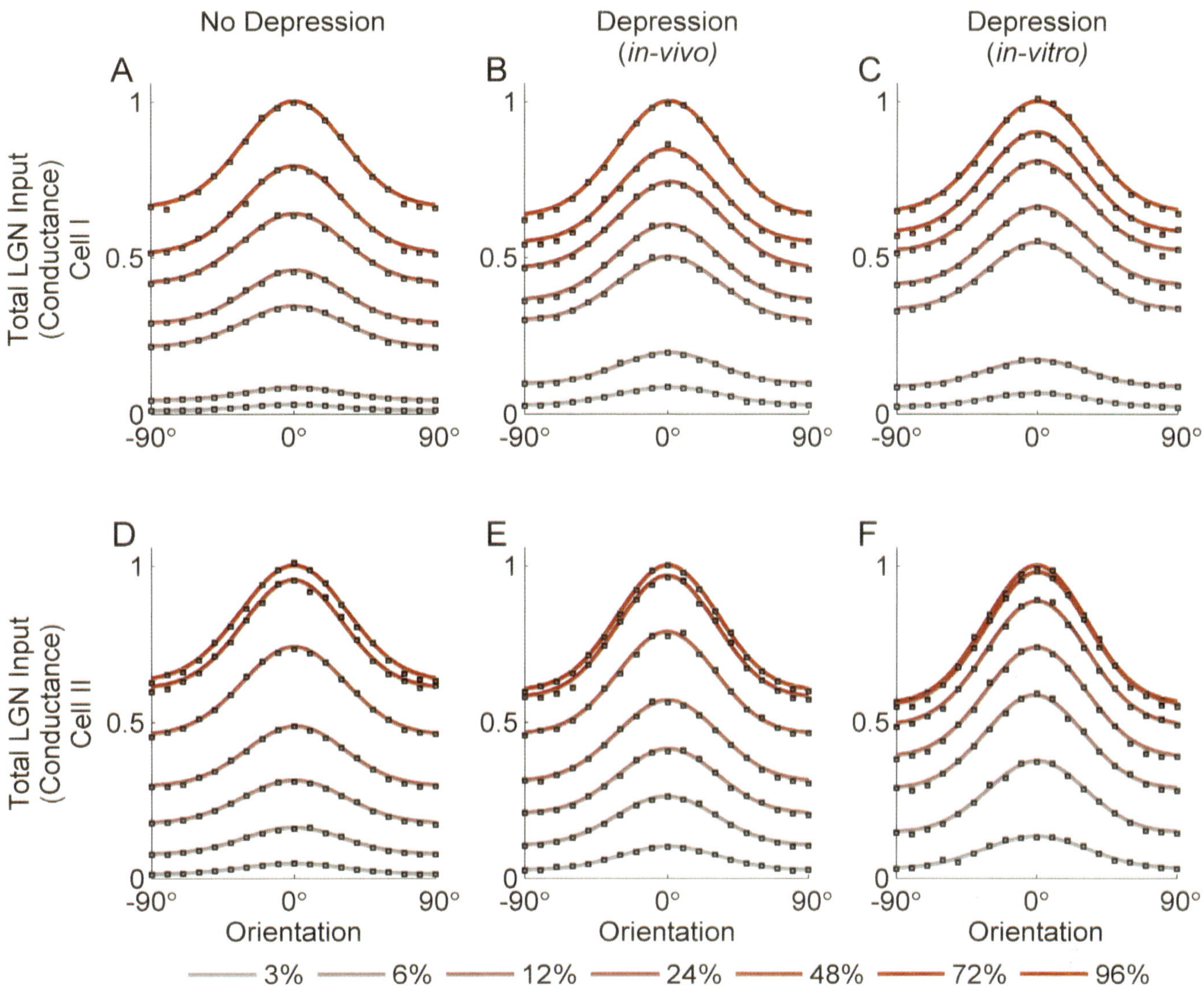

Figure 3. Orientation tuning of the peak LGN input to the simple cell (in terms of conductance) over a cycle in response to drifting grating stimuli of varying contrasts. Results are shown for two different models of LGN response time course, each based on the response time course of a measured LGN cell: Cell I (A–C) and Cell II (D–F). In each figure, the colored circles show peak input for 6 different contrast levels (3%, 6%, 12%, 24%, 48%, 72% and 96%) and 19 orientation angles (from −90° to 90° with steps of 10°). The colored smooth curves show fits of a Gaussian plus baseline to these tuning curves at the different contrasts. Each fit is normalized to the value of the fit at the preferred orientation at highest contrast (96%), which is set to 1. Orientation tuning curves are calculated for the cases: No Depression (A, D), Depression using *in-vivo* (B, E) fit parameters, Depression using *in-vitro* (C, F) fit parameters.

cycle. We then took v_m at each time equal to the corresponding value of c_m. We took the values of v_s across the cycle to be the corresponding values of c_s scaled so that, at the peak of the cycle, the value of v_s, relative to the peak v_m at 64% contrast and preferred orientation, was given by $f(c,o)$ (Eq. 12). That is, we used Eq. 12 to determine v_s at the peak of the cycle, relative to the peak v_m at 64% contrast and preferred orientation as determined by our simulations; and used our simulations to determine the relative values of v_s at other points in the cycle (relative to the v_s at the peak of the cycle). Then, using the v_m and v_s values at each point in the cycle, we used Eq. 11 to determine the normalized firing rates at each time across the cycle (normalized to the peak response across orientations and contrasts).

It is important to note that we are interested only in tuning properties and so we model normalized firing rates, ignoring absolute response levels. Given that (1) intracortical excitation does not alter mean voltage orientation tuning [6,7,29,30] and (2) our model of the voltage standard deviation implicitly includes the effects of intracortical excitation (because the voltage standard deviation at the cycle peak, relative to the peak mean voltage at 64% contrast, preferred orientation, is fit to empirical measurements of voltage noise in simple cells *in-vivo*), explicitly incorporating intracortical excitation into our model would not alter spiking orientation tuning. Hence, we neglect modeling intracortical excitation in determining the spike-rate tuning that would be induced by the LGN input. Note also that, if all conductances were multiplied by a factor k, then using the above procedure all spike rates would be multiplied by the factor k^p. Thus, only the relative conductances across contrasts and orientations, and not the absolute conductance amplitudes, influence the normalized spiking tuning that we present here.

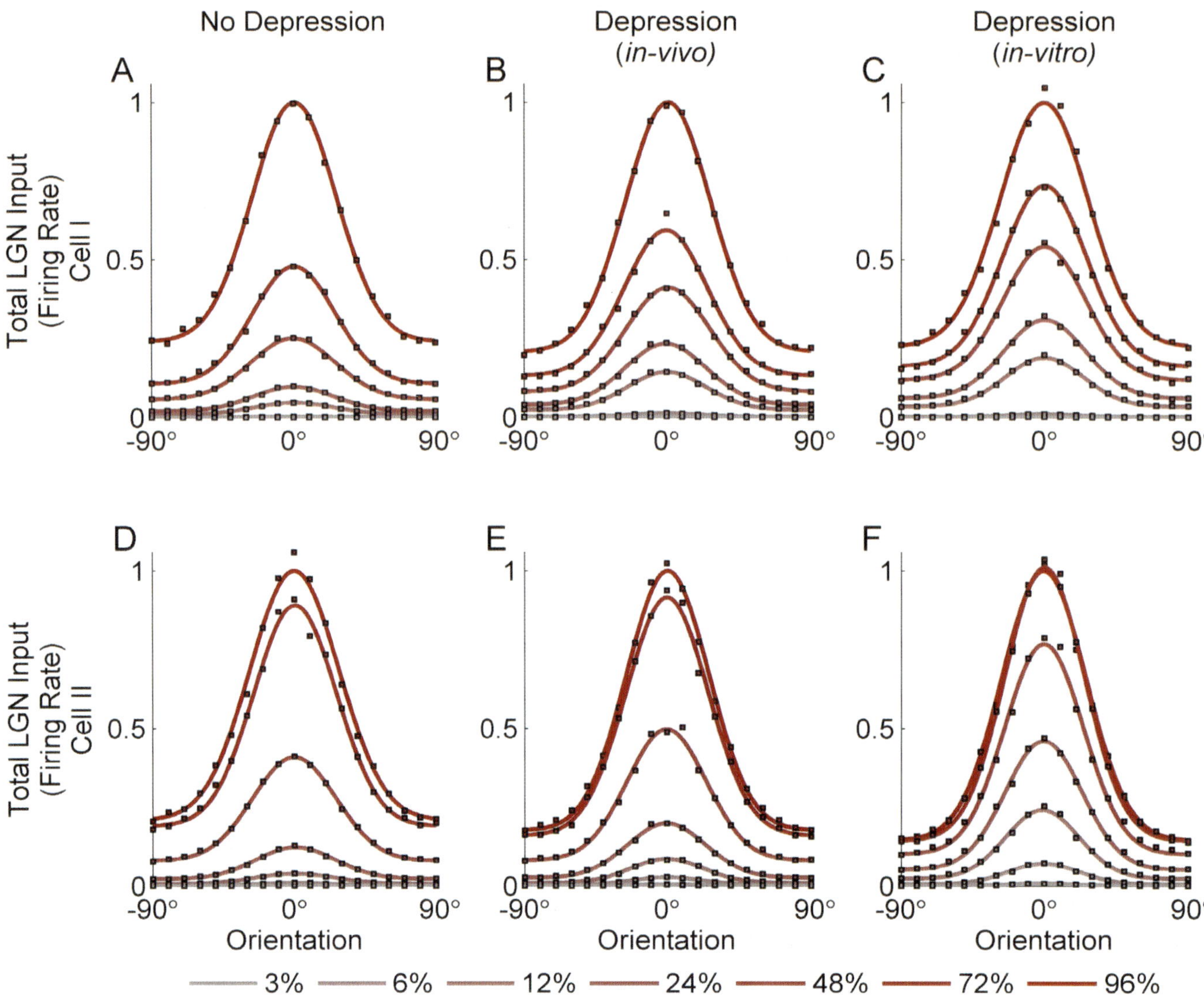

Figure 4. Orientation tuning of the peak LGN input to the simple cell (in terms of firing rate) over a cycle in response to drifting grating stimuli of varying contrasts. Results are shown for two different models of LGN response timecourse, each based on the response timecourse of a measured LGN cell: Cell I (A–C) and Cell II (D–F). In each figure, the colored circles show peak input for 6 different contrast levels (3%, 6%, 12%, 24%, 48%, 72% and 96%) and 19 orientation angles (from -90° to 90° with steps of 10°). The colored smooth curves show Gaussian fits to these tuning curves at the different contrasts. Each fit is normalized to the value of the fit at the preferred orientation at highest contrast (96%), which is set to 1. Orientation tuning curves are calculated for the cases: No Depression (A, D), Depression using *in-vivo* (B, E) fit parameters, Depression using *in-vitro* (C, F) fit parameters.

Quantifying orientation tuning width

We quantify orientation tuning as the half-width at half-height [17], where half-height is defined as half the distance between the maximum response and baseline (as shown in Supplementary Fig. 2 of [17]). Baseline is meant to indicate firing rate in the absence of a stimulus. We defined the baseline as the cortical-cell response when LGN-cell firing rates were set to their mean firing rates at 3% contrast, i.e. the weakest stimulus for which we had data. The rationale for this choice is that such weak stimuli typically modulate the firing rate of LGN cells linearly, without rectification. Consequently, the firing rate of LGN cells in the absence of a stimulus is approximately identical to their mean firing rate in response to a drifting grating with a 3% contrast. If the cortical cell's response to a stimulus orthogonal to the preferred was greater than the half-height, we set the half-width at half-height to be 90°.

Results

In order to assess depression of thalamocortical synapses *in-vivo*, Boudreau and Ferster [34] recorded intracellularly from V1 simple cells receiving direct input from the LGN, as judged by the short latency and low timing jitter of LGN-evoked PSP's. They delivered trains of electrical stimuli to the LGN, and examined the change over time in the resulting PSP amplitudes recorded in the simple cell. They observed that the second PSP amplitude (*i.e.*, in response to the second stimulus in the train) was strongly reduced relative to the first PSP amplitude, with relatively little further reduction for subsequent PSP's (see Fig. 1B). They tried to fit their data with a simple $''f-\tau''$ model, in which a synapse's strength is

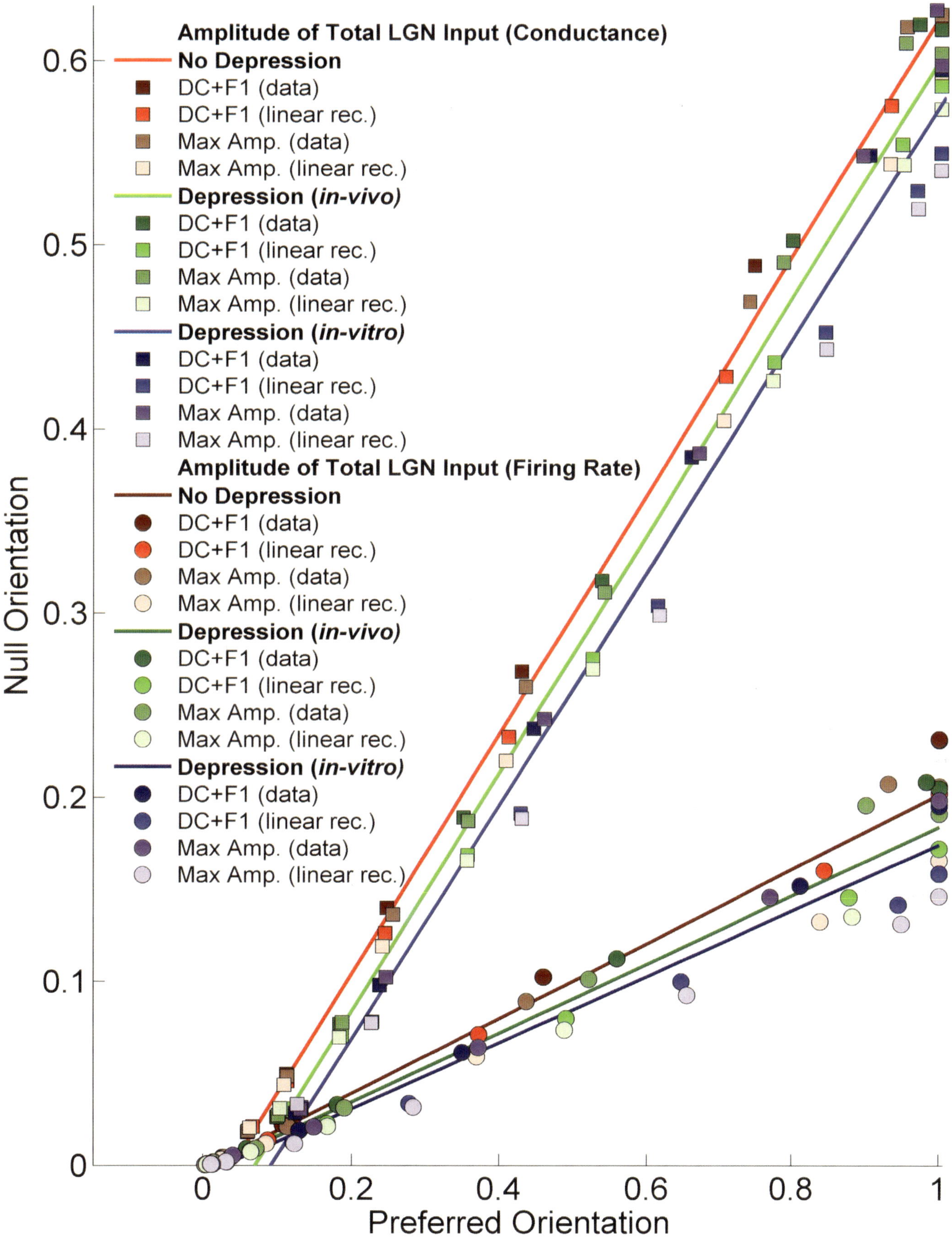
Amplitude of Total LGN Input (Conductance)
No Depression
DC+F1 (data)
DC+F1 (linear rec.)
Max Amp. (data)
Max Amp. (linear rec.)
Depression (in-vivo)
DC+F1 (data)
DC+F1 (linear rec.)
Max Amp. (data)
Max Amp. (linear rec.)
Depression (in-vitro)
DC+F1 (data)
DC+F1 (linear rec.)
Max Amp. (data)
Max Amp. (linear rec.)
Amplitude of Total LGN Input (Firing Rate)
No Depression
DC+F1 (data)
DC+F1 (linear rec.)
Max Amp. (data)
Max Amp. (linear rec.)
Depression (in-vivo)
DC+F1 (data)
DC+F1 (linear rec.)
Max Amp. (data)
Max Amp. (linear rec.)
Depression (in-vitro)
DC+F1 (data)
DC+F1 (linear rec.)
Max Amp. (data)
Max Amp. (linear rec.)
Null Orientation
Preferred Orientation
0
0.1
0.2
0.3
0.4
0.5
0.6
0
0.2
0.4
0.6
0.8
1

Figure 5. Amplitude of the conductance and the firing rate at the null orientation as a function of amplitude at the preferred orientation. The cases shown are: No Depression (red), Depression using *in-vivo* (green) or *in-vitro* (blue) fit parameters. Amplitudes are means across the 7 models of LGN timecourse, where for each model of LGN timecourse and depression the amplitude is scaled so that input to the preferred orientation at highest contrast is 1. Four different response measures are shown: either the actual experimental PSTH is used ("data") or a linear rectified approximation to it (see Materials and Methods); and there are two different measures of the size of this response (maximum amplitude over a cycle or DC+F1, where DC is mean over a cycle and F1 is Fourier amplitude of the first harmonic). Results from all contrast levels are pooled together and displayed for each of model of depression and response measure. Linear fits (minimizing sum-squared error) to each model are also shown (See color insets).

multiplied by $f<1$ after each spike and, between spikes, relaxes toward that synapse's maximal strength with time constant τ. Such models have been successfully used to model cortical synaptic depression as observed in many *in-vitro* experiments [23,45,46]. Boudreau and Ferster [34] observed that, because of the transient character of the synaptic depression observed *in-vivo*, this model underestimated the initial depression and overestimated the depression that occurred later in the train and so gave very poor fits.

In a different set of experiments, studying the climbing fiber synapse in cerebellum, Dittman and Regehr [44] showed that recovery from depression was accelerated by accumulation of presynaptic residual calcium. They suggested a modification to the $''f-\tau''$ model in which the recovery time, τ, is not constant but instead is calcium dependent. This dependence leads to maintenance of synaptic efficacy under conditions that would otherwise deplete the available transmitter pool.

We find that the [44] depression model allows good fits to the *in-vivo* experimental data on monosynaptic cells obtained by Boudreau and Ferster [34] (Fig. 1). From the time course of model response to presynaptic trains of stimuli at 20 Hz, 50 Hz and 100 Hz (Fig. 1A), we can extract the amplitude of response to each stimulus. The model amplitudes (Fig. 1B, 20 Hz (red), 50 Hz (green) and 100 Hz (blue)) show reasonable matches to the experimental observations and fall within an upper bound estimate of the experimental error (Fig. 1B, error bars) for all stimulus frequencies. The model successfully captures the large initial reduction in amplitude, evident on the 2nd stimulus of the train, and the small changes in amplitude over subsequent stimuli. For comparison, using parameters obtained from the $''f-\tau''$ model fit from *in-vitro* experiments, we observe a much more gradual decrease in amplitude with stimulus number (Fig. 1B, 100 Hz (brown)), as noted by [34], and we found that this was true of this model for any parameters that produced significant depression.

Hereafter, we will refer to the [44] model, which uses the depression parameters from the fit to the *in-vivo* geniculocortical data of [34], as the "*in-vivo*" model, and to the $''f-\tau''$ model, which uses the depression parameters from the fit of [23] to *in-vitro* geniculocortical data [35], as the "*in-vitro*" model.

The stimulus-induced depression observed by [34] was weak relative to that typically observed *in-vitro*. They speculated that this may be due to synapses already being partially depressed due to spontaneous activity, as had been suggested in the somatosensory thalamocortical system [48,49]. To test this, they reduced LGN spontaneous firing rates by about 65% by applying intraocular pressure. Consistent with pre-existing depression, they found that this increased the amplitude of response to the first stimulus in a 50 Hz train by 45±11% on average, but had little effect on responses to subsequent stimuli in the train. We replicated this experiment by lowering the LGN firing rates by the same amounts as in the experiments, as discussed in the Materials and Methods section. The results for the *in-vivo* model closely parallel the experimental observations (Fig. 1C). Reduced spontaneous activity (Fig. 1C, 50 Hz (black)) results in increased amplitude of response to the first stimulus and has little effect on the remaining stimuli compared to spontaneous activity obtained from the control condition (Fig. 1C, 50 Hz (green)). In Fig. 1 we assume that the simple cell receives LGN inputs with weights stochastically sampled from a Gabor function (see Materials and Methods), [20], but the fit does not depend on this choice: we obtain similar results if constant weights are assigned to all LGN ON and OFF-center inputs (not shown).

Having a successful model of the depression observed *in-vivo* in cat V1, we now use this to model the effects of depression on the total LGN input received by a layer 4 simple cell at various orientations and contrasts. We assume that the simple cell receives LGN inputs with weights stochastically sampled from a Gabor function [20]. We assume that all LGN inputs have the same periodic timecourse of response to a drifting sinusoidal luminance grating of a given contrast, except that the LGN inputs vary in the phase of their response according to their positions relative to the grating and the orientation of the grating. As a model of the timecourse of LGN response, we use the responses of a single measured LGN cell to gratings of various orientations and contrasts. We study the model for eight different choices of measured LGN cell and thus eight different models of the timecourse of LGN response. Alternatively, we could have let each LGN input be modeled by a different LGN cell, but this would have tended to average out the variations; we choose the more extreme alternative in order to see the largest range of possible variations in LGN input. To study the effect of depression at thalamocortical synapses, we simply model the net LGN input to a simple cell, and do not model any cortical mechanisms, such as inhibition, that might combine with this input to produce cortical responses. To characterize the tuning of the net LGN input, we use two measures, as described in Materials and Methods. First, we characterize the tuning of the total LGN-induced conductance as a direct measure of the net input. Second, to determine whether spike threshold effects might reveal stronger effects of synaptic depression on tuning, we estimate the tuning of the simple-cell firing rate responses that would be induced by this LGN input. Note that we are only interested in tuning, which is independent of intracortical excitation [6,7,29,30], and not the response amplitude, which depends on intracortical excitation [6,7,29,30], so we ignore amplitude and report only normalized responses (normalized to the response at optimal orientation and largest contrast studied).

Figs. 3 and 4 show the tuning of the peak LGN input conductance to a simple cell (Fig. 3) and of the firing rate this conductance would evoke in the simple cell (Fig. 4), for two models of LGN timecourse, each based on the response of a different measured LGN cell (cell 1: Fig. 3A-C and Fig. 4A–C; cell 2: Fig. 3D-F and Fig. 4D–F). For the conductance (Fig. 3), the input in response to the null orientation (defined as the orientation orthogonal to the preferred) grows strongly with contrast, so that the null input at high contrast is much larger than the input to the preferred orientation at low contrasts. This is true whether the synapses are modeled without depression (Fig. 3A,D) or with depression modeled as in the *in-vivo* model (Fig. 3 B,E) or the *in-vitro* model (Fig. 3 C,F). With depression, low-contrast input is

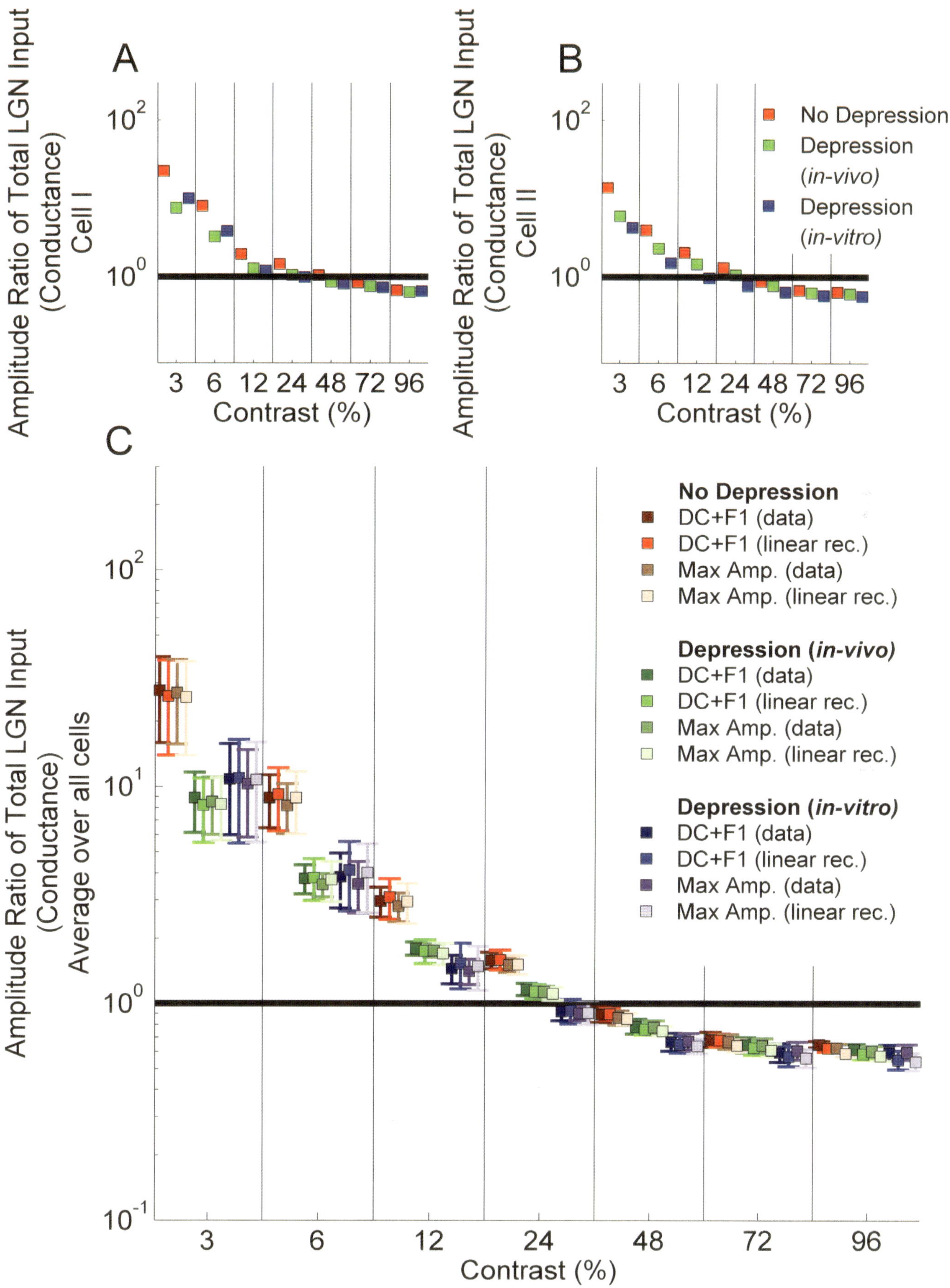
A
Amplitude Ratio of Total LGN Input
(Conductance)
Cell I
10^2
10^0
3 6 12 24 48 72 96
Contrast (%)
B
Amplitude Ratio of Total LGN Input
(Conductance)
Cell II
No Depression
Depression
(in-vivo)
Depression
(in-vitro)
C
Amplitude Ratio of Total LGN Input
(Conductance)
Average over all cells
10^{-1}
10^1
No Depression
DC+F1 (data)
DC+F1 (linear rec.)
Max Amp. (data)
Max Amp. (linear rec.)
Depression (in-vivo)
Depression (in-vitro)

Figure 6. Ratio of the amplitude of the tuning curve in Fig. 3 (normalized conductance) at the null orientation (the orientation orthogonal to the preferred) at 96% contrast to that at the preferred orientation (*x-axis*; 3%, 6%, 12%, 24%, 48%, 72% and 96%). Black horizontal line indicates amplitude ratio 1. The cases shown are: No Depression (red), Depression using *in-vivo* (green) fit parameters, Depression using *in-vitro* (blue) fit parameters. A) Amplitude ratios for Cell I of Fig. 2; B) Amplitude ratios for Cell II of Fig. 2; C) Amplitude ratios averaged over all 7 experimentally measured LGN cells (mean ± std error). In C, four different response measures are shown: either the actual experimental PSTH is used ("data") or a linear rectified approximation to it (see Materials and Methods); and there are two different measures of the size of this response (maximum amplitude over a cycle or DC+F1, where DC is mean over a cycle and F1 is Fourier amplitude of the first harmonic); see inset for colors corresponding to these 4 measures. All points between each pair of vertical bars represent the same contrast: for different response measures, results for each contrast are offset relative to each other for ease of visualization.

larger relative to high-contrast input than without depression. This corresponds to the fact that synaptic depression induces saturation of input at lower contrasts. That is, with depression, a given low contrast is a larger percentage of the saturating contrast and hence behaves, relative to the largest contrast, as does a higher contrast without depression (note that each panel in Fig. 3 is normalized so that 1 represents the preferred input to high contrast). However, for a curve with a given size of preferred input, the size of the null input is about the same with or without depression, though slightly reduced by depression. Results for firing rate tuning curves (Fig. 4) are similar in these respects, although the tuning curves for the firing rate are narrower and the null firing rate much lower relative to preferred firing rate than was the case for membrane potential (Fig. 3). Overall, as shown in Fig. 5, the ratio of null input to preferred input changes little across contrasts, both in terms of membrane potential and firing rate, and synaptic depression of either form causes only a very slight reduction in this ratio. Depression fit to the *in-vitro* data causes about twice the reduction in this ratio as does depression fit to the *in-vivo* model, but both reductions are slight.

To better assay the effect of the null-orientation response on orientation tuning, we examine the ratio of the response to the null orientation at the highest contrast to that at the preferred orientation at a given contrast (Fig. 6, membrane potential; Fig. 7, firing rate; contrast of preferred-orientation stimulus is given on the *x-axis*; different measures of response in figures discussed further below). As noted in the Introduction, in real neurons this ratio generally stays below 1 even for the lowest-contrast preferred-orientation stimulus. It must stay below 1 to explain the observation that cells show spike responses to the preferred orientation at the lowest responsive contrast but not to the null orientation even at the highest contrast. For the two LGN cells examined in Figs. 3,4 (Figs. 6A,B and Figs. 7A,B) and more generally on average across the eight LGN cells used as models of LGN time course (Figs. 6C, 7C), the results using *in-vivo* vs. *in-vitro* depression models are very close (see error bars in Figs. 6C, 7C). Depression improves the results (reduces the ratio) at any given preferred-orientation contrast, but ratios remain greater than 1 for low preferred-orientation contrasts under all depression models (for contrasts of 12% or less for the *in-vitro* depression model, and contrasts of 24% or less for the *in-vivo* depression model or for no depression). Although the contrast levels at which the ratio is less than 1 for firing rate responses (Fig. 7) are similar to those for conductance responses (Fig. 6), the range of the ratio for different contrasts is much broader for firing rate responses.

As discussed in the Introduction, the relative suppression of response to null-orientation stimuli, which is critical to observed orientation tuning, also manifests as a value significantly less than 1 for the ratio of the mean LGN-induced conductance to a null-orientation stimulus to that for a preferred-orientation stimulus, at least at high contrast. We examined this for our various models. We found that the ratio remains very close to 1 across all contrasts and regardless of the absence or, if present, the form of geniculocortical depression (Fig. 8). In this figure, at each contrast we averaged only over LGN cells for which the DC component of the null-orientation response and the DC component of the preferred-orientation response were both >0.05, in units in which the peak conductance to the highest-contrast preferred orientation is 1 (as in Fig. 3). When these mean responses were smaller, the ratios of the two responses could be poorly behaved, but the absolute difference between the two mean responses was never greater than 0.02 across the excluded cases.

Finally, we examined the dependence on contrast of the half-width at half-height (Materials and Methods) of the tuning curve (Fig. 9). Experimentally, half-width is invariant to stimulus contrast for firing rate responses [17,32,33,50], while for voltage responses it broadens moderately with contrast (this broadening, along with the changing input/output relationship due to decreasing voltage variance, produces the contrast-invariant spiking response) [17,19,50]. For conductance responses, the half-width increases dramatically with contrast, reaching a plateau near 90° for contrasts of 24% and above, reflecting the lack of suppression of the untuned component of the LGN input (Fig. 9A). This increase is slightly less with synaptic depression, with a greater reduction for *in-vitro* than for *in-vivo* depression, but the reductions due to depression are slight. As a result, firing-rate tuning widths increase significantly with contrast (Fig. 9B). The tuning widths are slightly lower with synaptic depression, but the increase in width with contrast is similar with or without depression.

Previous modeling efforts have used a linear rectified model of LGN input and have used the DC+F1 as a surrogate for the peak input [24]. To determine whether these approximations affect any of our results, in Figs. 5–9, we computed results both with and without these approximations. To model the response of an LGN cell, we considered the cycle-averaged PSTH (referred to as "data" in Fig. 6C, 7C), or a linear-rectified fit to this PSTH consisting of a sinusoidal modulation plus a constant, with negative values set to zero (see Materials and Methods). For each of these two models, we considered two measures of the total input to the simple cell: the peak input over a cycle, or the sum of the mean (DC) and first harmonic (F1) over a cycle, which would be equal to the peak if there were no higher harmonics. As can be seen in the figures, these alternative choices for measures of LGN response or of the summed LGN input make very little difference to the results.

Discussion

We find that synaptic depression as measured *in-vivo* in thalamocortical synapses [34] can be well fit by a model of depression that incorporates a calcium-dependent change in the time constant of recovery from depression [44]. Using this "*in-vivo*" model as well as an earlier, simpler model [45,46] fit to *in-vitro* data [35], we find that thalamocortical depression in either form has little impact on the orientation tuning of the LGN input to V1 simple cells or its contrast dependence, other than to induce response saturation at lower contrasts. Thus, the contrast-

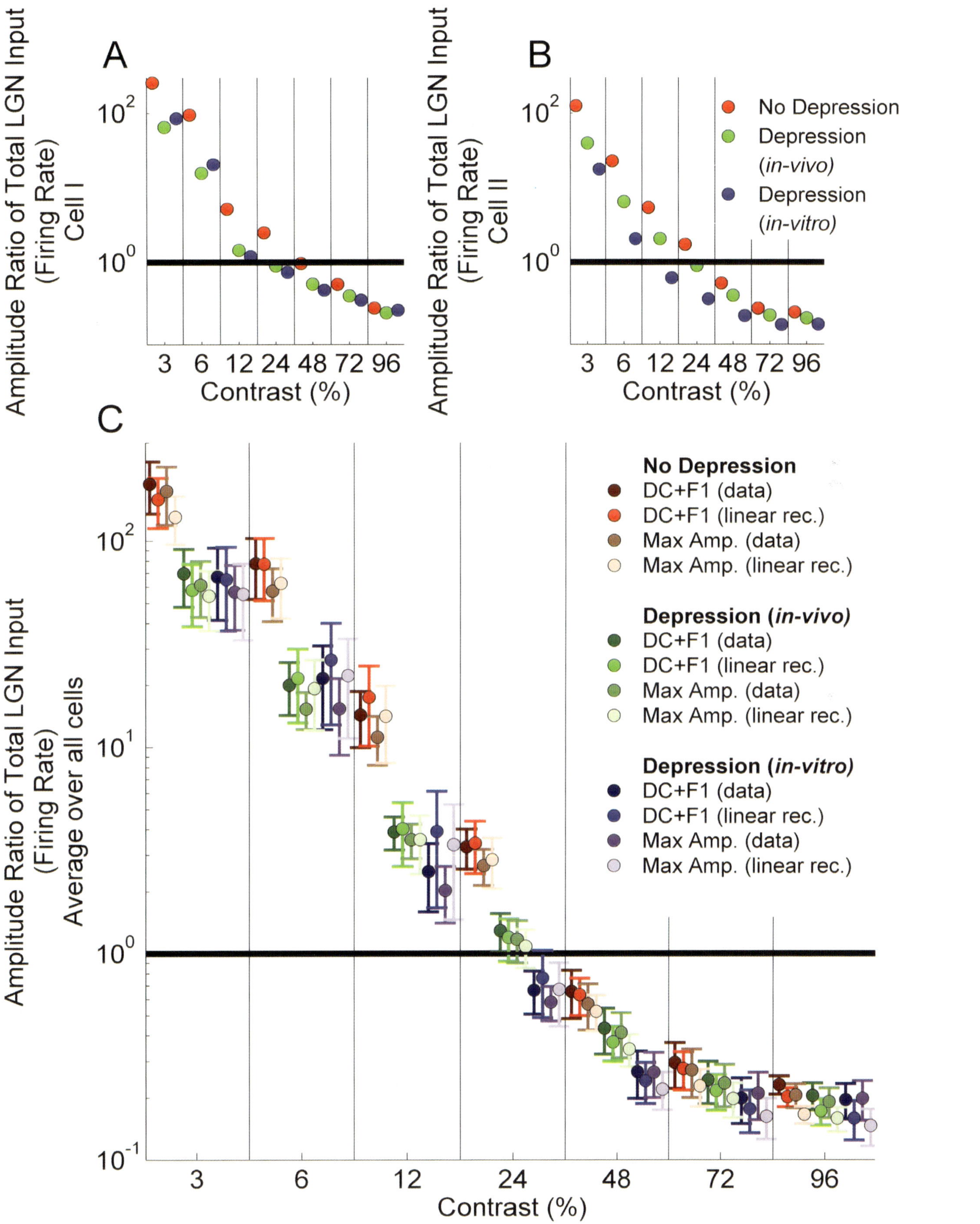
A
Amplitude Ratio of Total LGN Input
(Firing Rate)
Cell I
10^2
10^0
3 6 12 24 48 72 96
Contrast (%)
B
Amplitude Ratio of Total LGN Input
(Firing Rate)
Cell II
10^2
10^0
3 6 12 24 48 72 96
Contrast (%)
No Depression
Depression
(in-vivo)
Depression
(in-vitro)
C
Amplitude Ratio of Total LGN Input
(Firing Rate)
Average over all cells
10^2
10^1
10^0
10^{-1}
3 6 12 24 48 72 96
Contrast (%)
No Depression
DC+F1 (data)
DC+F1 (linear rec.)
Max Amp. (data)
Max Amp. (linear rec.)
Depression (in-vivo)
DC+F1 (data)
DC+F1 (linear rec.)
Max Amp. (data)
Max Amp. (linear rec.)
Depression (in-vitro)
DC+F1 (data)
DC+F1 (linear rec.)
Max Amp. (data)
Max Amp. (linear rec.)

Figure 7. Ratio of the amplitude of the orientation tuning curve in Fig. 4 (normalized firing rate) at the null orientation (the orientation orthogonal to the preferred) at 96% contrast to that at the preferred orientation at varying contrasts (*x-axis*; 3%, 6%, 12%, 24%, 48%, 72% and 96%). Black horizontal line indicates amplitude ratio 1. The cases shown are: No Depression (red), Depression using *in-vivo* (green) fit parameters, Depression using *in-vitro* (blue) fit parameters. A) Amplitude ratios for Cell I of Fig. 2; B) Amplitude ratios for Cell II of Fig. 2; C) Amplitude ratios averaged over all 7 experimentally measured LGN cells (mean ± std error). In C, four different response measures are shown: either the actual experimental PSTH is used ("data") or a linear rectified approximation to it (see Materials and Methods); and there are two different measures of the size of this response (maximum amplitude over a cycle or DC+F1, where DC is mean over a cycle and F1 is Fourier amplitude of the first harmonic); see inset for colors corresponding to these 4 measures. All points between each pair of vertical bars represent the same contrast: for different response measures, results for each contrast are offset relative to each other for ease of visualization.

invariance of the orientation tuning of simple cell responses [17,32,33,50] must depend on cortical mechanisms beyond the LGN synapse, e.g. feedforward inhibition driven by LGN excitation of cortical inhibitory cells [20,25,26,51] and/or effects of spike threshold and its interaction with voltage fluctuations [17,26,50].

Modeling synaptic depression

In our fit to the *in-vivo* data with the calcium-dependent recovery model, we found the exponential decay time constant for calcium to be $\tau_{Ca} = 3msec$, which is very low in comparison with/found by Dittman and Regehr [44], at the climbing fiber to purkinje cell synapse (or $\tau_{Ca} = 20msec$ when EGTA-AM was added to the presynaptic terminals). In addition to the difference in the synapses being studied, one possible contributor to the difference is temperature: Dittman and Regehr's experiments were conducted at 24 C, whereas Boudreau and Ferster's were at 38.3 C. A more accurate model of synaptic depression may also include the dependence of temperature as observed experimentally [52]. It also may be that the model, including the time constant necessary to fit the thalamocortical data, does not accurately represent the underlying biophysical mechanisms at the thalamocortical synapse, but is simply a phenomenological model that is able to fit the data.

The Role of Synaptic Depression in V1 Responses

We have found that synaptic depression causes little change in the ratio of null-orientation to preferred-orientation LGN input to a simple cell (Fig. 5) and thus has little effect on orientation tuning, other than to cause saturation to occur at lower contrasts as reported previously [23,27].

It is not surprising that synaptic depression causes similar suppression of response to all orientations at a given contrast, and thus has little effect on orientation tuning. Individual LGN cells are not tuned for the orientation of a drifting grating, and thus depression has the same effect on an individual LGN cell's output for any stimulus orientation. The LGN response is confined to and peaks within a particular portion of the stimulus cycle. Synaptic depression changes the temporal waveform over a cycle of the input from an LGN cell, relative to its firing rate, by suppressing later portions of the response relative to earlier portions (e.g., [23] (Fig. 5)). Orientation tuning arises from the fact that a preferred-orientation stimulus tends to drive all of a simple cell's LGN inputs to peak near the same phase of the stimulus cycle, whereas in response to a null grating LGN responses are dispersed across the stimulus cycle [20]. The total LGN input to a simple cell over time is predicted to be well approximated, as we have verified here, by the rectified sum of a mean (the zeroeth harmonic) and a sinusoid (the first harmonic or F1; the temporal modulation of the input at the same temporal frequency as the stimulus), in essence because the Gabor-function receptive field filters out higher harmonics in the time course of individual LGN cells [24]. The mean is untuned for orientation, and represents the sum of the means of the individual LGN inputs. The F1 is the orientation-tuned component, and represents the tendency of the LGN cells to all modulate their firing rates at roughly the same phase for preferred but not for null stimuli. For synaptic depression to differentially affect response to different orientations, the change in the LGN input waveform that it induces must either change the size of the DC relative to the F1 (*e.g.*, a thinner pulse of input has a smaller individual DC/F1 ratio) and/or change the tuning of the F1 (*i.e.*, lead to greater decrease in the net F1 for a given degree of phase desynchronization). Both effects are apparently small, even for strong depression.

Previous papers have studied the effects of synaptic depression on orientation selectivity. Carandini et al. [27] assumed perfect push-pull inhibition, i.e. that for each LGN cell driving excitatory input to a simple cell, an identical LGN cell except of opposite center type drives equal-strength inhibitory input. This eliminates the untuned component of the LGN input, leaving only the tuned component, so that in particular the input to a null-orientation stimulus is zero. Given a nearly-zero spike threshold, this solves the problem of achieving contrast-invariant orientation tuning [20], leaving synaptic depression simply to solve the problem of causing earlier contrast saturation in cortex than in LGN without altering orientation tuning.

Our results and conclusions significantly differ from Banitt et al. [28], who also studied the effect of synaptic depression on orientation tuning. First, we focused on the effects of thalamocortical synaptic depression as measured *in-vivo* by Boudreau and Ferster [34]. We fit our model to the full set of *in-vivo* data (including 20, 50, and 100 Hz pulse train data taking into account prior spontaneous activity, as well as the case of reduced spontaneous activity). The "moderate depression" model of Banitt et al. [28] was said to be fit to this *in-vivo* data, and in agreement with our findings it failed to suppress non-preferred responses. However their moderate depression model, while reasonably fitting the *in-vivo* data for 50 Hz pulse trains, failed to fit the data for 20 Hz pulse trains (their Fig. 6; conversely, their "strong depression" model in that figure reasonably fit the first two ISI's for 20 Hz *in-vivo* data, but failed to fit the 50 Hz *in-vivo* data); they did not illustrate model fits to 100 Hz *in-vivo* data. It also appears that their fitting to the *in-vivo* data was done assuming an undepressed state as the initial condition, rather than a partially depressed state due to prior spontaneous activity as in the data, as no mention of spontaneous activity was made for this protocol.

Second, Banitt et al. [28] primarily focused on a "strong depression" model that was said to be based on a fit to the *in-vitro* depression data of Stratford et al [35] (Fig. 1g). They reported that this strong depression could largely suppress depolarization at orientations far from the preferred and achieve contrast-invariant spiking tuning, unlike our findings using a depression model fit to the same *in-vitro* data. However, they appear to have used a different strong depression model to study orientation tuning than was used to fit the *in-vitro* data, and both appear to differ from the strong depression model as defined parametrically, even though all are identified as the same strong depression model. After a

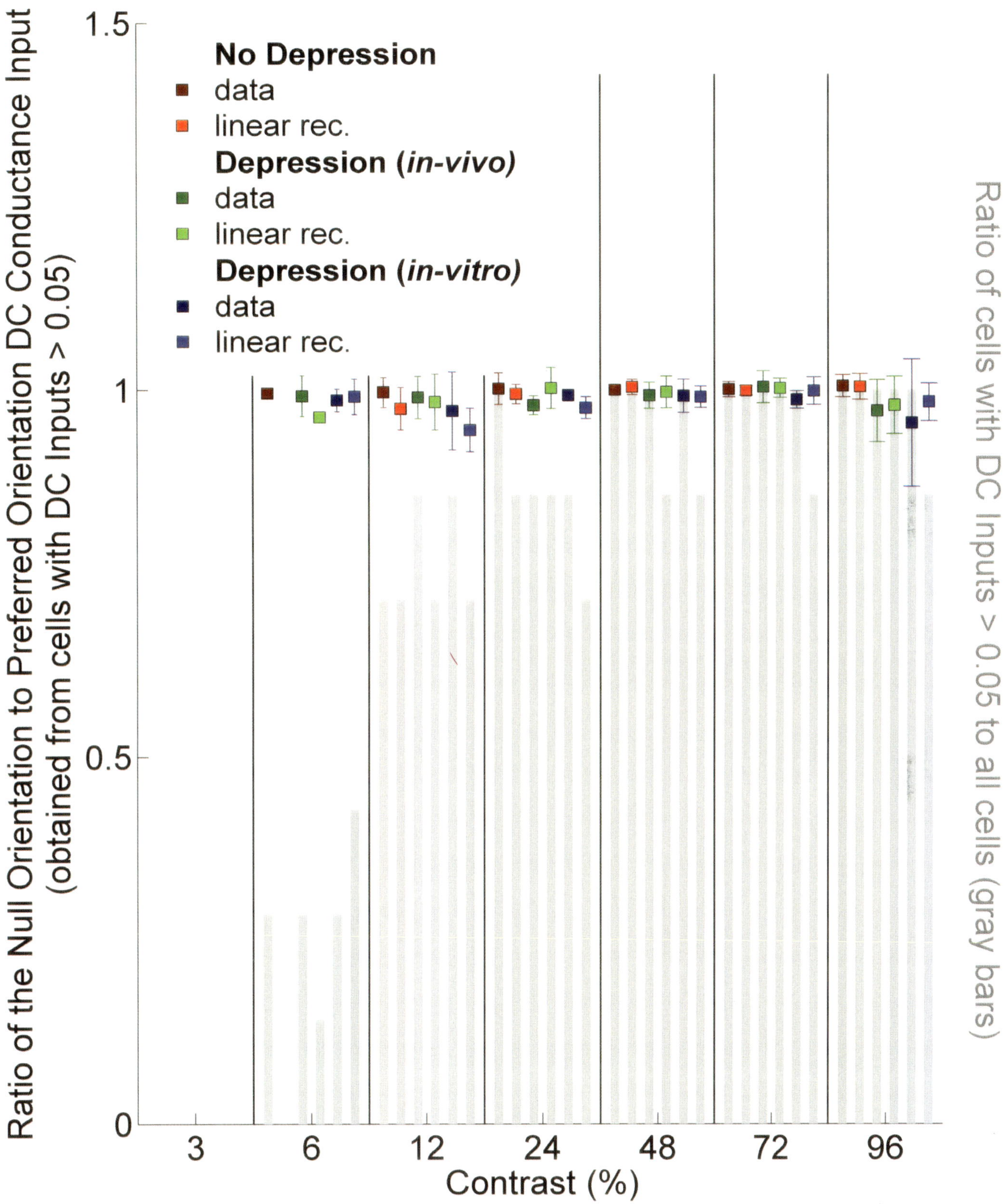

Figure 8. Ratio of the null orientation DC input to preferred orientation DC input averaged over LGN cells, across contrasts. Only cells for which both DC's were greater than 0.05 are included in the calculation; mean ratios (squares) and the standard deviations (error bars) are shown. The cases shown are: No Depression (red), Depression using *in-vivo* (green) or *in-vitro* (blue) fit parameters. For each case, two different response measures are shown: either the actual experimental PSTH is used ("data") or a linear rectified approximation to it (see Fig. 7 legend and Materials and Methods). For a given response measure and contrast (3%, 6%, 12%, 24%, 48%, 72% or 96%), ratio of number of cells that have both DC inputs >0.05 to total number of cells is shown as gray bars.

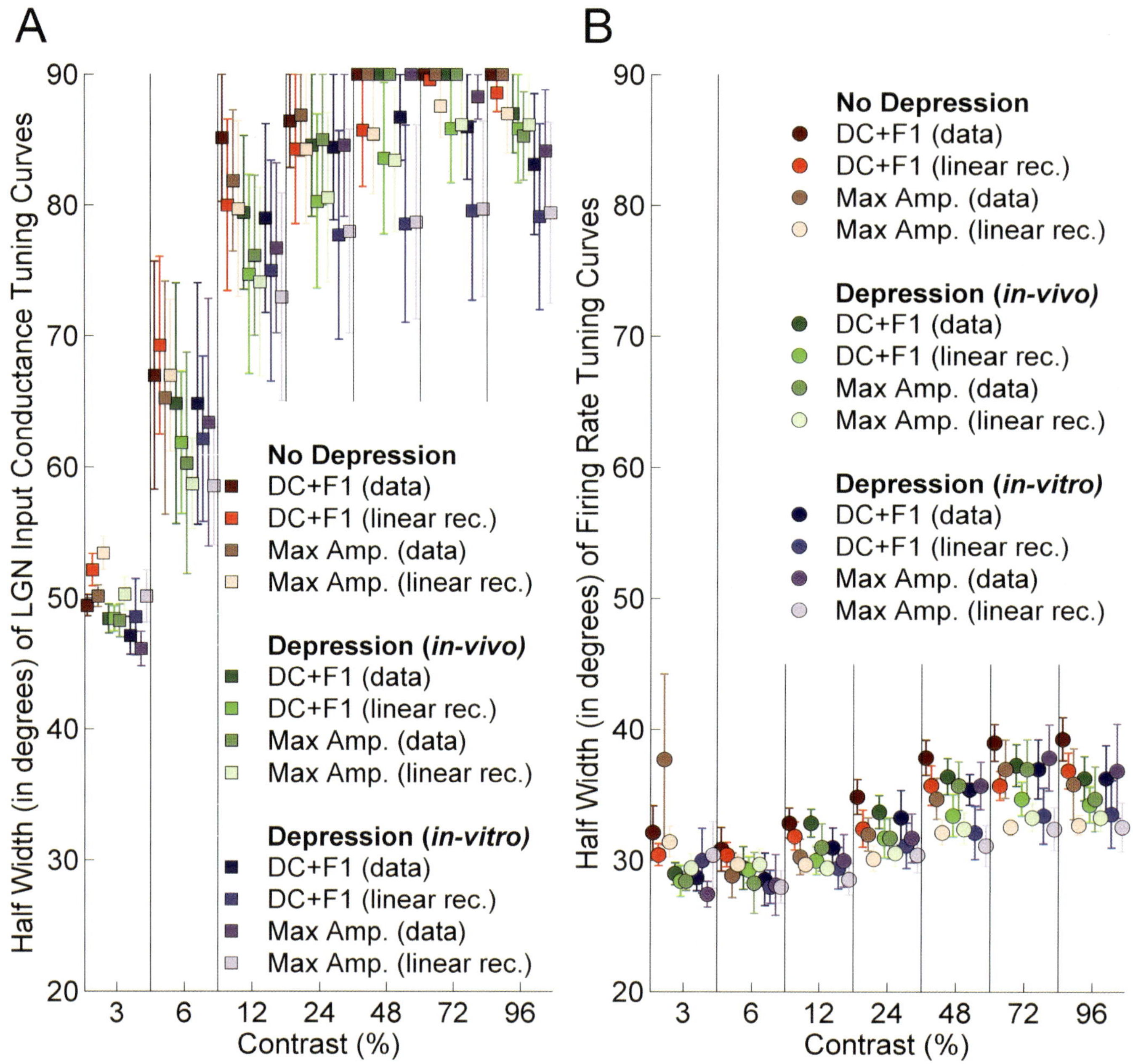

Figure 9. Half-width of tuning curves at half-height (i.e., difference between orientation giving peak response and orientation giving 50% of peak response) obtained from the tuning curves of total LGN input: A) Conductance B) Firing Rate. Each half-width is calculated at a specific contrast (*x-axis*; 3%, 6%, 12%, 24%, 48%, 72% and 96%). Half-widths are averaged over the experimentally measured LGN cells, mean ± std error (*y-axis*). If null-orientation response was greater than 50% of the peak response, the half-width is undetermined (half-width >90°, See Supplementary Fig. 2 of [17]; in such cases we set the half-width to 90°. Four different response measures are shown, as described in legend of Fig. 7. Conventions as in Fig. 7.

20 msec ISI beginning from an undepressed state, their model fit to the *in-vitro* data matched the observed depression to 62% of initial strength (their Fig. 3C); their model used in studying orientation tuning depressed to 44% of initial strength (their Fig. 6B); and it is easy to calculate that the parameters they gave for the strong depression model would produce synaptic depression to about 30% of initial strength, which should manifest as a similar level of EPSP depression (because their model was linear except for somatic voltage-dependent conductances and reversal potential effects, none of which should have led to significant deviations from linearity for the small depolarizations of an EPSP). These discrepancies were not noted or explained. It is also puzzling that their moderate depression model (their Fig. 9A) produced more hyperpolarized voltages than their strong depression model (their Fig. 8C) for non-preferred orientations at low contrasts (3% and 10%), even though their moderate depression model appeared to always produce less synaptic depression at the thalamocortical synapses than their strong depression model (*e.g.*, their Fig. 6). Without knowing the models they actually used to study orientation tuning, we find it difficult to compare their

findings to ours. In sum, we conclude that depression models matched to either *in-vivo* or *in-vitro* physiological data, which we have constructed, do not significantly impact orientation tuning.

Thalamocortical synaptic depression has also been postulated to contribute to other V1 response properties, including band-pass rather than low-pass responses to sinusoidal stimuli, nonlinear differences in the responses to broadband or transient stimuli vs. the responses to sinusoidal stimuli, contrast adaptation, and direction selectivity [53]; contrast-dependent changes in temporal frequency tuning [23] and in the temporal phase of response to drifting grating stimuli [23,53]; and the suppression of responses to preferred stimuli by superimposed mask stimuli [27]. It will be of interest to revisit these issues with a model matched to the thalamocortical depression observed *in-vivo*.

Applicability to Rodents

We have based our model on a large number of studies in cat V1 (see references in Introduction) that have established the classic "Hubel-Wiesel" model of the arrangement of LGN inputs to layer 4 simple cells, the dependence of spiking tuning for orientation and contrast on the tunings of the voltage mean and voltage standard deviation and on feedforward vs. intracortical input, and the properties of synaptic depression *in-vivo* and *in-vitro*. While we expect our basic finding, that synaptic depression does not significantly impact orientation tuning or its contrast dependence, will carry over to rodents, many of these details may differ in rodent V1. In particular, it is already known that ON-center and OFF-center excitatory inputs appear to be more strongly overlapping in rodent [54] vs. cat [10,14,55] simple cells, with spatially "intervening inhibition" playing an important role in segregating ON from OFF subregions in rodents [54]; cats have a "push-pull" arrangement between excitatory and inhibitory input, whereas in rodents the arrangement appears to be "push-push" [47,56]; and the difference between orientation tuning in LGN and V1 is much less marked in rodents than in cats [57]. Further investigation is needed to determine the degree to which the mechanisms of orientation selectivity and its contrast invariance differ between carnivores and rodents.

Origins of Contrast Invariance of Orientation Selectivity

As summarized in the Introduction, the origin of contrast-invariant orientation tuning in thalamic-recipient simple cells in middle layers of anesthetized cat V1, in response to drifting gratings, can be attributed to: (1) the Gabor-function arrangement of LGN inputs to a simple cell [5], which causes the net LGN input to be composed of an orientation-untuned DC and an orientation-tuned F1 [20,24]; (2) some degree of suppression of the voltage response to a null-orientation stimulus relative to that to a preferred-orientation stimulus, relative to the levels expected from LGN input alone [17,19]; and (3) contrast-dependent suppression of voltage noise, causing the mean voltage in response to a null stimulus to stay the same number of standard deviations from threshold across contrasts and thus preventing spiking response to the null orientation [17,19]. Sadogapan and Ferster [19] presented evidence that (3) is substantially due to a corresponding decrease in the variability of the LGN input to simple cells with increasing stimulus contrast. Several network mechanisms that could cause such variability of suppression have also been proposed [58–60]. The mechanism responsible for (2) is not known. One postulated mechanism for (2) is an untuned component of feedforward inhibition that grows with contrast [20,24,26,27], which might also contribute to (3) by decreasing input resistance. The present work demonstrates that thalamocortical synaptic depression matched to physiological measurements does not substantially contribute to (2) or more generally to contrast-invariant orientation tuning.

Supporting Information

Dataset S1 LGN Firing Rates (Hz). Each.csv file is from a single LGN cell. Each file contains a matrix. Rows: Time (Duration: 625 msec (1 cycle)). Columns: Contrast (Total 7:96%, 72%, 48%, 24%, 12%, 6%, 3%).

Author Contributions

Analyzed the data: AC KM. Contributed reagents/materials/analysis tools: AC KM. Contributed to the writing of the manuscript: AC KM.

References

1. Hubel DH, Wiesel TN (1962) Receptive fields, binocular interaction and functional architecture in the cat's visual cortex. J Physiol 160: 106–154.
2. Bullier J, Mustari MJ, Henry GH (1982) Receptive-field transformations between LGN neurons and S-cells of cat-striate cortex. J Neurophysiol 47: 417–438.
3. Tanaka K (1983) Cross-correlation analysis of geniculostriate neuronal relationships in cats. J Neurophysiol 49: 1303–1318.
4. Saul AB, Humphrey AL (1992) Evidence of input from lagged cells in the lateral geniculate nucleus to simple cells in cortical area 17 of the cat. J Neurophysiol 68: 1190–1208.
5. Reid RC, Alonso JM (1995) Specificity of monosynaptic connections from thalamus to visual cortex. Nature 378: 281–284.
6. Ferster D, Chung S, Wheat H (1996) Orientation selectivity of thalamic input to simple cells of cat visual cortex. Nature 380: 249–252.
7. Chung S, Ferster D (1998) Strength and orientation tuning of the thalamic input to simple cells revealed by electrically evoked cortical suppression. Neuron 20: 1177–1189.
8. Ferster D, Miller KD (2000) Neural mechanisms of orientation selectivity in the visual cortex. Annu Rev Neurosci 23: 441–471.
9. Alonso JM, Usrey WM, Reid RC (2001) Rules of connectivity between geniculate cells and simple cells in cat primary visual cortex. J Neurosci 21: 4002–4015.
10. Lampl I, Anderson JS, Gillespie DC, Ferster D (2001) Prediction of orientation selectivity from receptive field architecture in simple cells of cat visual cortex. Neuron 30: 263–274.
11. Hirsch JA, Martinez LM, Alonso JM, Desai K, Pillai C, et al. (2002) Synaptic physiology of the flow of information in the cat's visual cortex in vivo. J Physiol 540: 335–350.
12. Kara P, Pezaris JS, Yurgenson S, Reid RC (2002) The spatial receptive field of thalamic inputs to single cortical simple cells revealed by the interaction of visual and electrical stimulation. Proc Natl Acad Sci U S A 99: 16261–16266.
13. Martinez LM, Alonso JM, Reid RC, Hirsch JA (2002) Laminar processing of stimulus orientation in cat visual cortex. J Physiol 540: 321–333.
14. Martinez LM, Wang Q, Reid RC, Pillai C, Alonso JM, et al. (2005) Receptive field structure varies with layer in the primary visual cortex. Nat Neurosci 8: 372–379.
15. Priebe NJ, Ferster D (2005) Direction selectivity of excitation and inhibition in simple cells of the cat primary visual cortex. Neuron 45: 133–145.
16. Priebe NJ, Ferster D (2006) Mechanisms underlying cross-orientation suppression in cat visual cortex. Nat Neurosci 9: 552–561.
17. Finn IM, Priebe NJ, Ferster D (2007) The emergence of contrast-invariant orientation tuning in simple cells of cat visual cortex. Neuron 54: 137–152.
18. Priebe NJ, Ferster D (2012) Mechanisms of neuronal computation in Mammalian visual cortex. Neuron 75: 194–208.
19. Sadagopan S, Ferster D (2012) Feedforward origins of response variability underlying contrast invariant orientation tuning in cat visual cortex. Neuron 74: 911–923.
20. Troyer TW, Krukowski AE, Priebe NJ, Miller KD (1998) Contrast-invariant orientation tuning in cat visual cortex: thalamocortical input tuning and correlation-based intracortical connectivity. J Neurosci 18: 5908–5927.
21. Lauritzen TZ, Krukowski AE, Miller KD (2001) Local correlation-based circuitry can account for responses to multi-grating stimuli in a model of cat V1. J Neurophysiol 86: 1803–1815.
22. Krukowski AE, Miller KD (2001) Thalamocortical NMDA conductances and intracortical inhibition can explain cortical temporal tuning. Nat Neurosci 4: 424–430.

23. Kayser A, Priebe NJ, Miller KD (2001) Contrast-dependent nonlinearities arise locally in a model of contrast-invariant orientation tuning. J Neurophysiol 85: 2130–2149.
24. Troyer TW, Krukowski AE, Miller KD (2002) LGN input to simple cells and contrast-invariant orientation tuning: an analysis. J Neurophysiol 87: 2741–2752.
25. Lauritzen TZ, Miller KD (2003) Different roles for simple-cell and complex-cell inhibition in V1. J Neurosci 23: 10201–10213.
26. Palmer SE, Miller KD (2007) Effects of inhibitory gain and conductance fluctuations in a simple model for contrast-invariant orientation tuning in cat V1. J Neurophysiol 98: 63–78.
27. Carandini M, Heeger DJ, Senn W (2002) A synaptic explanation of suppression in visual cortex. J Neurosci 22: 10053–10065.
28. Banitt Y, Martin KA, Segev I (2007) A biologically realistic model of contrast invariant orientation tuning by thalamocortical synaptic depression. J Neurosci 27: 10230–10239.
29. Li YT, Ibrahim LA, Liu BH, Zhang LI, Tao HW (2013) Linear transformation of thalamocortical input by intracortical excitation. Nat Neurosci 16: 1324–1330.
30. Lien AD, Scanziani M (2013) Tuned thalamic excitation is amplified by visual cortical circuits. Nat Neurosci 16: 1315–1323.
31. Alitto HJ, Usrey WM (2004) Influence of contrast on orientation and temporal frequency tuning in ferret primary visual cortex. J Neurophysiol 91: 2797–2808.
32. Sclar G, Freeman RD (1982) Orientation selectivity in the cat's striate cortex is invariant with stimulus contrast. Exp Brain Res 46: 457–461.
33. Skottun BC, Bradley A, Sclar G, Ohzawa I, Freeman RD (1987) The effects of contrast on visual orientation and spatial frequency discrimination: a comparison of single cells and behavior. J Neurophysiol 57: 773–786.
34. Boudreau CE, Ferster D (2005) Short-term depression in thalamocortical synapses of cat primary visual cortex. J Neurosci 25: 7179–7190.
35. Stratford KJ, Tarczy-Hornoch K, Martin KA, Bannister NJ, Jack JJ (1996) Excitatory synaptic inputs to spiny stellate cells in cat visual cortex. Nature 382: 258–261.
36. Johnson DH, Swami A (1983) The transmission of signals by auditory-nerve fiber discharge patterns. J Acoust Soc Am 74: 493–501.
37. Jones K, Tubis A, Burns EM (1985) On the extraction of the signal-excitation function from a non-Poisson cochlear neural spike train. J Acoust Soc Am 78: 90–94.
38. Miller MI (1985) Algorithms for removing recovery-related distortion from auditory-nerve discharge patterns. J Acoust Soc Am 77: 1452–1464.
39. Bi Q (1989) A closed-form solution for removing the dead time effects from the poststimulus time histograms. J Acoust Soc Am 85: 2504–2513.
40. Berry MJ, 2nd, Meister M (1998) Refractoriness and neural precision. J Neurosci 18: 2200–2211.
41. Paninski L (2004) Maximum likelihood estimation of cascade point-process neural encoding models. Network 15: 243–262.
42. Worgotter F, Koch C (1991) A detailed model of the primary visual pathway in the cat: comparison of afferent excitatory and intracortical inhibitory connection schemes for orientation selectivity. J Neurosci 11: 1959–1979.
43. Jones JP, Palmer LA (1987) The two-dimensional spatial structure of simple receptive fields in cat striate cortex. J Neurophysiol 58: 1187–1211.
44. Dittman JS, Regehr WG (1998) Calcium dependence and recovery kinetics of presynaptic depression at the climbing fiber to Purkinje cell synapse. J Neurosci 18: 6147–6162.
45. Abbott LF, Varela JA, Sen K, Nelson SB (1997) Synaptic depression and cortical gain control. Science 275: 220–224.
46. Tsodyks MV, Markram H (1997) The neural code between neocortical pyramidal neurons depends on neurotransmitter release probability. Proc Natl Acad Sci U S A 94: 719–723.
47. Liu BH, Li YT, Ma WP, Pan CJ, Zhang LI, et al. (2011) Broad inhibition sharpens orientation selectivity by expanding input dynamic range in mouse simple cells. Neuron 71: 542–554.
48. Castro-Alamancos MA (2004) Absence of rapid sensory adaptation in neocortex during information processing states. Neuron 41: 455–464.
49. Castro-Alamancos MA, Oldford E (2002) Cortical sensory suppression during arousal is due to the activity-dependent depression of thalamocortical synapses. J Physiol 541: 319–331.
50. Anderson JS, Carandini M, Ferster D (2000) Orientation tuning of input conductance, excitation, and inhibition in cat primary visual cortex. J Neurophysiol 84: 909–926.
51. Hirsch JA, Martinez LM, Pillai C, Alonso JM, Wang Q, et al. (2003) Functionally distinct inhibitory neurons at the first stage of visual cortical processing. Nat Neurosci 6: 1300–1308.
52. Fuhrmann G, Cowan A, Segev I, Tsodyks M, Stricker C (2004) Multiple mechanisms govern the dynamics of depression at neocortical synapses of young rats. J Physiol 557: 415–438.
53. Chance FS, Nelson SB, Abbott LF (1998) Synaptic depression and the temporal response characteristics of V1 cells. J Neurosci 18: 4785–4799.
54. Liu BH, Li P, Sun YJ, Li YT, Zhang LI, et al. (2010) Intervening inhibition underlies simple-cell receptive field structure in visual cortex. Nat Neurosci 13: 89–96.
55. Ferster D (1988) Spatially opponent excitation and inhibition in simple cells of the cat visual cortex. J Neurosci 8: 1172–1180.
56. Tan AY, Brown BD, Scholl B, Mohanty D, Priebe NJ (2011) Orientation selectivity of synaptic input to neurons in mouse and cat primary visual cortex. J Neurosci 31: 12339–12350.
57. Scholl B, Tan AY, Corey J, Priebe NJ (2013) Emergence of orientation selectivity in the Mammalian visual pathway. J Neurosci 33: 10616–10624.
58. Rajan K, Abbott LF, Sompolinsky H (2010) Stimulus-dependent suppression of chaos in recurrent neural networks. Phys Rev E Stat Nonlin Soft Matter Phys 82: 011903.
59. Rubin DB, Miller KD (2011) Normalization in a simple circuit model of visual cortex explains stimulus-induced reduction in shared variability. Program No. 428.10. 2011 Neuroscience Meeting Planner. Washington, DC: Society for Neuroscience, 2011. Online.
60. Litwin-Kumar A, Doiron B (2012) Slow dynamics and high variability in balanced cortical networks with clustered connections. Nat Neurosci 15: 1498–1505.

Permissions

All chapters in this book were first published in PLOS ONE, by The Public Library of Science; hereby published with permission under the Creative Commons Attribution License or equivalent. Every chapter published in this book has been scrutinized by our experts. Their significance has been extensively debated. The topics covered herein carry significant findings which will fuel the growth of the discipline. They may even be implemented as practical applications or may be referred to as a beginning point for another development.

The contributors of this book come from diverse backgrounds, making this book a truly international effort. This book will bring forth new frontiers with its revolutionizing research information and detailed analysis of the nascent developments around the world.

We would like to thank all the contributing authors for lending their expertise to make the book truly unique. They have played a crucial role in the development of this book. Without their invaluable contributions this book wouldn't have been possible. They have made vital efforts to compile up to date information on the varied aspects of this subject to make this book a valuable addition to the collection of many professionals and students.

This book was conceptualized with the vision of imparting up-to-date information and advanced data in this field. To ensure the same, a matchless editorial board was set up. Every individual on the board went through rigorous rounds of assessment to prove their worth. After which they invested a large part of their time researching and compiling the most relevant data for our readers.

The editorial board has been involved in producing this book since its inception. They have spent rigorous hours researching and exploring the diverse topics which have resulted in the successful publishing of this book. They have passed on their knowledge of decades through this book. To expedite this challenging task, the publisher supported the team at every step. A small team of assistant editors was also appointed to further simplify the editing procedure and attain best results for the readers.

Apart from the editorial board, the designing team has also invested a significant amount of their time in understanding the subject and creating the most relevant covers. They scrutinized every image to scout for the most suitable representation of the subject and create an appropriate cover for the book.

The publishing team has been an ardent support to the editorial, designing and production team. Their endless efforts to recruit the best for this project, has resulted in the accomplishment of this book. They are a veteran in the field of academics and their pool of knowledge is as vast as their experience in printing. Their expertise and guidance has proved useful at every step. Their uncompromising quality standards have made this book an exceptional effort. Their encouragement from time to time has been an inspiration for everyone.

The publisher and the editorial board hope that this book will prove to be a valuable piece of knowledge for researchers, students, practitioners and scholars across the globe.

List of Contributors

Shen Chengfeng
Tianjin Centers for Disease Control and Prevention, Tianjin, China

Zhan Rui and Qian Lingjia
Beijing Institute of Basic Medical Sciences, Beijing, China

Wang Xinxing
Beijing Institute of Basic Medical Sciences, Beijing, China
Institute of Health and Environmental Medicine, Tianjin, China

Liu Wei and Wu Lei
Institute of Health and Environmental Medicine, Tianjin, China

Martine M. Veehof and Ernst T. Bohlmeijer
University of Twente, Department of Psychology, Health and Technology, Enschede, the Netherlands

Wendy T. M. Pots
University of Twente, Department of Psychology, Health and Technology, Enschede, the Netherlands
Dimence, Community Mental Health Center, Almelo, the Netherlands

Peter A. M. Meulenbeek
University of Twente, Department of Psychology, Health and Technology, Enschede, the Netherlands
GGNET, Community Mental Health Center, Warnsveld, the Netherlands

Jorinde Klungers
GGNET, Community Mental Health Center, Warnsveld, the Netherlands

Selver Demic and Sen Cheng
International Graduate School of Neuroscience, Bochum, Germany
Mercator Research Group "Structure of Memory", Bochum, Germany
Faculty of Psychology, Ruhr University Bochum, Bochum, Germany

Wendy A. Davis, Violetta Cetrullo, Timothy M. E. Davis and David G. Bruce
School of Medicine and Pharmacology, University of Western Australia, Crawley, Western Australia, Australia

Milan Dragovic and Sergio E. Starkstein
School of Psychiatry and Clinical Neuroscience, University of Western Australia, Crawley, Western Australia, Australia

Kang Chen, Wenhua Yan, Changyu Pan, Juming Lu, Jingtao Dou, Zhaohui Lu, JianmingBa, Baoan Wang and Yiming Mu
Department of Endocrinology, Chinese PLA General Hospital, Beijing, China

Yu Zheng
Department of Endocrinology, Chinese PLA General Hospital, Beijing, China
School of Medicine, Nankai University, Tianjin, China

Qihong Sun
Department of Endocrinology, Chinese PLA General Hospital, Beijing, China
Internal Medicine, Fushun Hospital of TCM, Liaoning, China

Xu Zhai, Peijing Rong, Jingjun Zhao and Hui Ben
Department of Physiology, Institute of Acupuncture and Moxibustion, China Academy of Chinese Medical Sciences, Beijing, China

Shaoyuan Li
Department of Physiology, Institute of Acupuncture and Moxibustion, China Academy of Chinese Medical Sciences, Beijing, China
Department of Anatomy, Xinxiang Medical University, Xinxiang, Henan, China

Shuxing Wang
Department of Physiology, Institute of Acupuncture and Moxibustion, China Academy of Chinese Medical Sciences, Beijing, China
Department of Anatomy, Xinxiang Medical University, Xinxiang, Henan, China
Department of Anesthesia, Critical Care, and Pain Medicine, Massachusetts General Hospital, Harvard Medical School, Boston, MA, United States of America
Primate Research Center, Guangdong Entomological Institute, Guangzhou, Guangdong, China
Guangdong Landau Biotechnology Co. Ltd, Guangzhou, Guangdong, China

Xing Wang
Department of Anatomy, Xinxiang Medical University, Xinxiang, Henan, China

Michael F. McCabe
Department of Anesthesia, Critical Care, and Pain Medicine, Massachusetts General Hospital, Harvard Medical School, Boston, MA, United States of America

Yiming Wang and Fangxian Chai
Department of Psychiatry, Hospital Affiliated to Guiyang Medical University, Guiyang, Guizhou, China

Songlin Tang
Department of Psychiatry, Hospital Affiliated to Guiyang Medical University, Guiyang, Guizhou, China
Department of Neurology, First People's Hospital of Shaoyang, Shaoyang, Hunan, China

Hongming Zhang
Department of Cardiology, The General Hospital of Jinan Military Region, Jinan, China

Xingde Liu
Department of Cardiology, Hospital Affiliated to Guiyang Medical University, Guiyang City, Guizhou, China

Adrienne O'Neil
IMPACT Strategic Research Centre, School of Medicine, Deakin University, Geelong, Australia
School of Public Health and Preventive Medicine, Monash University, Melbourne, Australia

Alyna Turner
IMPACT Strategic Research Centre, School of Medicine, Deakin University, Geelong, Australia
Department of Psychiatry, The University of Melbourne, Parkville, Victoria, Australia
School of Medicine and Public Health, The University of Newcastle, Callaghan, New South Wales, Australia

Michael Berk
IMPACT Strategic Research Centre, School of Medicine, Deakin University, Geelong, Australia
School of Public Health and Preventive Medicine, Monash University, Melbourne, Australia
Department of Psychiatry, The University of Melbourne, Parkville, Victoria, Australia
Department of Psychiatry, Orygen Youth Health Research Centre, The University of Melbourne, Parkville, Victoria, Australia
Florey Institute of Neuroscience and Mental Health, University of Melbourne, Parkville, Victoria, Australia

Fanying Chen
Mental Health Education And Counseling Center, Guiyang Medical University, Guiyang City, Guizhou, China

Norhayati Ibrahim, Noh Amit and Melia Wong Yuin Suen
Faculty of Health Sciences, National University of Malaysia (UKM), Kuala Lumpur, Malaysia

Chieko Matsubara, Hitoshi Murakami, Hidechika Akashi, Chiaki Miyoshi and Tamotsu Nakasa
Bureau of International Medical Cooperation, National Center for Global Health and Medicine, Shinjuku-ku, Tokyo, Japan

Koubun Imai
Department of Psychiatry, National Center for Global Health and Medicine, Shinjuku-ku, Tokyo, Japan

Tetsuya Mizoue
Department of Epidemiology and Prevention, National Center for Global Health and Medicine, Shinjuku-ku, Tokyo, Japan

Skye P. Barbic and Zachary Durisko
Social Aetiology of Mental Illness (SAMI) Canadian Institute of Health Research (CIHR) Training Program, Centre for Addiction and Mental Health, Toronto, Ontario, Canada

Paul W. Andrews
Department of Psychology, Neuroscience and Behaviour, McMaster University, Hamilton, Canada

Willem A. Nolen and Robert A. Schoevers
University of Groningen, University Medical Center Groningen (UMCG), Interdisciplinary Center Psychopathology and Emotion Regulation (ICPE)/ University Center Psychiatry (UCP), Groningen, The Netherlands
Vrije University Medical Center (VUMC), Department of Psychiatry and Extramuraal Geneeskundig Onderzoek (EMGO) Institute for Health and Care Research, Amsterdam, The Netherlands

Lynn Boschloo
University of Groningen, University Medical Center Groningen (UMCG), Interdisciplinary Center Psychopathology and Emotion Regulation (ICPE)/ University Center Psychiatry (UCP), Groningen, The Netherlands
Vrije University Medical Center (VUMC), Department of Psychiatry and Extramuraal Geneeskundig Onderzoek (EMGO) Institute for Health and Care Research, Amsterdam, The Netherlands

Brenda W. J. H. Penninx
University of Groningen, University Medical Center Groningen (UMCG), Interdisciplinary Center Psychopathology and Emotion Regulation (ICPE)/ University Center Psychiatry (UCP), Groningen, The Netherlands
Vrije University Medical Center (VUMC), Department of Psychiatry and Extramuraal Geneeskundig Onderzoek (EMGO) Institute for Health and Care Research, Amsterdam, The Netherlands

Leiden University Medical Center, Department of Psychiatry, Leiden, The Netherlands

Ralph Kupka
Vrije University Medical Center (VUMC), Department of Psychiatry and Extramuraal Geneeskundig Onderzoek (EMGO) Institute for Health and Care Research, Amsterdam, The Netherlands

Annet T. Spijker
PsyQ, Department of Mood Disorders, The Hague, The Netherlands

Erik Hoencamp
Parnassia Group, The Hague, The Netherlands
Leiden University, Institute of Psychology, Leiden, The Netherlands

Yuqi Cheng, Na Li, Fang Liu, Yan Bai and Xiufeng Xu
Department of Psychiatry, First Affiliated Hospital of Kunming Medical University, Kunming, PR China

Jian Xu
Department of Internal Medicine, First Affiliated Hospital of Kunming Medical University, Kunming, PR China

Chunrong Luo, Haijun Li and Hongjun Yu
Magnetic Resonance Imaging Center, the First Hospital of Kunming City, Kunming, PR China

Baoci Shan and Binbin Nie
Key Laboratory of Nuclear Analysis Techniques, Institute of High Energy Physics, Chinese Academy of Sciences, Beijing, PR China

Lin Xu
Key Laboratory of Animal Models and Human Disease Mechanisms, Chinese Academy of Sciences and Yunnan Province, Kunming Institute of Zoology, Kunming, PR China

Gemma Kok, Gerard van Rijsbergen, Hermien Elgersma and Claudi Bockting
Department of Clinical Psychology, University of Groningen, Groningen, The Netherlands

Huibert Burger
Department of General Practice, University of Groningen, University Medical Center Groningen, Groningen, The Netherlands
Interdisciplinary Center for Psychiatric Epidemiology, University of Groningen, University Medical Center Groningen, Groningen, The Netherlands

Heleen Riper and Pim Cuijpers
Department of Clinical Psychology and EMGO + Institute for Health and Care Research, VU University and VU University Medical Centre, Amsterdam, the Netherlands
Leuphana University, Lu¨neburg, Germany

Filip Smit
Department of Clinical Psychology and EMGO + Institute for Health and Care Research, VU University and VU University Medical Centre, Amsterdam, the Netherlands
Department of Epidemiology and Biostatistics, EMGO + Institute for Health and Care Research, VU University Medical Centre, Amsterdam, the Netherlands
Trimbos Institute (Netherlands Institute of Mental Health and Addiction), Utrecht, the Netherlands

Jack Dekker
Research Department, Arkin Mental Health Institute, Amsterdam, The Netherlands
Department of Clinical Psychology, VU University, Amsterdam, The Netherlands

Young Sup Woo, Tae-Youn Jun, Yang-Hwan Jeon, Hoo Rim Song and Tae-Suk Kim
Department of Psychiatry, The Catholic University of Korea School of Medicine, Seoul, Korea

Jung-Bum Kim
Department of Psychiatry, Keimyung University School of Medicine, Daegu, Korea

Min-Soo Lee
Department of Psychiatry, College of Medicine, Korea University, Seoul, Korea
Jae-Min Kim
Department of Psychiatry, Chonnam National University Medical School, Gwangju, Korea

Sun-Jin Jo
Department of Preventive Medicine, The Catholic University of Korea School of Medicine, Seoul, Korea

Vinay Nangia
Suraj Eye Institute, Nagpur, Maharashtra, India

Jost B. Jonas and Songhomitra Panda-Jonas
Suraj Eye Institute, Nagpur, Maharashtra, India
Department of Ophthalmology, Medical Faculty Mannheim of the Ruprecht-Karls-University Heidelberg, Mannheim, Germany

Prakash Behere
Suraj Eye Institute, Nagpur, Maharashtra, India

Department of Psychiatry, Datta Meghe Institute of Medical Sciences, Wardha, Maharashtra, India

Marcella Rietschel and Torsten Paul
Department of Genetic Epidemiology in Psychiatry, Central Institute of Mental Health, Medical Faculty Mannheim of the Ruprecht-Karls-University Heidelberg, Mannheim, Germany

Melonie Walcott, Ivan Herbey and Michael Saag
Division of Infectious Diseases, Department of Medicine, University of Alabama at Birmingham, Birmingham, Alabama, United States of America

Jessica S. Merlin
Division of Infectious Diseases, Department of Medicine, University of Alabama at Birmingham, Birmingham, Alabama, United States of America
Division of Gerontology, Geriatrics, and Palliative Care, University of Alabama at Birmingham, Birmingham, Alabama, United States of America

Christine Ritchie
Division of Geriatrics, Department of Medicine, University of California at San Francisco, San Francisco, California, United States of America
Jewish Home of San Francisco Center for Research on Aging, San Francisco, California, United States of America

Stefan G. Kertesz
Birmingham VA Medical Center, Birmingham, Alabama, United States of America
Division of Preventive Medicine, Department of Medicine, University of Alabama at Birmingham, Birmingham, Alabama, United States of America

Janet M. Turan and Eric Chamot
School of Public Health, University of Alabama at Birmingham, Birmingham, Alabama, United States of America

Tiina Pensola
Centre of Expertise for Health and Work Ability, Finnish Institute of Occupational Health, Helsinki, Finland

Svetlana Solovieva, Johanna Kausto, Rahman Shiri and Kirsti Husgafvel-Pursiainen
Centre of Expertise for Health and Work Ability, Finnish Institute of Occupational Health, Helsinki, Finland
Disability Prevention Centre, Finnish Institute of Occupational Health, Helsinki, Finland

Eira Viikari-Juntura
Disability Prevention Centre, Finnish Institute of Occupational Health, Helsinki, Finland

Markku Heliö vaara
National Institute for Health and Welfare, Helsinki, Finland

Alex Burdorf
Erasmus MC, University Medical Center Rotterdam, Rotterdam, The Netherlands

Masashige Saito
Department of Social Welfare, Nihon Fukushi University, Aichi, Japan

Katsunori Kondo
Center for Preventive Medical Science, Chiba University, Chiba, Japan

Naoki Kondo
Department of Health Economics and Epidemiology Research, The University of Tokyo, Tokyo, Japan

Aya Abe
Department of Empirical Social Security Research, National Institute of Population and Social Security Research, Tokyo, Japan

Toshiyuki Ojima
Department of Community Health and Preventive Medicine, Hamamatsu University School of Medicine, Shizuoka, Japan

Kayo Suzuki
Department of Social Studies, Aichi Gakuin University, Aichi, Japan

Michael A. Sugarman, Amy M. Loree, Boris B. Baltes and Emily R. Grekin
Wayne State University, Department of Psychology, Detroit, Michigan, United States of America

Irving Kirsch
Harvard Medical School, Boston, Massachusetts, United States of America

Peter A. Coventry and Linda Gask
Collaboration for Leadership in Applied Health Research and Care, Centre for Primary Care and Manchester Academic Health Science Centre, University of Manchester, Manchester, United Kingdom

Joanna L. Hudson
Health Psychology Section, Psychology Department, Institute of Psychiatry, King's College London, London, United Kingdom

Evangelos Kontopantelis and Peter Bower
NIHR School for Primary Care Research, Centre for Primary Care and Manchester Academic Health Science Centre, University of Manchester, Manchester, United Kingdom

Janine Archer and Karina Lovell
School of Nursing, Midwifery and Social Work, University of Manchester, Manchester, United Kingdom

Chris Dickens and David A. Richards
Institute of Health Service Research, University of Exeter Medical School, University of Exeter, Exeter, United Kingdom

Simon Gilbody
Mental Health Research Group, Department of Health Sciences and Hull York Medical School, University of York, York, United Kingdom

Waquas Waheed
Lancashire Care NHS Foundation Trust, Preston, United Kingdom

Aylin Cimenser
Harvard Medical School, Boston, Massachusetts, United States of America
Department of Physics, Boston University, Boston, Massachusetts, United States of America

Kenneth D. Miller
Center for Theoretical Neuroscience, College of Physicians and Surgeons, Columbia University, New York, New York, United States of America
Department of Neuroscience, College of Physicians and Surgeons, Columbia University, New York, New York, United States of America
Swartz Program in Theoretical Neuroscience, College of Physicians and Surgeons, Columbia University, New York, New York, United States of America

Index

S

T

W